# Henke's Med-Math

## Dosage Calculation, Preparation and Administration

FOURTH EDITION

# Henke's Med-Math
## Dosage Calculation, Preparation and Administration

▶ **Susan Buchholz**, RN, MSN
Assistant Professor
Georgia Perimeter College
Clarkston, Georgia

▶ **Sister Grace Henke**, SC, RN, MSN, EdD
Ethics Associate
Department of Ethics
Saint Vincent Catholic Medical Centers of New York
New York, New York

LIPPINCOTT WILLIAMS & WILKINS
A **Wolters Kluwer** Company
Philadelphia · Baltimore · New York · London
Buenos Aires · Hong Kong · Sydney · Tokyo

*Acquisitions Editor:* Margaret Zuccarini
*Editorial Assistant:* Helen Kogut
*Senior Project Editor:* Tom Gibbons
*Senior Production Manager:* Helen Ewan
*Art Director:* Carolyn O'Brien
*Manufacturing Manager:* William Alberti
*Indexer:* Victoria Boyle
*Compositor:* DPS/Cadmus
*Printer:* Quebecor

4th Edition
Copyright © 2003 by Lippincott Williams & Wilkins.

9  8  7  6  5  4  3  2

Library of Congress Cataloging-in-Publication Data

Buchholz, Susan, RN.
    Henke's med-math: dosage calculation, preparation, and administration/Susan Buchholz, Grace Henke.—4th ed.
        p. cm.
    Previous ed. cataloged under: Henke, Grace.
    Previous ed. published with title: Med-math.
    Includes index.
    ISBN 0-7817-3634-X (pbk.: alk. paper)
    1. Pharmaceutical arithmetic.   I. Henke, Grace.   II. Henke, Grace. Med-math.   III. Title.
    RS57 .H46 2002
    615.5'8'01513—dc21
                                                                                2002069527

Care has been taken to confirm the accuracy of the information presented and to describe generally accepted practices. However, the authors, editors, and publisher are not responsible for errors or omissions or for any consequences from application of the information in this book and make no warranty, express or implied, with respect to the content of the publication.

The authors, editors, and publisher have exerted every effort to ensure that drug selection and dosage set forth in this text are in accordance with the current recommendations and practice at the time of publication. However, in view of ongoing research, changes in government regulations, and the constant flow of information relating to drug therapy and drug reactions, the reader is urged to check the package insert for each drug for any change in indications and dosage and for added warnings and precautions. This is particularly important when the recommended agent is a new or infrequently employed drug.

Some drugs and medical devices presented in this publication have Food and Drug Administration (FDA) clearance for limited use in restricted research settings. It is the responsibility of the health care provider to ascertain the FDA status of each drug or device planned for use in his or her clinical practice.

# Reviewer List

**Susan Buchholz, RN, MSN**
Assistant Professor
Georgia Perimeter College
Clarkston, Georgia

**Kari R. Lane, RN, BSN, MSNc**
Nursing Instructor
Clinton Community College
Clinton, Iowa

**Linda McIntosh, RN, MSN, MS**
Clinical Instructor of Nursing
North Carolina A & T State University
Greensboro, North Carolina

**Victoria Lynne Oxner, RN, MSN**
Practical Nursing Chairperson/Instructor
Arkansas State University Mountain Home
Mountain Home, Arkansas

**Terri M. Perkins, RN, MN**
Instructor, ADN Faculty
Bellevue Community College
Bellevue, Washington

**Marsha K. Sharp, RN, MSN**
Assistant Professor of Nursing
Elizabethtown Community College
Elizabethtown, Kentucky

**Kathleen Stevens, RN, MN**
Instructional Resource Centre Coordinator
Centre for Nursing Studies
St. John's, Newfoundland, Canada

**Donna B. Vaughn, MS, RN**
Professor
Del Mar College
Corpus Christi, Texas

**Jo A. Voss, RN, MSN, CNS**
Instructor
South Dakota State University
Rapid City, South Dakota

# Preface

$2 + 2 = 4$

$3 - 1 = 2$

$3 \times 3 = 9$

$\dfrac{12}{4} = 3$

From our earliest years, addition, subtraction, multiplication, division, and all sorts of calculations play a major part in our lives.

"If I have two toys and you take one away, I'm not very happy," says the 2-year-old.

As elementary school students, we learn about the magic of multiplication and division: "If I get 5 dollars for allowance, in 10 weeks I will have $50!"

More advanced study takes place as we get older. "Is my grade-point average going to get me into Yale?"

Calculations become very practical in a job situation: "I'm only getting a 3% raise this year? That doesn't figure out to more money!"

In nursing, calculations of medications literally become a life-and-death skill. Too much or too little of a drug can help or harm. Any health care worker who works with medications must know how to accurately calculate dosages of drugs. Sister Grace Henke first wrote this book to ". . . help students in nursing and allied health fields learn to calculate, prepare, and administer drugs safely and confidently." As the co-author for the fourth edition, I want to challenge the reader to become an expert at dosage calculations, and I hope this book leads you to that goal.

## ▶ Text Organization

*Henke's Med-Math: Dosage Calculation, Preparation and Administration* has been designed to meet the needs of students in every type of nursing program. This text has also been widely used by other health care professionals who administer drugs, by practicing nurses in need of review, and by nurses returning to practice. Students in introductory courses should complete the chapters in order. Practicing nurses may wish to do the proficiency tests at the end of each dosage chapter to target areas of weakness for content review.

The first five chapters of this workbook lay the foundation for further study. Chapter 1 concentrates on the arithmetic needed to calculate doses. Chapter 2 identifies abbreviations used in prescriptions and explains how to interpret them. Chapter 3 clarifies information printed on drug labels and types of drug packaging. Chapter 4 explains dosage measurement systems and teaches students how to convert among systems when the physician's order differs from the available stock medication. Chapter 5 defines the forms in which drugs are manufactured and the equipment used in administration.

Chapters 6 to 11 concentrate on calculating doses through the application of simple rules for oral solid and liquid problems, injections from liquids and powders, intravenous medications, and pediatric doses. Numerous examples, self-tests, and proficiency tests enable students to achieve mastery of the material.

Chapters 12 and 13 present information and techniques for safe administration, including universal precautions, pregnancy categories, and legal and ethical considerations. Also included is information on how to administer drugs orally, parenterally, and topically.

## ▶ Key Features of the Text

- All dosage problems, presented as physicians' orders, simulate actual clinical experience.

- Simple to complex organization of the text assists the student in building a knowledge base and lasting understanding of important concepts and principles.

- Easy-to-learn formulas and a step-by-step approach aid the reader in solving problems.

- Plentiful self-tests and proficiency tests offer frequent and varied opportunities to translate text content into clinical application.

- "Learning Aid" feature provides key strategies to promote understanding.

- Rule and Example style of presentation highlights important rules of thumb, followed by their application, to clarify student learning.

- Answers to problems encourage the students to check their accuracy and promote immediate reinforcement of accurate solutions.

- Proficiency tests in every chapter provide ready-made material for student assignments. These tests are perforated and three-hole punched for each removal.

- Calculations for meters squared and milliunits, an explanation of the body surface nomogram, and patient-controlled analgesia (PCA) are included.

## ▶ New to This Edition

- Four-color design adds contrast and readability.

- Up-to-date drug labels ensure that information is current and accurate.

- Expanded glossary promotes student learning and includes common abbreviations.

- Intravenous calculations in two chapters provide content on basic, advanced, and special types of intravenous administration.

- Ratio and proportion method of solving problems is included.

- Formula method and ratio and proportion method are shown side-by-side.

- An enclosed CD-ROM contains math problems for students to practice calculations.

- Photographs enhance learning and show equipment, techniques, and medication administration.

- "Test Your Clinical Savvy" features clinical situations that promote critical thinking and practice safety in regards to potential medication errors.

- Easy to locate answer keys for proficiency tests and self-tests are included.

# ▶ Teaching Aid for Instructors

A fully-updated *Instructor's Manual and Testbank* is available for teachers who adopt this text for their course. The Instructor's Manual contains teaching aids for optimizing the teaching of dosage calculations and medication administration. The Testbank provides test items in addition to those found in the text.

   As you begin this workbook, I want to again quote the words of Sister Grace from the third edition:

"The maxim of drug therapy is: Give the
                            right drug to the
                            right patient in the
                            right dose at the
                            right time by the
                            right route.
It is my prayer that this workbook will prepare those who use it to achieve this goal."

I concur with Sister Grace and hope that you benefit from this edition of *Henke's Med-Math*.

*Susan Buchholz, RN, MSN*

# Acknowledgments

I'd like to thank Helen Kogut, senior editorial coordinator, and Margaret Zuccarini, senior acquisitions editor at Lippincott Williams & Wilkins, for the opportunity to write this book and for their invaluable assistance and editing skills. Thank you to Sister Grace for writing a wonderful book that teaches dosage calculations in such an organized way. Thanks go to my colleagues at Georgia Perimeter College in Atlanta, Georgia for their encouragement and support. During the editing process, the tragedy of September 11, 2001 occurred, and I want to continue to remember those families in our prayers. I'm grateful to God, my Christian faith, and my covenant community. Thank you to my family: Mary, Andrew, and Chelsea, who are my greatest blessing.

# Contents

CHAPTER 13

# Administration Procedures                    288

CHAPTER

1

# Arithmetic Needed for Dosage

When a physician's order differs from the fixed amount at which a drug is supplied, the dose needed must be calculated. Calculation requires knowledge of the systems of dosage measurements (see Chapter 4) and the ability to solve arithmetic. This chapter covers those common arithmetic functions needed for the safe administration of drugs.

Beginning students invariably express anxiety that they will miscalculate a dose and cause harm. Although *everyone* is capable of error, no one has to cause one. The surest way to prevent a mistake is to exercise care in performing basic arithmetic operations.

Do not skip this chapter!

Students who believe their skills are satisfactory should complete the self-tests and the proficiency exam. Answers to all problems are located at the end of the chapter.

Students with math anxiety and those with deficiencies in performing arithmetic should work through this chapter page by page. Examples and learning aids demonstrate how calculations are performed; self-tests provide practice and drill. The proficiency exam should be taken after mastering the content.

Why perform arithmetic operations when calculators are readily available? Solving the arithmetic forces one to think logically about the amount ordered and to evaluate the answer in relation to the dose. Mentally solving dosage problems increases speed and efficiency in preparing medications. There may be occasions when a problem that requires a calculator arises in the clinical area; however, all arithmetic problems in this chapter can be completed without a calculator.

## ▶ Multiplying Whole Numbers

The multiplication table (Fig. 1-1) is provided for review. Study the table for the numbers 1 through 12. You should achieve 100% accuracy without referring to the table.

**Example**    Multiply 8 by 7 (8 × 7)

1. Find column number 8.

2. Find row number 7.

3. Read across row 7 until you intersect column number 8. The answer is 56.

1

| 1 | 2 | 3 | 4 | 5 | 6 | ⑦ | 8 | 9 | 10 | 11 | 12 |
|---|---|---|---|---|---|---|---|---|----|----|----|
| 2 | 4 | 6 | 8 | 10 | 12 | 14 | 16 | 18 | 20 | 22 | 24 |
| 3 | 6 | 9 | 12 | 15 | 18 | 21 | 24 | 27 | 30 | 33 | 36 |
| 4 | 8 | 12 | 16 | 20 | 24 | 28 | 32 | 36 | 40 | 44 | 48 |
| 5 | 10 | 15 | 20 | 25 | 30 | 35 | 40 | 45 | 50 | 55 | 60 |
| 6 | 12 | 18 | 24 | 30 | 36 | 42 | 48 | 54 | 60 | 66 | 72 |
| 7 | 14 | 21 | 28 | 35 | 42 | 49 | 56 | 63 | 70 | 77 | 84 |
| ⑧ | 16 | 24 | 32 | 40 | 48 | ㊅ | 64 | 72 | 80 | 88 | 96 |
| 9 | 18 | 27 | 36 | 45 | 54 | 63 | 72 | 81 | 90 | 99 | 108 |
| 10 | 20 | 30 | 40 | 50 | 60 | 70 | 80 | 90 | 100 | 110 | 120 |
| 11 | 22 | 33 | 44 | 55 | 66 | 77 | 88 | 99 | 110 | 121 | 132 |
| 12 | 24 | 36 | 48 | 60 | 72 | 84 | 96 | 108 | 120 | 132 | 144 |

**FIGURE 1-1**

The multiplication table. The numbers going down the left side (from 1 to 12) are the column numbers. The numbers going across the top (from 1 to 12) are the row numbers. To multiply any two numbers from 1 to 12, find the column for one number, find the row for the other number, and read across the row until you intersect the column.

**SELF TEST 1**  **Multiplication**

*After studying the multiplication table, write the answers to these problems. Answers are given at the end of the chapter; if you do not achieve 100%, you need more study time.*

1. $2 \times 6 =$ _____

2. $9 \times 7 =$ _____

3. $4 \times 8 =$ _____

4. $5 \times 9 =$ _____

5. $12 \times 9 =$ _____

6. $8 \times 3 =$ _____

7. $11 \times 10 =$ _____

8. $2 \times 7 =$ _____

9. $8 \times 6 =$ _____

10. $8 \times 9 =$ _____

11. $3 \times 5 =$ _____

12. $6 \times 7 =$ _____

13. $4 \times 6 =$ _____

14. $9 \times 6 =$ _____

15. $8 \times 8 =$ _____

16. $7 \times 8 =$ _____

17. $2 \times 9 =$ _____

18. $8 \times 11 =$ _____

19. $4 \times 9 =$ _____

20. $3 \times 8 =$ _____

21. $12 \times 11 =$ _____

22. $9 \times 5 =$ _____

23. $9 \times 9 =$ _____

24. $7 \times 5 =$ _____

## ▶ Dividing Whole Numbers

The multiplication table is also helpful in dividing large numbers by smaller ones. Study the table for the division of numbers 2 through 12 (Fig. 1-2). Again, you should be able to achieve 100% accuracy without referring to the table; if not, study it again.

**Example**    Divide 108 by 12 ($108 \div 12$)

1. Find 12 (the smaller number) in the left column.

2. Read across that row until you find 108 (the larger number).

3. The number at the top of that column is the answer, 9.

Remember, because $9 \times 12 = 108$, then $108 \div 12 = 9$ (see Fig. 1-2).

| 1 | 2 | 3 | 4 | 5 | 6 | 7 | 8 | ⑨ | 10 | 11 | 12 |
|---|---|---|---|---|---|---|---|---|---|---|---|
| 2 | 4 | 6 | 8 | 10 | 12 | 14 | 16 | 18 | 20 | 22 | 24 |
| 3 | 6 | 9 | 12 | 15 | 18 | 21 | 24 | 27 | 30 | 33 | 36 |
| 4 | 8 | 12 | 16 | 20 | 24 | 28 | 32 | 36 | 40 | 44 | 48 |
| 5 | 10 | 15 | 20 | 25 | 30 | 35 | 40 | 45 | 50 | 55 | 60 |
| 6 | 12 | 18 | 24 | 30 | 36 | 42 | 48 | 54 | 60 | 66 | 72 |
| 7 | 14 | 21 | 28 | 35 | 42 | 49 | 56 | 63 | 70 | 77 | 84 |
| 8 | 16 | 24 | 32 | 40 | 48 | 56 | 64 | 72 | 80 | 88 | 96 |
| 9 | 18 | 27 | 36 | 45 | 54 | 63 | 72 | 81 | 90 | 99 | 108 |
| 10 | 20 | 30 | 40 | 50 | 60 | 70 | 80 | 90 | 100 | 110 | 120 |
| 11 | 22 | 33 | 44 | 55 | 66 | 77 | 88 | 99 | 110 | 121 | 132 |
| ⑫ | 24 | 36 | 48 | 60 | 72 | 84 | 96 | ⑽⑻ | 120 | 132 | 144 |

**FIGURE 1-2**

Division table. The numbers going down the left side (from 1 to 12) are the column numbers. The numbers going across the top (from 1 to 12) are the row numbers. To divide, find the divisor (the number performing the division) in the column. Read across the column to the dividend (the number to be divided). The number at the top of that column is the answer.

## SELF TEST 2   Division

*After studying the division of larger numbers by smaller numbers, write the answers to the following problems. Answers can be found at the end of the chapter.*

1. $63 \div 7 =$ _____
2. $24 \div 6 =$ _____
3. $36 \div 12 =$ _____
4. $42 \div 6 =$ _____
5. $35 \div 5 =$ _____
6. $96 \div 12 =$ _____
7. $12 \div 3 =$ _____
8. $27 \div 9 =$ _____

9. $49 \div 7 =$ _____
10. $18 \div 3 =$ _____
11. $72 \div 8 =$ _____
12. $48 \div 8 =$ _____
13. $28 \div 7 =$ _____
14. $21 \div 7 =$ _____
15. $24 \div 8 =$ _____
16. $84 \div 12 =$ _____

17. $81 \div 9 =$ _____
18. $32 \div 8 =$ _____
19. $36 \div 6 =$ _____
20. $18 \div 9 =$ _____
21. $21 \div 3 =$ _____
22. $48 \div 4 =$ _____
23. $144 \div 12 =$ _____
24. $56 \div 8 =$ _____

# ▶ Fractions

A *fraction* is a portion of a whole number. The top number is called the *numerator*. The bottom number is called the *denominator*.

**Example**

$\dfrac{1}{4}$  $\begin{array}{l} \rightarrow \text{numerator} \\ \rightarrow \text{denominator} \end{array}$

**Learning Aid**

The line between the numerator and the denominator is a division sign. Therefore, the fraction can be read as one divided by four.

## Types of Fractions

In a *proper* fraction, the numerator is smaller than the denominator.

**Example**    $\frac{2}{5}$ (Read as two-fifths.)

In an *improper* fraction, the numerator is larger than the denominator.

**Example**    $\frac{5}{2}$ (Read as five halves.)

A *mixed number* has a whole number plus a fraction.

**Example**    $1\frac{2}{3}$ (Read as one and two-thirds.)

In a *complex* fraction, both the numerator and the denominator are already fractions.

**Example**    $\dfrac{\frac{1}{2}}{\frac{1}{4}}$ (Read as one-half divided by one-fourth.)

**RULE**    **REDUCING FRACTIONS**

**Find the largest number that can be divided evenly into the numerator *and* the denominator.**

**Example**    *EXAMPLE 1:*

Reduce $\frac{4}{12}$

$$\frac{\overset{1}{\cancel{4}}}{\underset{3}{\cancel{12}}} = \frac{1}{3}$$

*EXAMPLE 2:*

Reduce $\frac{7}{49}$

$$\frac{\overset{1}{\cancel{7}}}{\underset{7}{\cancel{49}}} = \frac{1}{7}$$

> **Learning Aid**
>
> Check to see if the denominator is evenly divisible by the numerator. The number 7 can be evenly divided into 49.

Sometimes fractions are more difficult to reduce because the answer is not obvious.

**Example**    *EXAMPLE 1:*

Reduce $\frac{56}{96}$

$$\frac{56}{96} = \frac{\overset{1}{\cancel{8}} \times 7}{\underset{1}{\cancel{8}} \times 12} = \frac{7}{12}$$

> **Learning Aid**
>
> Your knowledge of the multiplication table can help you. Change the numbers to their multiples.

*EXAMPLE 2:*

Reduce $\frac{54}{99}$

$$\frac{54}{99} = \frac{\overset{1}{\cancel{9}} \times 6}{\underset{1}{\cancel{9}} \times 11} = \frac{6}{11}$$

Patience is required to reduce a very large fraction. It may be difficult to find the largest number that will divide evenly into the numerator and the denominator, and you may have to reduce several times.

**Example**

*EXAMPLE 1:*

Reduce $\frac{189}{216}$

Try to divide both by 3 $\quad \dfrac{\overset{63}{\cancel{189}}}{\underset{72}{\cancel{216}}} = \dfrac{63}{72}$

Then use multiples $\dfrac{63}{72} = \dfrac{\overset{1}{\cancel{9}} \times 7}{\underset{1}{\cancel{9}} \times 12} = \dfrac{7}{8}$

*EXAMPLE 2:*

Reduce $\frac{27}{135}$

Try to divide both by 3 $\quad \dfrac{\overset{9}{\cancel{27}}}{\underset{45}{\cancel{135}}} = \dfrac{\overset{1}{\cancel{9}}}{\underset{5}{\cancel{45}}} = \dfrac{1}{5}$

> ## Learning Aid
>
> Certain numbers are called prime numbers because they cannot be reduced further. Examples are 2, 3, 5, 7, and 11.
>
> In reducing, if the last number is even or a zero, try 2.
>
> If the last number is a zero or 5, try 5.
>
> If the last number is odd, try 3, 7, or 11.

---

## SELF TEST 3    Reducing Fractions

*Reduce these fractions to their lowest terms. Answers may be found at the end of the chapter. Be patient!*

1. $\dfrac{16}{24}$

2. $\dfrac{36}{216}$

3. $\dfrac{18}{96}$

4. $\dfrac{70}{490}$

5. $\dfrac{18}{81}$

6. $\dfrac{8}{48}$

7. $\dfrac{12}{30}$

8. $\dfrac{68}{136}$

9. $\dfrac{55}{121}$

10. $\dfrac{15}{60}$

## Multiplying Fractions

There are two ways to multiply fractions.

### First Way

Multiply the numerators across. Multiply denominators across. Reduce the answer to its lowest terms.

**Example**

$$\frac{2}{7} \times \frac{3}{4} = \frac{2 \times 3}{7 \times 4} = \frac{6}{28}$$

$$\frac{6}{28} = \frac{3 \times \overset{1}{\cancel{2}}}{14 \times \underset{1}{\cancel{2}}} = \frac{3}{14}$$

> **Learning Aid**
>
> In multiplying fractions, sometimes one way will be easier. Use whichever method is more comfortable for you.

### Second Way (When There Are Several Fractions)

Reduce by dividing numerators into denominators evenly. Multiply remaining numerators across. Multiply remaining denominators across. Check to see if further reductions can be made.

**Example**

EXAMPLE 1:

$$\frac{3}{14} \times \frac{7}{10} \times \frac{5}{12} = \frac{\overset{1}{\cancel{3}}}{\underset{2}{\cancel{14}}} \times \frac{\overset{1}{\cancel{7}}}{\underset{2}{\cancel{10}}} \times \frac{\overset{1}{\cancel{5}}}{\underset{4}{\cancel{12}}} = \frac{1}{16}$$

> **Learning Aid**
>
> $12 \div 3 = 4$
>
> $14 \div 7 = 2$
>
> $10 \div 5 = 2$

EXAMPLE 2:

$$1\frac{1}{2} \times \frac{4}{6} = \frac{\overset{1}{\cancel{3}}}{\underset{1}{\cancel{2}}} \times \frac{\overset{2}{\cancel{4}}}{\underset{2}{\cancel{6}}} = \frac{\cancel{3}}{\cancel{2}} = 1$$

> **Learning Aid**
>
> Mixed numbers must be changed to improper fractions. Multiply the whole number by the denominator and add the numerator.
>
> $1\frac{1}{2} = 1 \times 2 + 1 = \frac{3}{2}$

EXAMPLE 3:

$$\frac{4}{5} \times 6\frac{2}{3} = \frac{4}{\cancel{5}} \times \frac{\overset{4}{\cancel{20}}}{3} = \frac{16}{3}$$

> **Learning Aid**
>
> $6 \times 3 = 18 + 2 = \frac{20}{3}$

| SELF TEST 4 | Multiplying Fractions |
|---|---|

*Multiply these fractions. Answers may be found at the end of the chapter.*

**1.** $\frac{1}{6} \times \frac{4}{5} \times \frac{5}{2} =$

**2.** $\frac{4}{15} \times \frac{3}{2} =$

**3.** $1\frac{1}{2} \times 4\frac{2}{3} =$

**4.** $\frac{1}{5} \times \frac{15}{45} =$

**5.** $3\frac{3}{4} \times 10\frac{2}{3} =$

**6.** $\frac{7}{20} \times \frac{2}{14} =$

**7.** $\frac{9}{2} \times \frac{3}{2} =$

**8.** $6\frac{1}{4} \times 7\frac{1}{9} \times \frac{9}{5} =$

## Dividing Fractions

Fractions can be divided by inverting the number after the division sign then changing the division sign to a multiplication sign.

**Example**

*EXAMPLE 1:*

$$\frac{1}{75} \div \frac{1}{150} = \frac{1}{\cancel{75}} \times \frac{\overset{2}{\cancel{150}}}{1} = 2$$

*EXAMPLE 2:*

$$\frac{\frac{1}{4}}{\frac{3}{8}} = \frac{1}{4} \div \frac{3}{8} = \frac{1}{\cancel{4}} \times \frac{\overset{2}{\cancel{8}}}{3} = \frac{2}{3}$$

*EXAMPLE 3:*

$$\frac{1\frac{1}{5}}{\frac{2}{3}} = \frac{6}{5} \div \frac{2}{3} = \frac{\overset{3}{\cancel{6}}}{5} \times \frac{3}{\cancel{2}} = \frac{9}{5}$$

### Learning Aid

Complex fractions such as

$\frac{\frac{1}{4}}{\frac{3}{8}}$ may be read as $\frac{1}{4} \div \frac{3}{8}$

Remember, the long line represents a division sign.

| SELF TEST 5 | Dividing Fractions |
|---|---|

*Divide these fractions. This operation is important in calculating dosages correctly. Answers may be found at the end of the chapter.*

**1.** $\frac{1}{75} \div \frac{1}{150} =$

**2.** $\frac{1}{8} \div \frac{1}{4} =$

**3.** $2\frac{2}{3} \div \frac{1}{2} =$

**4.** $75 \div 12\frac{1}{2} =$

**5.** $\frac{7}{25} \div \frac{7}{75} =$

**6.** $\frac{1}{2} \div \frac{1}{4} =$

**7.** $\frac{3}{4} \div \frac{8}{3} =$

**8.** $\frac{1}{60} \div \frac{7}{10} =$

## *Changing Fractions to Decimals*

This can be accomplished by dividing the numerator by the denominator. Remember that the line between the numerator and the denominator is a division sign; hence, $\frac{1}{4}$ can be read as $1 \div 4$.

In division, the number being divided is called the *dividend;* the number that does the dividing is called the *divisor;* the answer is called the *quotient.*

$$\text{divisor} \rightarrow 16\overline{)640.} \leftarrow \text{dividend} \atop \phantom{x} \begin{array}{r} 40. \leftarrow \text{quotient} \\ \underline{64\phantom{0}} \\ 0 \end{array}$$

1. Look at the fraction $\frac{1}{4}$

   $\frac{1}{4}$ $\leftarrow$ numerator = dividend
   $\phantom{\frac{1}{4}}\leftarrow$ denominator = divisor

2. Write

   $4\overline{)1}$

3. If you have difficulty setting this up, you can continue the line for the fraction and place the number above the line into the box.

   $$\frac{1}{4} = \frac{\cancel{1}}{4\overline{)1}}$$

4. Once the division problem is set up, place a decimal point immediately after the dividend and also bring the decimal point up to the quotient.

   $$\begin{array}{r} \cancel{1}\phantom{x}. \leftarrow \text{quotient} \\ \hline 4\overline{)1.} \leftarrow \text{dividend} \end{array}$$

**Important! Failure to place decimal points carefully can lead to serious dosage errors.**

5. Carry out the division.

   $$\begin{array}{r} \cancel{1}\phantom{xx}.25 = 0.25 \\ \hline 4\overline{)1.00} \\ \underline{8\phantom{.00}} \\ 20 \\ \underline{20} \\ 0 \end{array}$$

> **Learning Aid**
>
> If the answer does not have a whole number, place a zero before the decimal. This prevents misreading the answer: .25 is incorrect; 0.25 is correct.
>
> The number of places to report your answer will vary depending on the way the stock drug comes and the equipment you use. For these exercises, carry answers to three places.

**Example**

*EXAMPLE 1:*

$$\frac{5}{16} = \frac{5}{16} \overset{0.312}{)5.000} = 0.312$$

$$\begin{array}{r} 4\,8 \\ \hline 20 \\ 16 \\ \hline 40 \\ 32 \\ \hline 8 \end{array}$$

*EXAMPLE 2:*

$$\frac{640}{8} = \frac{640}{8} \overset{80.}{)640.} = 80$$

*EXAMPLE 3:*

$$\frac{1}{75} = \frac{1}{75} \overset{.013}{)1.000} = 0.013$$

$$\begin{array}{r} 75 \\ \hline 250 \\ 225 \\ \hline 25 \end{array}$$

**Learning Aid**

Note that there is a space between the 8 and the decimal point in the answer. When this occurs, place a zero in the space to complete the answer.

---

**SELF TEST 6    Converting Fractions to Decimals**

*Divide these fractions to produce decimals. Answers will be found at the end of the chapter. Carry decimal places to three if necessary.*

1. $\frac{1}{6}$  

2. $\frac{6}{8}$  

3. $\frac{4}{5}$  

4. $\frac{9}{40}$  

5. $\frac{1}{8}$  

6. $\frac{1}{7}$  

## Decimals

Most medication orders are written in the metric system, which uses decimals.

### Reading Decimals

Count the number of places after the decimal point. As you read the decimal, you also create a fraction.

0.1 is read as one tenth ($\frac{1}{10}$).

0.01 is read as one hundredth ($\frac{1}{100}$).

0.001 is read as one thousandth ($\frac{1}{1000}$).

**Learning Aid**

The first number after the decimal point is the tenth place.
   The second number after the decimal point is the 100th place.
   The third number after the decimal point is the 1000th place.

**Example**

0.56 = fifty-six hundredths ($\frac{56}{100}$)

0.2 = two tenths ($\frac{2}{10}$)

0.194 = one hundred and ninety-four thousandths ($\frac{194}{1000}$)

0.31 = thirty-one hundredths ($\frac{31}{100}$)

1.6 = one and six tenths ($1\frac{6}{10}$)

17.354 = seventeen and three hundred and fifty-four thousandths ($17\frac{354}{1000}$)

**Learning Aid**

In reading decimals, read the number first, then count off the decimal places.
   Whole numbers preceding decimals are read in the usual way.

**SELF TEST 7    Reading Decimals**

*Write these decimals in longhand and as fractions. Answers may be found at the end of the chapter.*

1. 0.25 _____
2. 0.004 _____
3. 1.7 _____
4. 0.5 _____
5. 0.334 _____
6. 136.75 _____
7. 0.1 _____
8. 0.150 _____

## Dividing Decimals

Again, in division the number that is being divided is called the dividend; the number that does the dividing is called the divisor; and the answer is called the quotient.

$$0.312 \rightarrow \text{quotient}$$
$$\text{divisor} \rightarrow 16\overline{)5.000} \rightarrow \text{dividend}$$

Note that a decimal point is placed immediately after the dividend is written and also is moved up to the quotient.

**Example**    $\frac{13}{16}$ $16\overline{)13.}$

Division is then completed.

**Example**
$$16\overline{)\begin{matrix} 0.812 \\ 13.000 \end{matrix}}$$
$$\begin{matrix} 12\ 8 \\ \overline{\phantom{0}20} \\ \underline{16} \\ 40 \\ \underline{32} \\ 8 \end{matrix}$$

## Clearing the Divisor of Decimal Points

Before dividing one decimal by another, clear the divisor of decimal points. To do this, move the decimal point to the far right. Move the decimal point in the dividend *the same number of places* and bring the decimal point up to the quotient in the same place.

**Example**    EXAMPLE 1:

$$0.2\overline{)0.004} = 0.2\overline{)0.0\ 04}$$

Hence, $2\overline{)\begin{matrix}0.02\\00.04\end{matrix}}$

EXAMPLE 2:

$$4.3\overline{)5.427}\quad \text{becomes}\quad 43.\overline{)\begin{matrix}1.262\\54.270\end{matrix}}$$
$$\begin{matrix}\underline{43}\\11\ 2\\\underline{8\ 6}\\2\ 67\\\underline{2\ 58}\\90\\\underline{86}\\4\end{matrix}$$

**Learning Aid**

When dividing, the answer may not "come out even." Instructions are usually given as to how many places to carry out the answer. In Example 2, you could keep dividing and end up with an answer that is very long! (1.262093). In this example, the answer is carried out to three places.

| SELF TEST 8 | Division of Decimals |
|---|---|

*Do these problems in division of decimals. The answers may be found at the end of this chapter. If necessary, carry answer to three places.*

1. $24\overline{)0.0048}$

2. $0.004\overline{)0.1}$

3. $0.02\overline{)0.2}$

4. $7.8\overline{)140}$

5. $6\overline{)140}$

6. $0.025\overline{)10}$

## Rounding Off Decimals

How do you determine the number of places to carry out division? The answer depends on the way the drug is dispensed and the equipment needed to administer the drug. Some tablets can be broken into halves or fourths. Some liquids are prepared in units of measurement in tenths, hundredths, or thousandths. Some syringes are marked to the nearest tenth, hundredth, or thousandth place. As you become familiar with dosage, you will learn how far to round off answers. First review the general rule for rounding off decimals.

| RULE | **ROUNDING OFF DECIMALS** |
|---|---|

**When the number to be dropped is 5 or more, drop the number and add 1 to the previous number. When the last number is 4 or less, drop the number.** ■

**Example**

0.864 becomes 0.86        4.562 becomes 4.56

1.55 becomes 1.6          2.38 becomes 2.4

0.33 becomes 0.3

Suppose you want answers to the nearest tenth. Look at the number in the hundredth place and follow the rules for rounding off.

**Example**

0.12 becomes 0.1

0.667 becomes 0.7

1.46 becomes 1.5

Suppose you want answers to the nearest hundredth. Look at the number in the thousandth place and follow the rules for rounding off.

**Example**

0.664 becomes 0.66

0.148 becomes 0.15

2.375 becomes 2.38

Suppose you want answers to the nearest thousandth. Look at the number in the ten-thousandth place and follow the rules for rounding off.

**Example**

1.3758 becomes 1.376

0.0024 becomes 0.002

4.5555 becomes 4.556

## SELF TEST 9 | Rounding Decimals

*Round off these decimals as indicated. Answers may be found at the end of the chapter.*

| *Nearest Tenth* | *Nearest Hundredth* | *Nearest Thousandth* |
|---|---|---|
| 1. 0.25 = _____ | 6. 1.268 = _____ | 11. 1.3254 = _____ |
| 2. 1.84 = _____ | 7. 0.750 = _____ | 12. 0.0025 = _____ |
| 3. 3.27 = _____ | 8. 0.677 = _____ | 13. 0.4520 = _____ |
| 4. 0.05 = _____ | 9. 4.539 = _____ | 14. 0.7259 = _____ |
| 5. 0.63 = _____ | 10. 1.222 = _____ | 15. 0.3482 = _____ |

## Comparing the Value of Decimals

Understanding which decimal is larger or smaller is often a help in solving dosage problems. For example, will I need more than one tablet or less than one tablet?

**RULE** | **DETERMINING THE VALUE OF DECIMALS**

**The decimal with the higher number in the tenth place has the greater value.** ■

**Example**  Compare 0.25 with 0.5.

It is clear that 0.5 is greater because the number 5 is higher than the number 2.

## SELF TEST 10 | Value of Decimals

*In each pair, underline the decimal with the greater value. Answers may be found at the end of the chapter.*

1. 0.125 and 0.25      4. 0.1 and 0.2      7. 0.25 and 0.4

2. 0.04 and 0.1      5. 0.825 and 0.44      8. 0.7 and 0.350

3. 0.5 and 0.125      6. 0.9 and 0.5

## ▶ Percent

*Percent* means parts per hundred. Percent is a fraction with the number becoming the numerator and 100 becoming the denominator. Whole numbers, fractions, and decimals may be written as percent. Percents may be changed to decimals or to fractions.

**Example**  Whole number: 4% (four percent)

Decimal: 0.2% (two-tenths percent)

Fraction: $\frac{1}{4}$% (one-fourth percent)

## Percents That Are Whole Numbers

| Example |
|---------|

*EXAMPLE 1:*

Change to a fraction

$$4\% = \frac{4}{100} = \frac{1}{25}$$

*EXAMPLE 2:*

Change to a decimal

$$4\% = \frac{4}{100} \quad \begin{array}{r} .04 \\ 100 \overline{)4.00} \end{array} = 0.04$$

> **Learning Aid**
>
> Note that 4% means four parts per 100. The 100th place has two decimal points. A quick rule to change a percent to a decimal is to move the decimal point two places to the left.
>
> 4% = 0.04
>
> 25% = 0.25

## Percents That Are Decimals

These may be changed in three ways:

1. By using the quick rule (see Learning Aid)
   $$0.2\% = 00.2 = 0.002$$

> **Learning Aid**
>
> Quick rule: To remove a % sign, move the decimal point two places to the left.

2. By keeping the decimal

$$0.2\% = \frac{0.2}{100} \quad \begin{array}{r} 0.002 \\ )0.200 \end{array} = 0.002$$

3. By changing to a complex fraction

$$0.2\% = \frac{\frac{2}{10}}{100} =$$

$$\frac{2}{10} \div \frac{100}{1} =$$

$$\frac{2}{10} \times \frac{1}{100} = \frac{2}{1000}$$

$$\frac{\overset{1}{\cancel{2}}}{\underset{500}{\cancel{1000}}} = \frac{1}{500}$$

> **Learning Aid**
>
> Remember that the number after a division sign is inverted. The sign is changed to a multiplication sign.
>   Every whole number is understood to have a denominator of 1.
>
> $$\frac{2}{10} \div 100 = \frac{2}{10} \times \frac{1}{100}$$

## Percents That Are Fractions

| Example |
|---------|

*EXAMPLE 1:*

$$\frac{1}{4}\% = \frac{\frac{1}{4}}{100} = \frac{1}{4} \div \frac{100}{1}$$

$$\frac{1}{4} \div 100 = \frac{1}{4} \times \frac{1}{100} = \frac{1}{400}$$

EXAMPLE 2:

$$\frac{1}{2}\% = \frac{\frac{1}{2}}{100} = \frac{1}{2} \div \frac{100}{1}$$

$$\frac{1}{2} \times \frac{1}{100} = \frac{1}{200}$$

ALTERNATIVE WAY. Because $\frac{1}{2} = 0.5$, $\frac{1}{2}\%$ could also be written as 0.5%. By using the quick rule of moving the decimal point two places to the left to clear a percent, you have $00.5\% = 0.005$. Note that 0.005 is $\frac{5}{1000} = \frac{1}{200}$

---

**SELF TEST 11  Conversion of Percents**

Change these percents to both a **fraction** and a **decimal**. Answers may be found at the end of the chapter.

1. 10% _____ _____    7. 20% _____ _____

2. 0.9% _____ _____    8. 0.4% _____ _____

3. $\frac{1}{5}$ % _____ _____    9. $\frac{1}{10}$ % _____ _____

4. .01% _____ _____   10. 2 1/2% _____ _____

5. 2/3% _____ _____   11. 33% _____ _____

6. .45% _____ _____   12. 50% _____ _____

---

## ▶ Ratio and Proportion

A ratio indicates the relationship between two numbers. Ratios can be written as a fraction ($\frac{1}{10}$) or as two numbers separated by a colon (1:10). (Read as *one is to ten.*)

Proportion indicates a relationship between two ratios. Proportions can be written as fractions or as two ratios separated by a double colon.

**Example**   $\frac{2}{8} = \frac{10}{40}$ (Read as *two is to eight as ten is to forty*)

5:30 :: 6:36 (Read as *five is to thirty as six is to thirty-six*)

Proportions written with colons can be written as fractions; therefore 5:30 :: 6:36 becomes

$$\frac{5}{30} = \frac{6}{36}$$

### Solving Proportion With an Unknown

When one of the numbers in a proportion is unknown the letter $x$ is substituted. There are three steps in determining the value of $x$ in a proportion.

**Step 1.** Cross-multiply.

**Step 2.** Clear $x$.

**Step 3.** Reduce.

Let's see how this is done.

## Proportions Expressed as Decimals

Suppose you had to solve this proportion:

$$\frac{1}{0.125} = \frac{x}{0.25}$$

**Step 1.** Cross-multiply numerators and denominators.

$$0.125x = 0.25$$

> **Learning Aid**
>
> How to cross-multiply
>
> $$\frac{1}{0.125} \times \frac{x}{0.25}$$

**Step 2.** Clear $x$ by dividing both sides of the equation with the number preceding $x$.

$$x = \frac{0.25}{0.125}$$

> **Learning Aid**
>
> $$\frac{0.125x}{0.125} = \frac{0.25}{0.125}$$

**Step 3.** Reduce the number.

$$0.125 \overline{)0.250.} \qquad \overset{2.}{}$$
$$x = 2$$

> **Learning Aid**
>
> Remember the line between the two numbers in a fraction is a division sign.
>
> $$\frac{0.25}{0.125}$$
>
> Can be read as 0.25 divided by 0.125.

## Proportions Expressed as Two Ratios Separated by Colons

Suppose you had this proportion:

$4 : 3.2 :: 7 : x.$

**Step 1.** Cross-multiply the two outside numbers (called "extremes") and the two inside numbers (called "means").

$$4 : 3.2 :: 7 : x$$
$$4x = 22.4$$

**Step 2.** Clear $x$ by dividing both sides of the equation with the number preceding $x$.

$$x = \frac{22.4}{4}$$

> **Learning Aid**
>
> $$\frac{4x}{4} = \frac{22.4}{4}$$
>
> Remember that the line between two numbers in a fraction is a division sign. Read as 22.4 divided by 4.

**Step 3.** Reduce the number.

$$x = 5.6$$

**Learning Aid**

$$4\overline{)22.4} \atop 5.6$$

**Example**  $$\frac{45}{180}\diagdown\frac{3}{x}$$

$$45x = 540$$

$$x = 12$$

**Learning Aid**

$$45\overline{)540.} \atop 12.$$
$$\underline{45}$$
$$90$$
$$\underline{90}$$

**Example**  $$11x = 363$$
$$x = 33$$   $$11 : 121 :: 3 : x$$

**Learning Aid**

$$11\overline{)363.} \atop 33.$$
$$\underline{33}$$
$$33$$
$$\underline{33}$$

---

**SELF TEST 12**  **Solving Proportions**

*Solve these proportions. Answers may be found at the end of the chapter.*

1.  $\frac{120}{4.2} = \frac{16}{x}$

2.  $750 : 250 :: x : 5$

3.  $\frac{14}{140} = \frac{22}{x}$

4.  $2 : 5 :: x : 10$

5.  $\frac{81}{3} = \frac{x}{15}$

6.  $0.125 : 0.5 :: x : 10$

---

## Ratio and Proportion in Dosage

When the amount of drug ordered by a physician differs from the stock, ratio and proportion are used to solve the problem.

**Example**  Order: 0.5 mg of a drug

Stock: A liquid labeled 0.125 mg per 4 mL

We know the liquid comes as 0.125 mg in 4 mL. We want 0.5 mg. We don't know what amount of liquid will contain 0.5 mg. We have three pieces of information. We need the fourth, which is X.

This arithmetic operation can be set up and solved as a fraction-ratio or as two ratios separated by colons.

*Fraction-Ratio*

$$\frac{0.5}{0.125} \diagup\!\!\!\!\times \frac{X}{4}$$

$$0.125X = 2.0$$

$$\downarrow$$

$$\frac{0.125X}{0.125} = \frac{2.0}{0.125}$$

$$\downarrow$$

$$X = \frac{2.0}{0.125}$$

$$\downarrow$$

$$X = 2.0 \qquad \begin{array}{r} 16. \\ 0.125\overline{)2.000.} \\ \underline{1\ 25} \\ 750 \\ \underline{750} \end{array}$$

*Two Ratios Using Colons*

$$0.5 : 0.125 :: X : 4$$

$$0.125X = 2.0$$

$$\downarrow$$

$$\frac{0.125X}{0.125} = \frac{2.0}{0.125}$$

$$\downarrow$$

$$X = \frac{2.0}{0.125}$$

$$\downarrow$$

$$X = 2.0 \qquad \begin{array}{r} 16. \\ 0.125\overline{)2.000.} \\ \underline{1\ 25} \\ 750 \\ \underline{750} \end{array}$$

**Learning Aid**

Clear *X* by dividing both sides of the equation with the number preceding *X*.

**Learning Aid**

Remember the line between the two numbers in a fraction is a division sign. Read as 2.0 divided by 0.125.

    In the examples shown above, several steps are needed to solve ratio and proportion. This procedure can be simplified.

    In Chapter 6 we will learn the formula method, which is derived from ratio and proportion.

*Name:* _____

*These arithmetic operations are needed to calculate doses. Answers are on page 326. If you have difficulty in any area, study the related materials again. Your instructor can provide other practice tests if necessary from the* Instructors' Manual.

**A.** Multiply

   **a)** $\begin{array}{r} 647 \\ \times\,38 \\ \hline \end{array}$    **b)** $\frac{8}{9} \times \frac{12}{32}$    **c)** $\begin{array}{r} 0.56 \\ \times\,0.17 \\ \hline \end{array}$

**B.** Divide. If necessary report decimals two places.

   **a)** $82\overline{)793}$   **b)** $5\frac{1}{4} \div \frac{7}{4}$   **c)** $0.015\overline{)0.3}$

**C.** Change to a decimal. If necessary report decimals two places.

   **a)** $\frac{1}{18}$   **b)** $\frac{3}{8}$

**D.** Change to a fraction and reduce to lowest terms.

   **a)** 0.35   **b)** 0.08

**E.** In each set, which number has the greater value?

   **a)** _____ 0.4 and 0.162

   **b)** _____ 0.76 and 0.8

   **c)** _____ 0.5 and 0.83

   **d)** _____ 0.3 and 0.25

**F.** Reduce these fractions to their lowest terms as decimals. Report to one decimal place.

   **a)** $\frac{20}{12}$   **b)** $\frac{7}{84}$   **c)** $\frac{6}{13}$

**G.** Round off these decimals as indicated.

   **a)** nearest tenth      5.349 _____

   **b)** nearest hundredth   0.6284 _____

   **c)** nearest thousandth   0.9244 _____

**H.** Change these percents to a fraction.

   **a)** $\frac{1}{3}\%$   **b)** 0.8%

**I.** Solve these ratios.

   **a)** $\frac{32}{128} = \frac{4}{X}$

   **b)** $8 : 72 :: 5 : X$

   **c)** $\frac{0.4}{0.12} = \frac{X}{8}$ (nearest whole number)

# Answers

## Self-Test 1 Multiplication

| | | | | | |
|---|---|---|---|---|---|
| **1.** 12 | **5.** 108 | **9.** 48 | **13.** 24 | **17.** 18 | **21.** 132 |
| **2.** 63 | **6.** 24 | **10.** 72 | **14.** 54 | **18.** 88 | **22.** 45 |
| **3.** 32 | **7.** 110 | **11.** 15 | **15.** 64 | **19.** 36 | **23.** 81 |
| **4.** 45 | **8.** 14 | **12.** 42 | **16.** 56 | **20.** 24 | **24.** 35 |

## Self-Test 2 Division

| | | | | | |
|---|---|---|---|---|---|
| **1.** 9 | **5.** 7 | **9.** 7 | **13.** 4 | **17.** 9 | **21.** 7 |
| **2.** 4 | **6.** 8 | **10.** 6 | **14.** 3 | **18.** 4 | **22.** 12 |
| **3.** 3 | **7.** 4 | **11.** 9 | **15.** 3 | **19.** 6 | **23.** 12 |
| **4.** 7 | **8.** 3 | **12.** 6 | **16.** 7 | **20.** 2 | **24.** 7 |

## Self-Test 3 Reducing Fractions

**1.** $\frac{16}{24} = \frac{4}{6} = \frac{2}{3}$   (divide by 4, then 2)

Alternatively: $\frac{16}{24} = \frac{2}{3}$ (divide by 8)

**2.** $\frac{36}{216} = \frac{6}{36} = \frac{1}{6}$   (divide by 6, then 6)

**3.** $\frac{18}{96} = \frac{9}{48} = \frac{3}{16}$   (divide by 2, then 3)

**4.** $\frac{70}{490} = \frac{7}{49} = \frac{1}{7}$   (divide by 10, then 7)

**5.** $\frac{18}{81} = \frac{2}{9}$   (divide by 9)

**6.** $\frac{8}{48} = \frac{1}{6}$   (divide by 8)

**7.** $\frac{12}{30} = \frac{6}{15} = \frac{2}{5}$   (divide by 2, then 3)

Alternatively: $\frac{12}{30} = \frac{2}{5}$   (divide by 6)

**8.** $\frac{68}{136} = \frac{34}{68} = \frac{1}{2}$   (divide by 2, then 34)

**9.** $\frac{55}{121} = \frac{5}{11}$   (divide by 11)

**10.** $\frac{15}{60} = \frac{1}{4}$   (divide by 15)

Alternatively: $\frac{15}{60} = \frac{3}{12} = \frac{1}{4}$ (divide by 5, then 3)

## Self-Test 4 (Two Ways to Solve) Multiplying Fractions

**First Way**

**1.** $\frac{1}{6} \times \frac{4}{5} \times \frac{5}{2} = \frac{20}{60} = \frac{1}{3}$

**2.** $\frac{4}{15} \times \frac{3}{2} = \frac{\overset{2}{\cancel{12}}}{\underset{5}{\cancel{30}}} = \frac{2}{5}$

(Divide by 6)

**3.** $1\frac{1}{2} \times 4\frac{2}{3} = \frac{3}{2} \times \frac{14}{3} = \frac{\overset{7}{\cancel{42}}}{\underset{1}{\cancel{6}}} = 7$

**Second Way**

**1.** $\frac{1}{\underset{3}{\cancel{6}}} \times \frac{\overset{\overset{1}{\cancel{2}}}{\cancel{4}}}{\underset{1}{\cancel{5}}} \times \frac{\overset{1}{\cancel{5}}}{\underset{1}{\cancel{2}}} = \frac{\overset{1}{\cancel{2}}}{\underset{3}{\cancel{6}}} = \frac{1}{3}$

**2.** $\frac{\overset{2}{\cancel{4}}}{\underset{5}{\cancel{15}}} \times \frac{\overset{1}{\cancel{3}}}{\cancel{2}} = \frac{2}{5}$

**3.** $1\frac{1}{2} \times 4\frac{2}{3} = \frac{\overset{1}{\cancel{3}}}{\underset{1}{\cancel{2}}} \times \frac{\overset{7}{\cancel{14}}}{\underset{1}{\cancel{3}}} = 7$

First Way

$$4.\ \frac{1}{5} \times \frac{15}{45} = \frac{\cancel{15}^{3}}{\cancel{225}_{45}} = \frac{3}{45} = \frac{1}{15}$$

(Divide by 5)

$$5.\ 3\frac{3}{4} \times 10\frac{2}{3} = \frac{15}{4} \times \frac{32}{3}$$

(Too confusing! Use the second way.)

$$6.\ \frac{7}{20} \times \frac{2}{14}$$

(Too difficult. Use the second way.)

$$7.\ \frac{9}{2} \times \frac{3}{2} = \frac{27}{4}$$

(Cannot reduce)

$$8.\ 6\frac{1}{4} \times 7\frac{1}{9} \times \frac{9}{5} = \frac{25}{4} \times \frac{64}{9} \times \frac{9}{5}$$

(Too difficult. Use the second way.)

Second Way

$$4.\ \frac{1}{5} \times \frac{\cancel{15}^{1}}{\cancel{45}_{3}} = \frac{1}{15}$$

$$5.\ \frac{\cancel{15}^{5}}{\cancel{4}_{1}} \times \frac{\cancel{32}^{8}}{\cancel{3}_{1}} = 40$$

$$6.\ \frac{\cancel{7}^{1}}{\cancel{20}_{10}} \times \frac{\cancel{2}^{1}}{\cancel{14}_{2}} = \frac{1}{20}$$

$$8.\ \frac{\cancel{25}^{5}}{\cancel{4}_{1}} \times \frac{\cancel{64}^{16}}{\cancel{9}_{1}} \times \frac{\cancel{9}^{1}}{\cancel{5}_{1}} = 80$$

## Self-Test 5 Dividing Fractions

$$1.\ \frac{1}{75} \div \frac{1}{150} = \frac{1}{\cancel{75}_{1}} \times \frac{\cancel{150}^{2}}{1} = 2$$

$$2.\ \frac{1}{8} \div \frac{1}{4} = \frac{1}{8} \times \frac{\cancel{4}^{1}}{1} = \frac{1}{2}$$

$$3.\ 2\frac{2}{3} \div \frac{1}{2} = \frac{8}{3} \times \frac{2}{1} = \frac{16}{3}$$

$$4.\ 75 \div 12\frac{1}{2} = 75 \div \frac{25}{2} = \frac{\cancel{75}^{3}}{1} \times \frac{2}{\cancel{25}_{1}} = 6$$

$$5.\ \frac{7}{25} \div \frac{7}{75} = \frac{\cancel{7}^{1}}{\cancel{25}_{1}} \times \frac{\cancel{75}^{3}}{\cancel{7}_{1}} = 3$$

$$6.\ \frac{1}{2} \div \frac{1}{4} = \frac{1}{\cancel{2}_{1}} \times \frac{\cancel{4}^{2}}{1} = 2$$

$$7.\ \frac{3}{4} \div \frac{8}{3} = \frac{3}{4} \times \frac{3}{8} = \frac{9}{32}$$

$$8.\ \frac{1}{60} \div \frac{7}{10} = \frac{1}{\cancel{60}_{6}} \times \frac{\cancel{10}^{1}}{7} = \frac{1}{42}$$

## Self-Test 6 Converting Fractions to Decimals

**1.** $\dfrac{1}{6}$ $\begin{array}{r} .166 \\ 6\overline{\smash{)}1.000} \\ \underline{6} \\ 40 \\ \underline{36} \\ 40 \\ \underline{36} \\ 4 \end{array}$ $= 0.166$

**2.** $\dfrac{\overset{3}{\cancel{6}}}{\underset{4}{8}} = \dfrac{3}{4}$ $\begin{array}{r} .75 \\ 4\overline{\smash{)}3.00} \\ \underline{2\,8} \\ 20 \\ \underline{20} \\ 0 \end{array}$ $= 0.75$

**3.** $\dfrac{4}{5}$ $\begin{array}{r} .8 \\ 5\overline{\smash{)}4.0} \\ \underline{4\,0} \\ 0 \end{array}$ $= 0.8$

**4.** $\dfrac{9}{40}$ $\begin{array}{r} .225 \\ 40\overline{\smash{)}9.000} \\ \underline{8\,0} \\ 1\,00 \\ \underline{80} \\ 200 \\ \underline{200} \\ 0 \end{array}$ $= 0.225$

**5.** $\dfrac{1}{8}$ $\begin{array}{r} .125 \\ 8\overline{\smash{)}1.000} \\ \underline{8} \\ 20 \\ \underline{16} \\ 40 \\ \underline{40} \\ 0 \end{array}$ $= 0.125$

**6.** $\dfrac{1}{7}$ $\begin{array}{r} .142 \\ 7\overline{\smash{)}1.000} \\ \underline{7} \\ 30 \\ \underline{28} \\ 20 \\ \underline{14} \\ 6 \end{array}$ $= 0.142$

## Self-Test 7 Reading Decimals

**1.** Twenty-five hundredths ($\frac{25}{100}$)

**2.** Four thousandths ($\frac{4}{1000}$)

**3.** One and seven tenths ($1\frac{7}{10}$)

**4.** Five tenths ($\frac{5}{10}$)

**5.** Three hundred thirty-four thousandths ($\frac{334}{1000}$)

**6.** One hundred thirty-six and seventy-five hundredths ($136\frac{75}{100}$)

**7.** One tenth ($\frac{1}{10}$)

**8.** One hundred fifty thousandths ($\frac{150}{1000}$). The zero at the end of 0.150 is not necessary. The number could be read as fifteen hundredths ($\frac{15}{100}$).

## Self-Test 8 Division of Decimals

**1.** $\begin{array}{r} 0.0002 \\ 24\overline{\smash{)}0.0048} \end{array}$  No decimals in the divisor, so no need to move the decimal in the dividend.

**2.** $0.004\overline{\smash{)}0.100}$  Now it is $\begin{array}{r} 25. \\ 4\overline{\smash{)}100.} \end{array}$

**3.** $0.02\overline{\smash{)}0.20}$  Now it is $\begin{array}{r} 10. \\ 2\overline{\smash{)}20.} \end{array}$

**4.** $7.8\overline{\smash{)}140.0}$  Now it is $\begin{array}{r} 17.948 \\ 78\overline{\smash{)}1400.000} \\ \underline{78} \\ 620 \\ \underline{546} \\ 74\,0 \\ \underline{70\,2} \\ 3\,80 \\ \underline{3\,12} \\ 680 \\ \underline{624} \\ 56 \end{array}$

**5.** $\begin{array}{r} 23.333 \\ 6\overline{\smash{)}140.000} \\ \underline{12} \\ 20 \\ \underline{18} \\ 20 \\ \underline{18} \\ 20 \\ \underline{18} \\ 20 \\ \underline{18} \\ 20 \\ \underline{18} \\ 2 \end{array}$

**6.** $0.025\overline{\smash{)}10.000}$  Now it is $\begin{array}{r} 400. \\ 25\overline{\smash{)}10000.} \end{array}$

Note that because there are two places between the 4 and the decimal, you had to add 2 zeros.

## Self-Test 9 Rounding Decimals

| Nearest Tenth | Nearest Hundredth | Nearest Thousandth |
|---|---|---|
| **1.** 0.3 | **6.** 1.27 | **11.** 1.325 |
| **2.** 1.8 | **7.** 0.75 | **12.** 0.003 |
| **3.** 3.3 | **8.** 0.68 | **13.** 0.452 |
| **4.** 0.1 | **9.** 4.54 | **14.** 0.726 |
| **5.** 0.6 | **10.** 1.22 | **15.** 0.348 |

## Self-Test 10 Value of Decimals

| | | |
|---|---|---|
| **1.** 0.25 | **4.** 0.2 | **7.** 0.4 |
| **2.** 0.1 | **5.** 0.825 | **8.** 0.7 |
| **3.** 0.5 | **6.** 0.9 | |

## Self-Test 11 Conversion of Percents

**1.** Fraction $\quad 10\% = \dfrac{\overset{1}{\cancel{10}}}{\underset{10}{\cancel{100}}} = \dfrac{1}{10}$

Decimal $\quad 10\% = \dfrac{10}{100} \enspace \overset{.1}{\overline{)10.0}} = 0.1$

Quick rule decimal $\quad 1\underset{\frown}{0}.\% = 0.1$

**2.** Fraction $\quad 0.9\% = \dfrac{\frac{9}{10}}{100} = \frac{9}{10} \div 100 = \frac{9}{10} \times \frac{1}{100} = \frac{9}{1000}$

Decimal $\quad 0.9\% = \dfrac{0.9}{100} \enspace \overset{.009}{\overline{)0.900}} = 0.009$

Quick rule decimal $\quad \underset{\frown}{0}0.9 = 0.009$

**3.** Fraction $\quad \frac{1}{5}\% = \dfrac{\frac{1}{5}}{100} = \frac{1}{5} \div 100 = \frac{1}{5} \times \frac{1}{100} = \frac{1}{500}$

Decimal $\quad \frac{1}{5}\% = \frac{1}{5} \div 100 = \dfrac{1}{500} \enspace \overset{.002}{\overline{)1.000}} = 0.002$

Quick rule decimal $\quad \frac{1}{5}\% = \frac{1}{5} \enspace \overset{.2}{\overline{)1.0}} = 0.2\%$

$\underset{\frown}{0}0.2 = 0.002$

**4.** Fraction $\quad .01\% = \dfrac{\frac{1}{100}}{100} = \frac{1}{100} \div \frac{100}{1} = \frac{1}{100} \times \frac{1}{100} = \frac{1}{10000}$

Decimal $\quad .01\% = \dfrac{0.01}{100} \enspace \overset{0.0001}{\overline{)\ .0100}} = .0001$

Quick rule decimal $\quad \underset{\frown}{0}0.01\% = 0.0001$

5. Fraction  $\dfrac{2}{3}\% = \dfrac{\frac{2}{3}}{100} = \dfrac{2}{3} \div \dfrac{100}{1} = \dfrac{2}{3} \times \dfrac{1}{100} = \dfrac{2}{300} = \dfrac{1}{150}$

Decimal  $\dfrac{2}{3}\% = \dfrac{2}{3} \div \dfrac{100}{1} = \dfrac{2}{3} \times \dfrac{1}{100} = \dfrac{2}{300} \;\overset{.0066}{\overline{)2.000}} = .0066$

Quick rule decimal  $\dfrac{2}{3}\% = \dfrac{2}{3} \overset{.66}{\overline{)2.00}} = 0.66\% = 00.66 = .0066$

6. Fraction  $.45\% = \dfrac{\frac{45}{100}}{100} = \dfrac{45}{100} \div \dfrac{100}{1} = \dfrac{45}{100} \times \dfrac{1}{100} = \dfrac{45}{10000} = \dfrac{9}{2000}$

Decimal  $.45\% = \dfrac{.45}{100} \overset{.0045}{\overline{)0.4500}} = .0045$

Quick rule decimal  $00.45\% = .0045$

7. Fraction  $\dfrac{\overset{1}{\cancel{20}}}{\underset{5}{\cancel{100}}} = \dfrac{1}{5}$

Decimal  $20\% = \dfrac{20}{100} \overset{0.2}{\overline{)20.0}}$

Quick rule decimal  $20.\% = 0.2$

8. Fraction  $0.4\% = \dfrac{\frac{4}{10}}{100} = \dfrac{4}{10} \div \dfrac{100}{1} = \dfrac{\overset{1}{\cancel{4}}}{10} \times \dfrac{1}{\underset{25}{\cancel{100}}} = \dfrac{1}{250}$

Decimal  $0.4\% = \dfrac{0.4}{100} \overset{0.004}{\overline{)0.400}} = 0.004$

Quick rule decimal  $00.4\% = 0.004$

9. Fraction  $\dfrac{1}{10}\% = \dfrac{\frac{1}{10}}{100} = \dfrac{1}{10} \div \dfrac{100}{1} = \dfrac{1}{10} \times \dfrac{1}{100} = \dfrac{1}{1000}$

Decimal  $\dfrac{1}{10}\% = \dfrac{1}{10} \div \dfrac{100}{1} = \dfrac{1}{10} \times \dfrac{1}{100} = \dfrac{1}{1000} \overset{0.001}{\overline{)1.000}} = 0.001$

Quick rule decimal  $\dfrac{1}{10}\% = \dfrac{1}{10} \overset{0.1}{\overline{)1.0}} = 0.1\% = 00.1 = 0.001$

10. Fraction  $2\dfrac{1}{2}\% = 2.5\% = \dfrac{\frac{2.5}{1000}}{100} = \dfrac{2.5}{1000} \div \dfrac{100}{1} = \dfrac{2.5}{1000} \times \dfrac{1}{100} = \dfrac{25}{10000} = \dfrac{5}{2000} = \dfrac{1}{400}$

Decimal  $2.5\% = \dfrac{2.5}{100} \overset{0.025}{\overline{)2.50}} = .025$

Quick rule decimal  $002.5\% = .025$

11. Fraction  $33\% = \dfrac{33}{100}$

Decimal  $33\% = \dfrac{33}{100} \overset{.33}{\overline{)33.00}} = .33$

Quick rule decimal  $33.\% = .33$

**12.** Fraction   $50\% = \frac{50}{100} = \frac{1}{2}$

Decimal   $50\% = \frac{50}{100}$  $\overset{.5}{100\overline{)50.0}} = .5$

Quick rule decimal   $\underset{\curvearrowleft}{50.}\% = .5$

## Self-Test 12 Solving Proportions

**1.**   $\frac{120}{4.2} = \frac{16}{x}$     $\overset{0.56}{120\overline{)67.20}}$

$120x = 67.2$     $\underline{60\ 0}$

$x = 0.56$     $7\ 20$

     $\underline{7\ 20}$

**2.** $750 : 250 :: x : 5$

$250x = 750 \times 5$     $\frac{750 \times 5}{250} \overset{3}{\underset{1}{}} = 15$

$x = 15$

**3.** $\frac{14}{140} = \frac{22}{x}$

$14x = 22 \times 140$     $\frac{22 \times 140}{14} \overset{10}{\underset{1}{}} = 220$

$x = 220$

**4.** $2 : 5 :: x : 10$

$5x = 20$

$x = 4$

**5.** $\frac{81}{3} = \frac{x}{15}$     $\frac{81 \times 15}{3} \overset{5}{\underset{1}{}} = 405$

$3x = 81 \times 15$

$x = 405$

**6.** $0.125 : 0.5 :: x : 10$     $\frac{0.125}{0.500} \overset{1}{\underset{4}{}} \times 10 = \frac{10}{4} \overset{2.5}{4\overline{)10.0}}$

$0.5x = 0.125 \times 10$

$x = 2.5$

# Interpreting the Language of Prescriptions

CONTENT TO MASTER

▶ Abbreviating times and routes of administration

▶ Understanding military time: the 24-hour clock

▶ Abbreviating metric, household, and apothecary measures

▶ Understanding SI units

▶ Reading prescriptions

▶ Terms and abbreviations for drug preparations

Misreading abbreviations leads to medication errors. When you are unsure of the abbreviation, of the handwriting, or have a question regarding a medication order, do not attempt to prepare the dose. *Clarify the order with the person who wrote the order.*

Here are three medication orders that will make sense to you after studying material in this chapter:

Morphine sulfate 15 mg SC stat and 10 mg q 4 h prn

Chloromycetin 0.01% Ophth Oint OS bid

Ampicillin 1 g IVPB q 6 h

## ▶ Time of Administration of Drugs

The abbreviations for times of drug administration are based on Latin words. They are included here under *Learning Aid* for your information, but it is not necessary for you to study or learn the Latin words. Learn the abbreviations, their meanings, and the sample times that indicate how the abbreviations are interpreted.

| Time Abbreviation | Meaning | Learning Aid | |
|---|---|---|---|
| ac | Before meals | Latin, *ante cibum* | |
| | | **Sample time** | 7:30 AM, 11:30 AM, 4:30 PM |
| pc | After meals | Latin, *post cibum* | |
| | | **Sample time** | 10 AM, 2 PM, 6 PM |
| | | | *(continued)* |

(Continued)

| Time Abbreviation | Meaning | Learning Aid |
|---|---|---|
| qd | Every day, daily | Latin, *quaque die* |
| | | **Sample time**    10 AM |
| bid | Twice a day | Latin, *bis in die* |
| | | **Sample time**    10 AM, 6 PM |
| tid | Three times a day | Latin, *ter in die* |
| | | **Sample time**    10 AM, 2 PM, 6 PM |
| qid | Four times a day | Latin, *quater in die* |
| | | **Sample time**    10 AM, 2 PM, 6 PM, 10 PM |
| qh | Every hour | Latin, *quaque hora* |
| | | Because the drug is given every hour, it will be given 24 times in one day. |
| hs | At bedtime, hour of sleep | Latin, *hora somni* |
| | | **Sample time**    10 PM |
| qn | Every night | Latin, *quaque nocte* |
| | | **Sample time**    10 PM |
| stat | Immediately | Latin, *statim* |
| | | **Sample time**    Now! |

The following time abbreviations are based on a 24-hour day. To determine the number of times a medication will be given in a day, divide 24 by the number given in the abbreviation.

| Time Abbreviation | Meaning | Learning Aid |
|---|---|---|
| q2h or q2° | Every 2 hours | The drug will be given 12 times in a 24-hour period (24 ÷ 2). |
| | | **Sample times**    even hours at 2 AM, 4 AM, 6 AM, 8 AM, 10 AM, 12 noon, 2 PM, 4 PM, 6 PM, 8 PM, 10 PM, 12 midnight |
| q4h or q4° | Every 4 hours | The drug will be given six times in a 24-hour period (24 ÷ 4). |
| | | **Sample time**    2 AM, 6 AM, 10 AM, 2 PM, 6 PM, 10 PM |

*(continued)*

(Continued)

| Time Abbreviation | Meaning | Learning Aid |
|---|---|---|
| q6h or q6° | Every 6 hours | The drug will be given four times in a 24-hour period (24 ÷ 6)<br><br>**Sample times**   6 AM, 12 noon, 6 PM, 12 midnight |
| q8h or q8° | Every 8 hours | The drug will be given three times in a 24-hour period (24 ÷ 8)<br><br>**Sample times**   6 AM, 2 PM, 10 PM |
| q12h or q12° | Every 12 hours | The drug will be given twice in a 24-hour period (24 ÷ 12)<br><br>**Sample times**   6 AM, 6 PM |

There are four additional time abbreviations that require explanation. They are as follows:

| Time Abbreviation | Meaning | Learning Aid |
|---|---|---|
| qod | Every other day | Latin, *quaque otra die*<br><br>This abbreviation is interpreted by the days of the **month:** the nurse writes on the medication record:<br><br>qod odd days of the month<br><br>**Sample time**   10 AM on the first, third, fifth day, and so on<br><br>The nurse might write:<br><br>qod even days of the month<br><br>**Sample time**   10 AM on the second, fourth, sixth day, and so on |
| prn | As needed | Latin, *pro re nata*<br><br>***This abbreviation is usually combined with a time abbreviation.***<br><br>**Example**   q4h prn (every 4 hours as needed).<br><br>This permits the nurse to assess the patient and make a nursing judgment about whether or not to administer the medication.<br><br>**Sample**   acetaminophen 650 mg po q4h prn (650 milligrams of acetaminophen by mouth, every 4 hours as needed for pain)<br><br>The nurse assesses the patient for pain every 4 hours; if the patient has pain, the nurse may administer the drug. This abbreviation has three administration implications:<br><br>1. The nurse **must wait** 4 hours before giving the next dose.<br>2. Once 4 hours has elapsed, the dose may be given any time thereafter.<br>3. Sample times are not given because the nurse does not know when the patient will need the drug. |

*(continued)*

(Continued)

| Time Abbreviation | Meaning | Learning Aid |
|---|---|---|
| tiw | Three times per week | Latin, *ter in vicis*<br>Time relates to days of the **week**.<br>**Sample time**　10 AM on Monday, Wednesday, Friday<br>Do not confuse with tid (three times per **day**). |
| biw | Twice per week | Latin, *bis in vicis*<br>Time relates to days of the **week**.<br>**Sample time**　10 AM on Monday, Thursday<br>Do not confuse with bid (twice per **day**). |

**SELF TEST 1** **Abbreviations**

*After studying the abbreviations for times of administration, give the meaning of the following terms. Include sample times. Answers are given at the end of the chapter.*

1. tid _____
2. qn _____
3. pc _____
4. qod _____
5. bid _____
6. hs _____
7. stat _____
8. qid _____

9. q4h _____
10. ac _____
11. qd _____
12. q8h _____
13. qh _____
14. prn _____
15. q4h prn _____

## Military Time: The 24-Hour Clock

Confusion about times of administration can arise by misinterpreting handwriting as AM or PM. To prevent error, many institutions have converted from the traditional 12-hour clock to a 24-hour clock, referred to as military time.

The 24-hour clock begins at midnight as 0000. The hours from 1 AM to 12 noon are the same as traditional time; colons and the terms AM and PM are omitted. For example:

| Traditional | Military |
|---|---|
| 12 midnight | 0000 |
| 1 AM | 0100 |
| 5 AM | 0500 |
| 7:30 AM | 0730 |
| 11:45 AM | 1145 |
| 12:00 noon | 1200 |

**Learning Aid**

In military time, minutes are written in tenths, hours Dhs or thousandths.

The hours from 1 PM continue numerically; 1 PM becomes 1300. For example:

| Traditional | Military |
|---|---|
| 1 PM | 1300 |
| 2:30 PM | 1430 |
| 5 PM | 1700 |
| 7:15 PM | 1915 |
| 10:45 PM | 2245 |
| 11:59 PM | 2359 |

**Learning Aid**

To change traditional time to military time from 1 PM on, add 12.

**SELF TEST 2**   **Military Time**

A. Change these traditional times to military time. Answers may be found at the end of the chapter.

1. 2 PM _____
2. 9 AM _____
3. 4 PM _____
4. 12 noon _____
5. 1:30 AM _____
6. 9.15 PM _____
7. 4:50 AM _____
8. 6:20 PM _____

B. Change these military times to traditional times. Answers may be found at the end of this chapter.

1. 0130 _____
2. 1745 _____
3. 1100 _____
4. 2015 _____
5. 1910 _____
6. 0600 _____
7. 2450 _____
8. 1000 _____

**Learning Aid**

To change military time to traditional time from 1300 on, subtract 12.

# ▶ Routes of Administration

Some of these abbreviations are based on Latin words, whereas others are not. Again, the Latin words are included for your information, but it is not necessary to study them. Alternative abbreviations are given in parentheses.

| Route Abbreviation | Meaning | Learning Aid |
|---|---|---|
| AD | Right ear | Latin, *aures dextra* |
| AL | Left ear | Latin, *aures laeva* |
| AU | Each ear | Latin, *aures utrae* |
| HHN | Hand-held nebulizer | Medication is placed in a device that produces a fine spray for inhalation. |
| IM | Intramuscularly | The injection is given at a 90° angle into a muscle. |
| IV | Intravenously | The injection is given into a vein. |

*(continued)*

(Continued)

| Route Abbreviation | Meaning | Learning Aid |
|---|---|---|
| IVP | Intravenous push | Medication is injected directly in a vein. |
| IVPB | Intravenous piggyback | Medication prepared in a small volume of fluid is attached to an IV (which is already infusing fluid into a patient's vein) at specified times (Fig. 2-1). |
| MDI | Metered-dose inhaler | An aerosol device delivers medication by inhalation. |
| NGT (ng) | Nasogastric tube | Medication is placed in the stomach through a tube in the nose. |
| OD | In the right eye | Latin, *oculus dextra* |
| OS | In the left eye | Latin, *oculus sinister* |
| OU | In both eyes | Latin, *oculi utrique* |
| po (PO) | By mouth | Latin, *per os* |
| pr (PR) | In the rectum | Latin, *per rectum* |
| SC (SQ) | Subcutaneously | The injection is usually given at a 45° angle into subcutaneous tissue. |
| SL | Sublingual, under the tongue | Latin, *sub lingua* |
| S & S | Swish and swallow | By using tongue and cheek muscles, the patient coats his/her mouth with a liquid medication. |

⊐ 1 mL        **Carpuject®**
              **with Luer Lock**

**Demerol®** ⒸⒾⒾ
meperidine
hydrochloride
injection, USP

Warning: May be habit forming.

**75 mg/mL**

For IM, SC or Slow IV Use

Sterile Aqueous Injection 7.5%
pH adjusted with NaOH or HCl.
For usual dosage and route of administration, see
package insert.
**Store at room temperature up to 25°C (77°F).**
Caution: Federal (USA) law prohibits dispensing
without prescription.
Demerol® is a registered trademark of Sanofi
Pharmaceuticals, Inc.

©Abbott 1997    08-8409-2/R1-11/97   Printed in USA
Abbott Laboratories, North Chicago, IL 60064, USA

**FIGURE 2-1**

Label states the routes of administration. Meperidine HCL, may be administered intramuscularly (IM), subcutaneously (SC), or slowly intravenous (IV). (Courtesy of Abbott Laboratories)

## SELF TEST 3 | Abbreviations (Routes)

*After studying the abbreviations for route of administration, give the meaning of the following terms. Answers are given at the end of the chapter.*

1. SL _____
2. OU _____
3. NGT _____
4. IV _____
5. po _____

6. OD _____
7. IVPB _____
8. OS _____
9. IM _____
10. pr _____

11. S&S _____
12. SC _____
13. AU _____
14. AL _____

# ▶ Metric and SI Abbreviations

Metric abbreviations in dosage relate to a drug's weight or volume and are the most common measures in dosage. The International System of Units (Système International d'Unités; SI) was adapted from the metric system in 1960. Most developed countries except the United States have adopted SI nomenclature to provide a standard language of measurement.

Differences between metric and SI systems do not occur in dosage. The meaning and abbreviations for weight and volume are the same. Weight measures are based on the gram: volume measures are based on the liter.

Study the meaning of the abbreviations listed in the following table. Under *Learning Aid*, one equivalent is given for each abbreviation to help you understand what kinds of quantities are involved. It is not yet necessary to study the equivalents (equivalents are discussed in Chapter 4). The preferred abbreviation is listed first; variations are given in parentheses.

| Metric Abbreviation | Meaning | Learning Aid |
|---|---|---|
| cc | Cubic centimeter | This is a measure of volume usually reserved for measuring gases. However, you may still find it used as a liquid measure. (One cubic centimeter is approximately equal to 16 drops from a medicine dropper.) |
| g (gm, Gm) | Gram | This is a solid measure of weight. (One gram is approximately equal to the weight of two paper clips.) |
| kg (Kg) | Kilogram | This is a weight measure. (One kilogram equals 2.2 pounds.) |
| L | Liter | This is a liquid measure. (One liter is a little more than a quart.) |
| $\mu$g (mcg) | Microgram | This is a measure of weight. (One thousand micrograms make up 1 milligram: 1000 $\mu$g = 1 mg) |
| mEq | Milliequivalent | No equivalent necessary. Drugs are prepared and ordered in this weight measure. |
| mg | Milligram | This is a measure of weight. (One thousand milligrams make up 1 gram: 1000 mg = 1 g) |
| mL (ml) | Milliliter | This is a liquid measure. The terms *cubic centimeter* (cc) and *milliliter* (mL) are interchangeable in dosage (1 cc = 1 mL). |
| unit (U) | Unit | This is a measure of biologic activity. Nurses do not calculate this measure. |

**Example**  penicillin potassium 300,000 units

*Important:* It is considered safer to write the word *unit* rather than use the abbreviation because the *U* could be read as a zero and a medication error might result.

*After studying metric abbreviations, write the meaning of the following terms. Answers can be found at the end of the chapter.*

**1.** 0.3 g _____   **6.** 0.25 mg _____

**2.** 150 mcg _____   **7.** 14 kg _____

**3.** 80 U _____   **8.** 20 mEq _____

**4.** 0.5 mL _____   **9.** 1.5 L _____

**5.** 1.7 cc _____   **10.** 50 $\mu$g _____

## ▶ Apothecary Abbreviations

Apothecary measures were common in the United States as far back as colonial times. Today apothecary measures are discouraged for several reasons: equivalency with the metric system is not exact; the system requires Roman numbers and fractions; apothecary symbols can be misinterpreted. Several apothecary terms are still in use.

minim   abbreviated m; is about the size of one drop. The term is found on some syringes. In *Figure 2-2* note two sets of marks. The upper lines indicate doses to 3 cc. The lower lines indicate minims. On this syringe 1 cc = 16 minims.

dram   abbreviated dr; is a liquid measure slightly less than a household teaspoon. 1 dr = 4 mL. In *Figure 2-3* note that the medication cup has measures in metric, household, and apothecary systems. If the answer to a dosage calculation was 12 mL, one could pour 3 drams.

grain   abbreviated gr; comes from the Latin word *granum*. This solid measure was based on the weight of a grain of wheat in medieval times. There is no commonly accepted equivalent to the grain in the metric system. In *Figure 2-4* note that an aspirin tablet is labeled 325 mg (5 gr). In written prescriptions, the metric gram (g; gm; Gm) can be confused with the apothecary grain (gr).

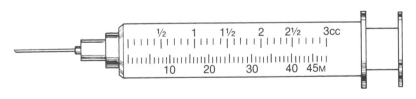

**FIGURE 2-2**

A 3-mL (cc) syringe calibrated in tenths of a milliliter and in minims.

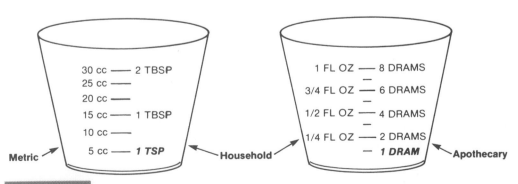

**FIGURE 2-3**

A medicine cup with metric, household, and apothecary equivalents. Two sides of the cup are shown.

| ASPIRIN | Lot: 52896<br>Exp. Date:<br>03/01 |
| --- | --- |
| *325 mg (5 gr)* | |
| *100 tablets* | N10590 |

drop    abbreviated gtt; from the Latin word *guttae*. This liquid measure was based on a drop of water; 1 gtt = 1 m. The term gtt is used in ordering eye medications. Ex. Timoptic 0.25% Ophth Sol 1 gtt ou bid.

i       means one in Roman numerals, which are represented by using letters of the alphabet. Roman numbers never have more than three of the same digit in a row. Ex. ii = 2; iii = 3; V = 5; X = 10.

---

**SELF TEST 5   Abbreviations (Apothecary)**

*After studying apothecary abbreviations still used in prescriptions, write the meaning of the following terms. Answers can be found at the end of the chapter.*

**1.** m x _____    **6.** gr i _____

**2.** ii dr _____    **7.** 2 gtt _____

**3.** 5 gr _____    **8.** 10 gr _____

**4.** gtt iii _____    **9.** m v _____

**5.** dr i _____

---

## ▶ Household Abbreviations

Physicians may use these common household measures to order drugs. Metric equivalents are included in the *Learning Aid* column for your information.

| Household<br>Abbreviation | Meaning | Learning Aid |
| --- | --- | --- |
| pt | Pint | One pint is approximately equal to 500 milliliters (1 pt ≅ 500 mL). |
| | | One quart is approximately equal to 1 liter, which is equal to 1000 milliliters (1 qt ≅ 1 L = 1000 mL). |
| qt | Quart | One-half quart is approximately equal to 1 pint ($\frac{1}{2}$ qt ≅ 1 pt = 500 mL). |
| tbsp | Tablespoon | One tablespoon equals 15 milliliters (1 tbsp = 15 mL). |
| tsp | Teaspoon | One teaspoon equals 5 milliliters (1 tsp = 5 mL). |
| oz | Ounce | One ounce equals 30 milliliters (1 oz = 30 mL). |

**Example**    6 tsp = 1 oz = 30 mL
3 tsp = $\frac{1}{2}$ oz = 15 mL
2 tbsp = 1 oz = 30 mL = 6 tsp
(see Fig. 2-3)

| SELF TEST 6 | Abbreviations (Household) |
| --- | --- |

*After studying household measures, write the meaning of the following terms. Answers can be found at the end of the chapter.*

**1.** 3 tsp _____    **3.** $\frac{1}{2}$ qt _____    **5.** 1 pt _____

**2.** 1 oz _____    **4.** 1 tsp _____    **6.** 2 tbsp _____

## ▶ Terms and Abbreviations for Drug Preparations

The following abbreviations and terms are used to describe selected drug preparations.

| Term Abbreviation | Meaning | Learning Aid |
| --- | --- | --- |
| cap, caps | Capsule | Medication is encased in a gelatin shell. |
| CR<br>LA<br>SA<br>SR<br>DS | Controlled-release<br>Long-acting<br>Sustained-action<br>Slow-release<br>Double-strength | These abbreviations indicate that the drug has been prepared in a form that allows extended action. Therefore, the drug is given less frequently. |
| EC | Enteric-coated | The tablet is coated with a substance that will not dissolve in the acid secretions of the stomach; instead, it dissolves in the more alkaline secretions of the intestines. |
| el, elix | Elixir | A drug is dissolved in a hydroalcoholic sweetened base. |
| sol | Solution | The drug is contained in a clear liquid preparation. |
| sp | Spirit | An alcoholic solution of a volatile substance (eg, spirit of ammonia). |
| sup, supp | Suppository | A solid, cylindrically shaped drug that can be inserted into a body opening (eg, the rectum or vagina). |
| susp | Suspension | Small particles of drug are dispersed in a liquid base and must be shaken before being poured; gels and magmas are also suspensions. |
| syr | Syrup | A sugar is dissolved in a liquid medication and flavored to disguise the taste. |
| tab, tabs | Tablet | Medication is compressed or molded into a solid form; additional ingredients are used to shape and color the tablet. |
| tr, tinct. | Tincture | This is a liquid alcoholic or hydroalcoholic solution of a drug. |
| ung, oint. | Ointment | This is a semisolid drug preparation that is applied to the skin (for external use only). |
| KVO | Keep vein open | **Example order** 1000 mL dextrose 5% in water IVKVO. The nurse is to continue infusing this fluid. |
| D/C | Discontinue | **Example order** D/C ampicillin |
| NKA | No known allergies | This is an important assessment that is noted on the medication record of a patient. |

## SELF TEST 7  Abbreviations (Drug Forms)

*After studying the abbreviations for drug forms, write out the meaning of the following terms. Answers can be found at the end of the chapter.*

**1.** elix _____

**2.** DS _____

**3.** NKA _____

**4.** caps _____

**5.** susp _____

**6.** tab _____

**7.** SR _____

**8.** D/C _____

**9.** supp _____

**10.** tr _____

## PROFICIENCY TEST 1  Abbreviations

*Name:* _____

*Aim for 90% or better on this test. There are 50 items, each worth 2 points. If you have any difficulty, study the content again. Answers will be found on page 328.*

1. bid _____
2. hs _____
3. prn _____
4. OU _____
5. po _____
6. pr _____
7. SL _____
8. S&S _____
9. tiw _____
10. mL _____
11. q4h _____
12. cc _____
13. SC _____
14. AU _____
15. g _____
16. PC _____
17. qd _____

18. stat _____
19. q12h _____
20. tid _____
21. OS _____
22. kg _____
23. qn _____
24. qh _____
25. OD _____
26. mEq _____
27. AC _____
28. qid _____
29. mg _____
30. IM _____
31. qod _____
32. biw _____
33. NGT _____
34. q8h _____

35. L _____
36. mcg _____
37. q6h _____
38. $\mu$g _____
39. U _____
40. tsp _____
41. AD _____
42. gr _____
43. IV _____
44. susp _____
45. tbsp _____
46. IVPB _____
47. m _____
48. Gm _____
49. q2h _____
50. q3h _____

**PROFICIENCY TEST 2** | Reading Prescriptions

*Name:* _____

*Now that you have studied the language of prescriptions, you are ready to interpret medication orders! Write the following orders in longhand. Give sample times.*

1. Nembutal 100 mg hs prn po _____

2. Propranolol hydrochloride 40 mg po bid _____
   _____

3. Ampicillin 1 g IVPB q6h _____
   _____

4. Demerol 50 mg IM q4h prn for pain _____
   _____

5. Tylenol 325 mg tabs ii po stat _____
   _____

6. Pilocarpine gtt ii OU q3h _____
   _____

7. Scopolamine 0.8 mg SC stat _____
   _____

8. El Digoxin 0.25 mg po qd _____
   _____

9. Kaochlor 30 mEq po bid _____
   _____

10. Liquaemin sodium 6000 units SC q4h _____
    _____

11. Tobramycin 70 mg IM q8h _____
    _____

12. Prednisone 10 mg po qod _____
    _____

13. Milk of magnesia 1 tbsp po hs qn _____
    _____

14. Septra DS tab i qd po _____
    _____

15. Morphine sulfate 15 mg SC stat and 10 mg q4h prn _____
    _____

## PROFICIENCY TEST 3 | Interpreting Written Prescription Orders

*Name:* _____

*These are actual prescriptions written by physicians. Interpret each in longhand. Remember that if an order is not clear, you must check with the person who wrote the order.*

| | |
|---|---|
| 1. Calare 100 mg po TID | 1. |
| 2. Ativan 1mg IVP x Ī now | 2. |
| 3. 10 meq KCl in 100cc NS over 1h X1 | 3. |
| 4. Tylenol #3 ĪĪ Tabs po q4° prn Pain | 4. |
| 5. Heparin 25,000 IU in 250ª D5W @ 500 u/Hr. | 5. |
| 6. Ticlid 250mg Ī PO BID. | 6. |
| 7. lopenor 25mg po BID. | 7. |
| 8. Benadryl 25mg po qm | 8. |

# Answers

## Self-Test 1 Abbreviations

1. Three times a day. (**Sample times:** 10 AM, 2 PM, 6 PM)
2. Every night. (**Sample time:** 10 PM)
3. After meals. (**Sample times:** 10 AM, 2 PM, 6 PM)
4. Every other day. (**Sample times:** odd days of month at 10 AM)
5. Twice a day. (**Sample times:** 10 AM, 6 PM)
6. Hour of sleep. (**Sample time:** 10 PM)
7. Immediately. (**Sample time:** whatever the time is now)
8. Four times a day. (**Sample times:** 10 AM, 2 PM, 6 PM, 10 PM)
9. Every 4 hours. (**Sample times:** 2 AM, 6 AM, 10 AM, 2 PM, 6 PM, 10 PM)
10. Before meals. (**Sample times:** 7:30 AM, 11:30 AM, 4:30 PM)
11. Every day. (**Sample time:** 10 AM)
12. Every 8 hours. (**Sample times:** 6 AM, 2 PM, 10 PM)
13. Every hour.
14. Whenever necessary. (**Sample times:** No time routine can be written.)
15. Every 4 hours as needed. (**Sample times:** No time routine is written because we do not know when the drug will be needed.)

## Self-Test 2 Military Time

A.
1. 1400
2. 0900
3. 1600
4. 1200
5. 0130
6. 2115
7. 0450
8. 1820

B.
1. 1:30 AM
2. 5:45 PM
3. 11 AM
4. 8:15 PM
5. 7:10 PM
6. 6 AM
7. 12:50 PM
8. 10 AM

## Self-Test 3 Abbreviations (Routes)

1. Sublingual; under the tongue
2. Both eyes
3. Nasogastric tube
4. Intravenously
5. By mouth
6. Right eye
7. Intravenous piggyback
8. Left eye
9. Intramuscularly
10. Rectally
11. Swish and swallow
12. Subcutaneously
13. Both ears
14. Left ear

## Self-Test 4 Abbreviations (Metric)

1. Three-tenths of a gram
2. One hundred fifty micrograms
3. Eighty units
4. Five-tenths of a milliliter
5. One and seven-tenths of a cubic centimeter
6. Twenty-five hundredths of a milligram
7. Fourteen kilograms
8. Twenty milliequivalents
9. One and five-tenths liters
10. Fifty micrograms

## Self-Test 5 Abbreviations (Apothecary)

1. 10 minims
2. 2 drams
3. 5 grains

4. 3 drops
5. 1 dram
6. 1 grain

7. 2 drops
8. 10 grains
9. 5 minims

## Self-Test 6 Abbreviations (Household)

1. Three teaspoons
2. One ounce

3. One-half quart
4. One teaspoon

5. One pint
6. Two tablespoons

## Self-Test 7 Abbreviations (Drug Forms)

1. Elixir
2. Double-strength
3. No known allergies
4. Capsules

5. Suspension
6. Tablet
7. Slow-release
8. Discontinue

9. Suppository
10. Tincture

CHAPTER

3

# Drug Labels and Packaging

## ▶ Drug Labels

An understanding of drug labels and the ways in which drugs are packaged provides a background for dosage and administration. This information can be self-taught and does not require class time. Students find it helpful to see and touch samples.

Labels that contain specific facts are found on drugs to be administered in the form in which they are packaged. This form may be solid or liquid. Occasionally some information such as route of administration, usual dose, and storage may not be on the label because the container is too small. When further information is needed, a professional reference should be consulted.

Here is a sample drug label:

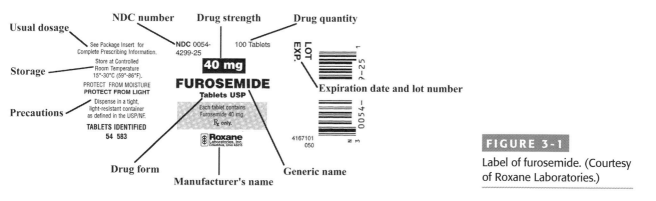

**FIGURE 3-1**

Label of furosemide. (Courtesy of Roxane Laboratories.)

*NDC NUMBER.* The National Drug Code (NDC) is a number used by the pharmacist to identify the drug and the method of packaging.

NDC in Figure 3-1 is 0054-4299-25. The letters NSN mean National Supply Number, a code for ordering the drug.

*TOTAL AMOUNT OF DRUG IN THE CONTAINER.* This information is found at the top of the label to the left or the right or at the bottom.

Figure 3-1 indicates 100 tablets.

*TRADE NAME.* The term *trade name,* which is also referred to as a brand name or proprietary name, may be identified by the symbol ® that follows the name. Several companies may manufacture the same drug using different trade names. Trade names may be capitalized on the labels, or they may have an initial capital only. *They are always written with the first letter capitalized.*

In Figure 3-1 Lasix ® is the trade or brand name.—It is not on this label.

*GENERIC NAME.* The generic name is the official accepted name of a drug, as listed in the United States Pharmacopeia (USP). A drug may have several trade names but only one official generic name. The generic name is not capitalized.

The generic name given in Figure 3-1 is furosemide.

*STRENGTH OF THE DRUG.* Solid drugs are given in metric weights; liquids are stated as a solution of drug in solvent.

In Figure 3-1 the strength is 40 mg.

*FORM OF THE DRUG.* The label specifies the type of preparation in the container.

Figure 3-1 indicates the drug is dispensed in tablets.

*USUAL DOSAGE.* This states how much drug is given at a single time or over a 24-hour period and also identifies who should receive the drug.

Figure 3-1 label states: see package insert for prescribing information.

*ROUTE OF ADMINISTRATION.* The label specifies how the drug is to be given: orally, parenterally (an injection of some type), or topically (applied to skin or mucous membranes). *When the label does not specify the route, the drug is in an oral form.*

In Figure 3-1 the route is oral.

*STORAGE.* This information describes the conditions necessary to protect the drug from losing its potency (effectiveness). Some drugs come in a dry form and must be dissolved, that is, reconstituted. The drug may be stored one way when dry and another way after reconstitution.

Figure 3-1 states to store at controlled room temperature 15–30°C (59°–86°F).

*PRECAUTIONS.* These are specific instructions related to safety, effectiveness, and/or administration that must be noted and followed.

Figure 3-1. Federal law prohibits dispensing without prescription.

Protect from moisture.

Protect from light.

Dispense in a tight, light-resistant container.

*MANUFACTURER'S NAME.* Any questions about the drug should be directed to this company.

Figure 3-1. Roxane Laboratories, Inc.

*EXPIRATION DATE.* The drug cannot be used after the last day of the month indicated.

Not shown in Figure 3-1.

*LOT NUMBER.* This number indicates the batch of drug from which this stock came.

Not shown in Figure 3-1.

*ADDITIVES.* The manufacturer may have used substances to bind the drug, to aid in dissolving the drug, to produce a specific pH, and so on. This information may be found on the label or in the literature accompanying the drug.

Not shown in Figure 3-1.

- Some drugs are dispensed in a dry (powder) form and must be reconstituted (dissolved).

- The drug label or drug insert provides specific directions about dissolving the powder.

- The amount and type of liquid to be used to dissolve the drug and the resulting solution are stated by the manufacturer.

**Example**   Amoxicillin (Polymox) comes in powder form. Prepare suspension at time of dispensing. Add 88 ml water to the bottle. For ease in preparation, add the water in two portions. Shake well after each addition. This provides 150 mL of suspension. Dosage is 125 mg of Amoxicillin per 5 mL of solution.

## SELF TEST 1    Drug Labels

*Read the label in Figure 3-2 and give the information requested. Answers are given at the end of the chapter.*

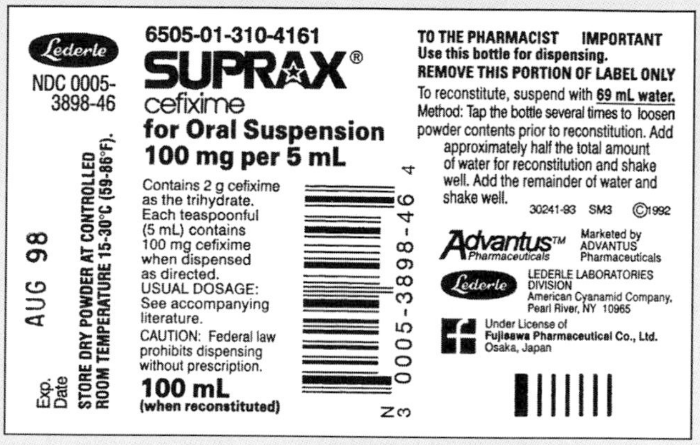

**FIGURE 3-2**

Label of cefixime for oral suspension (Suprax).
(Sample—for educational use only.)

1. NDC number _____

2. Total amount of drug in the container _____

3. Trade name _____

4. Generic name _____

5. Strength of the drug _____

6. Form of the drug _____

7. Usual dosage _____

8. Route of administration _____

9. Storage _____

_____

10. Directions for preparation _____

_____

11. Precautions _____

_____

12. Manufacturer _____

13. Expiration date _____

*(continued)*

*Read the label in Figure 3-3 and answer the following questions. Answers are located at the end of the chapter.*

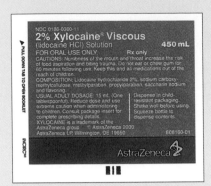

NDC 0186-0360-11
**2% Xylocaine® Viscous**
(lidocaine HCl) Solution          **450 mL**
FOR ORAL USE ONLY.          Rx only
CAUTIONS: Numbness of the mouth and throat increase the risk
of food aspiration and biting trauma. Do not eat or chew gum for
60 minutes following use. Keep this and all medications out of the
reach of children.
COMPOSITION: Lidocaine hydrochloride 2%, sodium carboxy-
methylcellulose, methylparaben, propylparaben, saccharin sodium
and flavoring.
USUAL ADULT DOSAGE: 15 mL (One      Dispense in child-
tablespoonful). Reduce dose and use    resistant packaging.
extreme caution when administering     Shake well before using.
to children. Consult package insert for  Squeeze bottle to
complete prescribing details.          dispense contents.
XYLOCAINE is a trademark of the
AstraZeneca group    © AstraZeneca 2000
AstraZeneca LP, Wilmington, DE 19850       608160-01

AstraZeneca

**FIGURE 3-3**

Label of lidocaine HCl (2% Xylocaine Viscous). (Courtesy of Astra Zeneca Pharmaceuticals.)

**14.** What is the trade name? _____

**15.** What is the generic name? _____

**16.** By what route(s) may this drug be given? _____

**17.** In what form is the drug dispensed? _____

**18.** What is the strength of the drug? _____

**19.** What is the total amount of drug in the container? _____

**20.** What is the usual adult dose? _____

_____

**21.** Give seven cautions on the label regarding this drug. _____

_____

_____

_____

_____

*When a medication container holds a single drug,* the written prescription indicates the dose in milligrams or grams, and calculation may be necessary.

**Example**

**a.** Tylenol 0.6 g po q 4 h prn for temperature ↑ 101°

*Label: Tylenol 325 mg tablets*

**b.** Prednisone 20 mg po bid

*Label: Prednisone 10 mg tablets*

**c.** Digoxin 0.5 mg po qd

*Label: Digoxin 0.25 mg*

**d.** Cefrozil 0.5 g po q 8°

*Label: 125 mg/5 mL*

*Some medication labels indicate more than one drug* in the dose form. These combination drugs are ordered by the number of tablets to give or the amount of liquid to pour.

**Example**

a. Order: Tylenol #3 tabs ii po q 4 h prn for pain

  *Label: acetaminophen 300 mg/codeine 30 mg tablet*

b. Order: Robitussin DM 1 tsp po qid

  *Label: guaifenesin 100 mg/dextromethorphan 10 mg per 5 mL*

c. Order: Talwin Compound 1 tab po q 6 h

  *Label: aspirin 325 mg/pentazocine 12.5 mg*

d. Order: Phenergan VC Syrup 2 tsp po q 6 h while awake

  *Label: phenylephrine 5 mg/promethazine 6.25 mg per 5 mL*

# ❱ Drug Packaging

In the future, innovative delivery systems will revolutionize the ways in which drugs are administered. In this chapter, however, we focus on the common types of containers that nurses handle as they prepare medications.

There are two types of packaging: *unit-dose* and *multidose*. Each type may contain a solid or liquid form of the drug for oral, parenteral, or topical use. Most institutions use a combination of unit-dose and multidose.

## Unit-Dose Packaging

In an institutional setting, each dose is individually wrapped and labeled, and a 24-hour supply is prepared by the pharmacy and dispensed. A major value of unit-dose packaging is that two professionals check the drug and the dose—the pharmacist and the nurse—thereby decreasing the possibility of error.

It should be stressed that unit-dose packaging does not relieve responsibility to *check the label three times* and to calculate the amount of drug needed. Unit-dose drugs come in different strengths, and there is always a chance of error when trade names are ordered instead of generic names. A dose may consist of one unit packet, two or more unit packets, or a fraction of one packet.

**Example**

A nurse has a unit-dose 100 mg tablet. If an order calls for 50 mg, only half the tablet would be administered.

A nurse may have an order for 75 mg. Unit packets contain 25 mg tablets.

The nurse would administer 3 tablets.

*FOR THE ORAL ROUTE.* For oral administration, unit-dose packaging may consist of:

1. Plastic bubble, foil, or paper wrappers containing tablets or capsules (Fig. 3-4*A*).

2. Plastic or glass containers that hold a single dose of a liquid or powder. The powder is reconstituted to a liquid form by following the directions given on the label (see Fig. 3-4*B*).

3. A sealed medication cup containing one dose of a liquid. The nurse removes the cover and the dose is ready to administer (see Fig. 3-4*C*).

*FOR THE PARENTERAL ROUTE.* These drugs are given by injection. The route must be specified in the order (eg, IM, SC, IVPB). Drugs in such containers are sterile, and sterile technique is used for their preparation and administration. The drugs may come in a solid or liquid form.

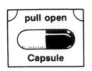
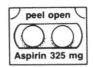
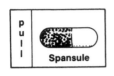
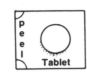
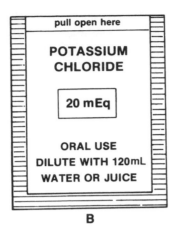
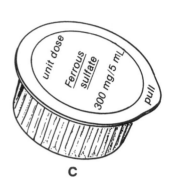

**FIGURE 3-4**

(*A*) Unit-dose tablets and capsules in foil wrappers. (*B*) Unit-dose powder in a sealed packet; it is placed in a container and diluted before giving. (*C*) Sealed cup containing one dose of a liquid medication ready to administer.

1. An *ampule* (ampoule) is a glass container that holds a single sterile dose of drug. The container has a narrow neck that must be broken to reach the drug. A sterile syringe is used to withdraw the medication (Fig. 3-5). The drug in the ampule may come as a liquid, a powder, or a crystal. Directions must be followed to reconstitute the solid forms. Once the glass is broken, any portion of the drug not used must be discarded because the drug cannot be kept sterile.

2. A *vial* is a glass or plastic container with a sealed rubber top. Medication in the container can be kept sterile. The container may have a sterile liquid or a sterile powder that must be reconstituted with a sterile diluent and syringe. *Single-dose vials* do not contain a preservative or a bacteriostatic agent. Therefore, any medication remaining after the dose is prepared should be discarded (see Fig. 3-5).

3. Flexible *plastic bags* or *glass vials* may hold sterile medication for intravenous use. The fluid is administered with the use of IV tubing that is connected to a needle or catheter placed in the patient's blood vessel (Fig. 3-6).

4. *Prefilled syringes* contain liquid, sterile medication that is ready to administer without further preparation. This type of unit-dose packaging is expensive but life saving in an emergency when speed is essential.

5. *Prefilled cartridges* are actually small vials, with a needle attached, that fit into a metal or plastic holder and eject one unit-dose of a sterile drug in liquid form (see Fig. 3-7).

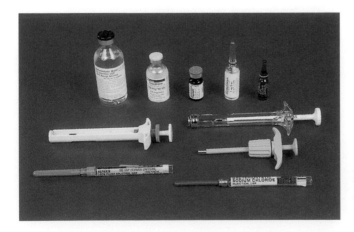

**FIGURE 3-5**

Parenteral route: (*top row*) vials and ampules; (*middle-bottom row*) prefilled cartridges and holders.

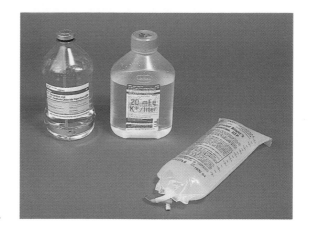

**FIGURE 3-6**

Plastic or glass containers hold medication for IV use.

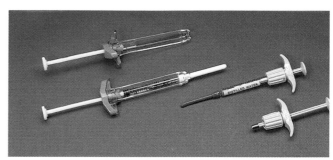

A

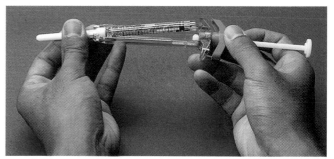

B

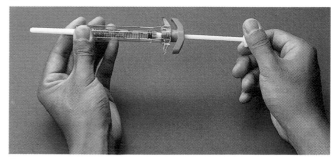

C

**FIGURE 3-7**

(*A*) Prefilled cartridges. (*B*) Inserting cartridge into injector device. (*C*) Cartridge is screwed into device, ready to administer drug.

*FOR TOPICAL ADMINISTRATION.* Drugs are applied to the skin or mucous membranes to achieve a local effect. They may be absorbed into the circulation, thereby achieving a systemic effect.

1. *Transdermal patches* or *pads* are adhesive bandages placed on the skin. They hold a drug form that is slowly absorbed into the circulation over a period ranging from hours to several days (Fig. 3-8).

2. *Lozenges and pastilles* are disklike solids that are slowly dissolved in the mouth (eg, cough drops). Some drugs are prepared in a gum and are released by chewing (eg, nicotine).

3. *Suppositories* in foil or plastic wrappers are molded forms that can be inserted into the rectum or vagina. They hold medication in a substance, such as cocoa butter, that melts at body temperature and releases the drug (Fig. 3-9). Suppositories may be used for unconscious patients or those unable to swallow.

4. *Plastic, disposable, squeezable containers* hold prepared solutions for the vagina (douches) or enema solutions that are administered rectally. The containers for enemas have a lubricated nozzle for ease in insertion. As the container is squeezed, the solution is forced out (Fig. 3-10).

## Multidose Packaging

In the institutional setting, each unit may receive large stock containers of medications from which doses are poured. This type of packaging reduces the pharmacy's workload but requires more time to prepare and increases the possibility of error.

*FOR THE ORAL ROUTE.* Stock bottles contain a liquid or a solid form such as tablets, capsules, or powders. When powders are reconstituted, the date and time of preparation must be written on the label and storage directions and expiration must be carefully noted. Powders, once dissolved, begin losing potency. Large stock bottles hold medication that is dispensed over a period of days (Fig. 3-11*A*).

*FOR THE PARENTERAL ROUTE.* Large-volume vials contain a sterile liquid or powder to be reconstituted using sterile technique. The data and time of preparation must be written on the label and the expiration and storage noted (see Fig. 3-11*B*).

*FOR TOPICAL ADMINISTRATION.* Care must be exercised to avoid contaminating these containers because they will be used over an extended period. Whenever possible, label the container with the patient's name and reserve its use for that one patient. The following types of containers may be used:

1. *Metal or plastic tubes* that contain ointments or creams to be applied to the skin or mucous membranes are squeezed to release the medication (Fig. 3-12*A*).

2. To avoid contamination medication is removed from *jars for creams, ointments, and pastes* by using a sterile tongue blade or sterile glove.

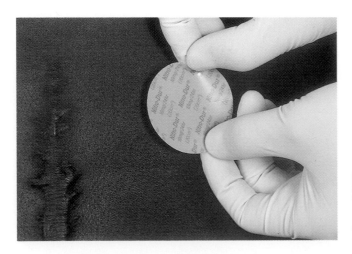

**FIGURE 3-8**

Transdermal patches or pads are placed on the skin. Drugs prepared in this manner include estrogen, fentanyl, testosterone, and nitroglycerin.

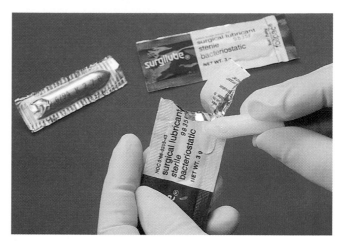

A

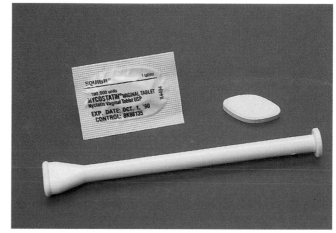

B

## FIGURE 3-9

(A) Rectal suppository. (B) Vaginal suppository and applicator.

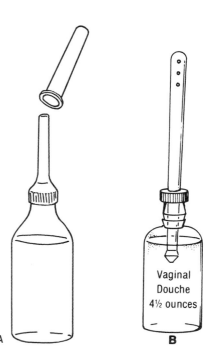

A

B

## FIGURE 3-10

Unit-dose containers for rectal enema (A) and vaginal irrigation (B).

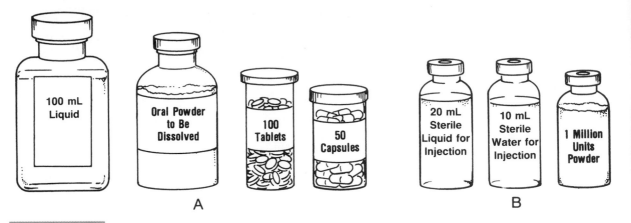

FIGURE 3-11

Multidose containers: (*A*) for the oral route; (*B*) for the parenteral route.

3. To prevent cross-contamination, *dropper bottles* for eyes, ear, or nose medications should be labeled with one patient's name. The nurse must be careful to avoid touching mucous membranes with the dropper, because contamination of the dropper could result in the growth of pathogens. There are two kinds of droppers: monodrop containers that are squeezed to release the medication and those in which the dropper can be removed from the bottle. Separate, packaged droppers are available to administer medications. These are calibrated, that is, marked in milliliters (see Fig. 3-12*B,C*).

Eye medications are labeled "ophthalmic" or "for the eye." Ear drugs are labeled "otic" or "auric" or "for the ear." Drugs for nasal administration are labeled "nose drops." Routes must never be interchanged.

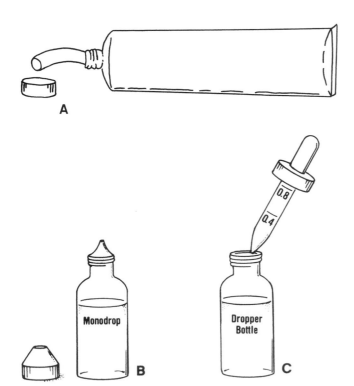

FIGURE 3-12

Topical multidose containers: (*A*) tubes for creams or ointments; (*B*) monodrop containers—the dropper is attached; (*C*) removable dropper is sometimes calibrated for liquid measures.

4. *Lozenges and pastilles* may be packaged in multidose as well as unit-dose containers.

5. *Metered-dose inhalers* (MDI) are aerosol devices that consist of two parts: a canister under pressure and a mouthpiece. The canister contains multiple drug doses in a liquid form or as a microfine powder or crystal. The mouthpiece fits on the canister. Finger pressure on the mouthpiece opens a valve on the canister that discharges one dose. The physician's order will state the number of inhalations or "puffs" to be taken (Fig. 3-13). Medications for inhalation also may be packaged as liquids in vials or bottles or as capsules containing powder to be used with a hand-held nebulizer (HHN) or with an intermittent positive-pressure breathing apparatus (IPPB).

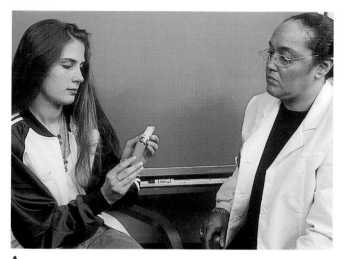

A

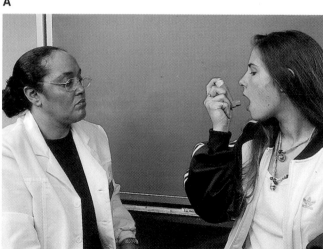

B

**FIGURE 3-13**

(*A*) Preparing the inhaler for use. (*B*) Administering medication.

**SELF TEST 2** | **Drug Packaging**

*Match Column A with the letters in Column B to identify the meaning of terms used in drug packaging. Answers may be found at the end of the chapter.*

*Column A*

1. _____ Unit dose
2. _____ Ampule
3. _____ Parenteral
4. _____ Prefilled cartridge
5. _____ Reconstitution
6. _____ Topical
7. _____ Transdermal patch
8. _____ Vial
9. _____ Lozenge
10. _____ Cocoa butter

*Column B*

a. Dissolving a powder into solution

b. Glass container with a sealed rubber top

c. Route of administration to skin or mucous membranes

d. Individually wrapped and labeled drugs

e. Disklike solid that dissolves in the mouth

f. Suppository ingredient that melts at body temperature

g. General term for an injection route

h. Adhesive bandage applied to the skin that gradually releases a drug

i. Small vial, with a needle attached, that fits into a syringe holder

j. Glass container that must be broken to obtain the drug

*Complete these statements related to the drug packaging. Answers may be found at the end of the chapter.*

11. Date and time of reconstitution must be written _____

_____

_____

12. The best way to avoid cross-contamination of a multidose tube of ointment is to _____

_____

13. To remove medication from a jar of paste, the nurse should use _____

_____

14. Dropper bottles for eye medications will be labeled _____

_____

15. Doses of medication that require use of a metered-dose inhaler are ordered in _____

_____

16. Medications for the ear will be labeled _____

*(continued)*

**SELF TEST 2    Drug Packaging (Continued)**

**17.** The term "multidose" refers to _____

_____

**18.** The type of drug packaging that decreases the possibility of error is termed_____

_____

**19.** Drugs administered topically for a local effect may be absorbed and produce another effect

that is called _____

_____

_____

**20.** The word "lozenge" describes _____

_____

_____

*Name:* _____

*Complete these questions. Answers will be found on page 329.*

1. Explain the difference between each of these pairs.

   a. 1. unit dose _____

      2. multidose _____

   b. 1. ampule _____

      2. vial _____

   c. 1. topical _____

      2. parenteral _____

   d. 1. trade name _____

      2. generic name _____

   e. 1. prefilled _____

      2. reconstituted _____

2. Choose the correct answer.

   _____ a. A major advantage of the unit-dose system of drug administration is that

      1. the drug supply is always available.

      2. no error is possible.

      3. drugs are less expense then stock bottles.

      4. the pharmacist provides a second professional check.

   _____ b. A major disadvantage of ampules over vials is that ampules

      1. are only glass.

      2. when opened cannot be kept sterile.

      3. contain only liquids.

      4. cannot be used for injections.

   _____ c. Which information is not found on the label for a drug to be given IVPB?

      1. expiration date.

      2. indications (uses).

      3. generic name.

      4. averge dose.

*(continued)*

_____ **d.** An order reads Valium 5 mg po now. A nurse correctly chooses diazempam. What name does diazempam represent?

   **1.** generic

   **2.** chemical

   **3.** trade

   **4.** proprietary

_____ **e.** Which drug form is safest to administer to an unconcious patient?

   **1.** suppository

   **2.** syrup

   **3.** capsule

   **4.** aerosole

**3.** Match the following:

   **1.** _____ Avoid cross-contamination          **a.** Topical application

   **2.** _____ Removing medication from a jar      **b.** Auric

   **3.** _____ Eye medication                       **c.** Slow absorption over time

   **4.** _____ Puffs ordered                        **d.** Reconstitution

   **5.** _____ Date and time label                  **e.** Use a tongue blade

   **6.** _____ Lozenge                              **f.** Cough drop

   **7.** _____ Parenteral                           **g.** Individual nose droppers

   **8.** _____ Local effect                         **h.** Ophthalmic

   **9.** _____ Transdermal                          **i.** Inhalation

   **10.** _____ Ear medication                      **j.** IM, SC, IV

*Name:* _____

*Read the label and answer the questions. Answers will be found on page 329.*

NDC 0173-0378-35

*Glaxo Pharmaceuticals*

**Fortaz**®
(ceftazididime for
injection)

**1g**

Equivalent to 1 g of ceftazidime

For IM or IV use.

Caution: Federal law prohibits
dispensing without prescription.

See package insert for Dosage and Administration.
Before constitution store between 15° and 30°C
(59° and 86°F) and protect from light.
IMPORTANT: The vial is under reduced pressure. Addition of diluent
generates a positive pressure.
Before constituting, see Instructions for Constitution.
After constitution solutions maintain potency for 24
hours at room temperature (not exceeding 25°C[77°F])
or for 7 days under refrigeration. Constituted solutions
in sterile water for injection may be frozen. See package
insert for details. Color changes do not affect potency.
This vial contains 118 mg of sodium carbonate. The
sodium content is approximately 54 mg (2.3 mEq).

Glaxo Pharmaceuticals
Division of Glaxo Inc.
Research Traingle Park, NC 27709
Manufactured in England  5/93

4043081

Table 5: Preparation of Fortaz Solutions

| Size | Amount of Diluent to Be Added (mL) | Approximate Available Volume (mL) | Approximate Ceftazidime Concentration (mg/mL) |
|---|---|---|---|
| Intramuscular | | | |
| 500-mg vial | 1.5 | 1.8 | 280 |
| 1-gram vial | 3.0 | 3.6 | 280 |
| Intravenous | | | |
| 500-mg vial | 5.0 | 5.3 | 100 |
| 1-gram vial | 10.0 | 10.6 | 100 |
| 2-gram vial | 10.0 | 11.5 | 170 |
| Infusion pack | | | |
| 1-gram vial | 100* | 100 | 10 |
| 2-gram vial | 100* | 100 | 20 |
| Pharmacy bulk package | | | |
| 6-gram vial | 26 | 30 | 200 |

* **Note:** Addition should be in two stages (see Instructions for Constitution).

**COMPATIBILITY AND STABILITY:**
**Intramuscular:** Fortaz®, when constituted as directed with sterile water for injection, bacteriostatic water for injection, or 0.5% or 1%
lidocaine hydrochloride injection, maintains satisfactory potency for 24 hours at room temperature or for 7 days under refrigeration.
Solutions in sterile water for injection that are frozen immediately after constitution in the original container are stable for 3 months when
stored at -20°C. Once thawed, solutions should not be refrozen. thawed solutions may be stored for up to 8 hours at room temperature or
for 4 days in a refrigerator.

Reproduced with permission of GlaxoSmithKline.

1. Trade name _____

2. Generic name _____

3. Route of administration _____

4. Total volume when reconstituted _____

5. Strength of reconstituted solution _____

6. Directions to reconstitute _____

   _____

   _____

   _____

7. Drug form as dispensed _____

*(continued)*

8. Storage _____

   _____

   _____

9. Expiration date _____

10. Usual dose _____

11. Cautions _____

   _____

   _____

# Answers

## Self-Test 1 Drug Labels

1. 0005-3898-46
2. 100 mL when reconstituted
3. Suprax®
4. cefixime
5. 100 mg per 5 mL
6. dry powder
7. See accompanying literature
8. oral
9. Dry powder at controlled room temperature 15–30°C (59–86°F). See accompanying literature for liquid storage after reconstitution.
10. To reconstitute, suspend with 69 mL water. Tap the bottle several times to loosen the powder. Add approximately half the total amount of water for reconstitution and shake well. Add the remainder of water and shake well.
11. Federal law prohibits dispensing without a prescription.
    See accompanying literature.
    Use this bottle for dispensing.
    Remove this portion of label only.
12. Advantus Pharmaceuticals
13. August 1998
14. 2% Xylocaine Viscous
15. lidocaine HCL
16. oral only
17. as a solution
18. 2% = 2 grams in 100 mL
19. 450 mL
20. 15 mL (one tablespoon)
21. Numbness of the mouth and throat increases the risk of food aspiration or biting trauma; do not eat or chew gum for 60 minutes following use; keep this and all medications out of the reach of children; dispense out of the reach of children; dispense in a child-resistant package, shake well before using; squeeze bottle to dispense contents; federal law prohibits dispensing without a prescription.

## Self-Test 2 Drug Packaging

1. d
2. j
3. g
4. i
5. a
6. c
7. h
8. b
9. e
10. f
11. On the label of any powder that nurse dissolves. Powders begin to lose their potency as soon as they are placed in solution. By writing the date and time on the label, the nurse will be able to check for expiration time.
12. Label the tube with one patient's name and restrict its use to that one patient.
13. A sterile tongue blade or sterile gloves to prevent contamination of the jar contents.
14. "Ophthalmic" or "for the eye"
15. Number of inhalations or puffs
16. "Otic" or "auric"
17. Large stock containers that hold many doses of a drug
18. Unit-dose
19. A systemic effect; the drug reaches the circulation and is carried to other parts of the body.
20. A disklike solid that is slowly dissolved in the mouth (eg, a cough drop)

# Metric, Apothecary and Household Systems of Measurement

Medication orders are written in metric terms. In this chapter we will learn solid and liquid measures in the metric system and their equivalents.

In preparing liquid doses, knowledge of apothecary and household equivalents may aid in pouring exact amounts. Medicine cups are marked in metric, apothecary, and household measures; syringes are marked in metric and apothecary lines.

## ▶ Metric System

### Measures of Weight

Solid measures in the metric system are

Gram: abbreviated g or gm

Milligram: abbreviated mg

Microgram: abbreviated $\mu$g or mcg ($\mu$g, which uses the Greek letter mu [$\mu$], is printed; mcg is written)

Kilogram: abbreviated kg

### Weight Equivalents

The basic weight equivalents in the metric system are

1 g = 1000 mg

1 mg = 1000 $\mu$g (mcg)

Note that the gram is larger than a milligram. It takes 1000 mg to equal the weight of 1 g. A milligram is itself larger than a microgram; it takes 1000 $\mu$g to equal the weight of 1 mg. These relationships can be indicated using the symbol >, which means "is greater than":

$g > mg > \mu g$

Read: A gram is greater than a milligram, which is greater than a microgram.

## Converting Solid Equivalents

The nurse will have to calculate how much of a drug to give if the supply on hand is not in the same weight measure as the medication order.

**Example**   Order: 0.25 g

Supply: tablets labeled 125 mg

We know the equivalent 1 g = 1000 mg. Therefore, we could change 0.25 g to milligrams by multiplying the number of grams by 1000.

$$\begin{array}{r} 0.25 \\ \times\ 1000 \\ \hline 250.00 \end{array}$$

The order, then, is that 0.25 g = 250 mg.

There is a shortcut. In decimals, the thousandth place is three numbers after the decimal point. We can change grams to milligrams by moving the decimal point three places to the right, which produces the same answer as multiplying by 1000. We can also change milligrams to grams by moving the decimal point three places to the left, which is the same as dividing by 1000. This is the method we will learn.

**RULE**   **CHANGING GRAMS TO MILLIGRAMS**

**To multiply by 1000, move the decimal point three places to the right.** ■

**Example**   *EXAMPLE 1:*

0.25g = _____ mg

0.250 = 250

0.25g = 250 mg

*EXAMPLE 2:*

0.1g = _____ mg

0.100 = 100

0.1g = 100 mg

**Grams to Milligrams Quick Rule:** Some students have difficulty deciding whether to move decimal points to the left or the right. Here is a method that might be helpful.

1. Write the order first.

2. Write the equivalent measure needed.

3. Use an arrow to show which way the decimal point should move.

4. The open part of the arrow always faces the *larger* measure.

5. In the equivalent 1 g = 1000 mg, the gram is the larger measure. It takes 1000 mg to make 1 g.

**Example**

*EXAMPLE 1:*

Order: 0.25 g

Supply: 125 mg

You want to convert grams to milligrams

0.25 g >____mg

The arrow is telling you to move the decimal point three places to the right.

0.250 = 250

Hence, 0.25 g = 250 mg

*EXAMPLE 2:*

Order: 1.5 g

Supply: 500 mg

You want to convert grams to milligrams

1.5g > ____ mg

1.500 = 1500

Hence, 1.5 g = 1500 mg

## SELF TEST 1    Grams to Milligrams

*Try these conversions from grams to milligrams. Answers may be found at the end of the chapter.*

**1.** 0.3 g = _____ mg    **5.** 5 g = _____ mg

**2.** 0.001 g = _____ mg    **6.** 0.4 g = _____ mg

**3.** 0.02 g = _____ mg    **7.** 0.08 g = _____ mg

**4.** 1.2 g = _____ mg    **8.** 0.275 g = _____ mg

## RULE    CHANGING MILLIGRAMS TO GRAMS

**To divide by 1000, move the decimal point three places to the left.** ◼

**Example**

*EXAMPLE 1:*

100 mg =____ g

100. = 0.1

100 mg = 0.1 g

*EXAMPLE 2:*

8 mg =____ g

008. = 0.008

8 mg = 0.008 g

**Milligrams to Grams Quick Rule:** The arrow method also works to convert milligrams to grams. Remember the steps:

1. Write the order first.
2. Write the equivalent measure needed.
3. Use an arrow to show which way the decimal point should move.
4. The open part of the arrow always faces the *larger* measure.
5. In the equivalent 1 g = 1000 mg, the gram is the larger measure.

**Example**

*EXAMPLE 1:*

Order: 15 mg

Supply: 0.03 g

You want to convert milligrams to grams

15 mg < g

The arrow tells you to move the decimal point three places to the left.

015. = 0.015

15 mg = 0.015 g

*EXAMPLE 2:*

Order: 500 mg

Supply: 1 g

You want to convert mg to g

500 mg =____ g

500 mg < g

The arrow tells you to move the decimal point three places to the left.

500. = 0.5

500 mg = 0.5 g

---

**SELF TEST 2   Milligrams to Grams**

*Try these conversions from milligrams to grams. Answers may be found at the end of the chapter.*

1. 4 mg = _____ g     5. 250 mg = _____ g
2. 120 mg = _____ g     6. 1 mg = _____ g
3. 40 mg = _____ g     7. 50 mg = _____ g
4. 75 mg = _____ g     8. 600 mg = _____ g

---

The second major weight equivalent in the metric system is

1 mg = 1000 $\mu$g   *Remember:* $\mu$g is *written* mcg.

Some medications are so powerful that minute microgram doses are sufficient to produce a therapeutic effect. It is easier to write orders in micrograms as whole numbers than to use milligrams written as decimals.

| RULE | CHANGING MILLIGRAMS TO MICROGRAMS |
|------|-----------------------------------|

**To multiply by 1000, move the decimal point three places to the right.** ■

**Example**

*EXAMPLE 1:*

0.1 mg =_____ μg

0.100 = 100

0.1 mg = 100 μg

*EXAMPLE 2:*

0.25 mg =_____ μg

0.250 = 250

0.25 mg = 250 μg

**Milligrams to Micrograms Quick Rule:** Some students have difficulty deciding whether to move decimal points to the left or the right.

1. Write the order first.

2. Write the equivalent measure needed.

3. Use an arrow to show which way the decimal point should move.

4. The open part of the arrow always faces the *larger* measure.

5. In the equivalent 1 mg = 1000 μg, the milligram is the larger measure. It takes 1000 μg to make 1 mg.

**Example**

*EXAMPLE 1:*

Order: 0.1 mg

Supply: 200 μg

You want to convert milligrams to micrograms.

0.1 mg >_____ μg

The arrow is telling you to move the decimal point three places to the right.

0.100 = 100

Hence: 0.1 mg = 100 μg

*EXAMPLE 2:*

Order: 0.3 mg

Supply: 600 μg

You want to convert milligrams to micrograms.

0.3 mg >_____ μg

0.300 = 300

Hence, 0.3 mg = 300 μg

| SELF TEST 3 | Milligrams to Micrograms |
|---|---|

*Try these conversions from milligrams to micrograms. Use either method. Answers may be found at the end of the chapter.*

**1.** 0.3 mg = _____ μg     **5.** 1.2 mg = _____ μg

**2.** 0.001 mg = _____ μg     **6.** 0.4 mg = _____ μg

**3.** 0.02 mg = _____ μg     **7.** 5 mg = _____ μg

**4.** 0.08 mg = _____ μg     **8.** 0.7 mg = _____ μg

## RULE     CHANGING MICROGRAMS TO MILLIGRAMS

**To divide by 1000, move the decimal point three places to the left.** ■

**Example**

*EXAMPLE 1:*

300 μg = _____ mg

300. = 0.3

300 μg = 0.3 mg

*EXAMPLE 2:*

50 μg = _____ mg

050. = 0.05

50 μg = 0.05 mg

**Micrograms to Milligrams Quick Rule:** The arrow method also works to convert micrograms to milligrams. Remember the steps.

**1.** Write the order first.

**2.** Write the equivalent measure needed.

**3.** Use an arrow to show which way the decimal point should move.

**4.** The open part of the arrow always faces the *larger* measure.

**5.** In the equivalent 1 mg = 1000 μg, the milligram is the larger measure.

**Example**

*EXAMPLE 1:*

Order: 100 μg

Supply: 0.1 mg

You want to convert micrograms to milligrams.

100 μg < mg

The arrow tells you to move the decimal point three places to the left.

100. = 0.1

100 μg = 0.1 mg

*EXAMPLE 2:*

Order: 50 $\mu$g

Supply: 0.1 mg

You want to convert micrograms to milligrams.

50 $\mu$g =____ mg

$\mu$g < mg

The arrow tells you to move the decimal point three places to the left.

$\underset{\frown}{0}50.$ = 0.05

50 $\mu$g = 0.05 mg

---

## SELF TEST 4  Micrograms to Milligrams

*Try these conversions from micrograms to milligrams. Answers may be found at the end of the chapter.*

**1.** 800 $\mu$g = _____ mg

**2.** 4 $\mu$g = _____ mg

**3.** 14 $\mu$g = _____ mg

**4.** 25 $\mu$g = _____ mg

**5.** 1 $\mu$g = _____ mg

**6.** 200 $\mu$g = _____ mg

**7.** 50 $\mu$g = _____ mg

**8.** 750 $\mu$g = _____ mg

---

## SELF TEST 5  Mixed Conversions

*Now try mixed conversions in metric weight measures. Be careful when reading and take the time to think and apply the rules you have learned. Answers may be found at the end of the chapter.*

**1.** 0.3 mg = _____ g

**2.** 0.03 g = _____ mg

**3.** 15 $\mu$g = _____ mg

**4.** 0.1 g = _____ mg

**5.** 100 $\mu$g = _____ mg

**6.** 50 mg = _____ g

**7.** 0.014 g = _____ mg

**8.** 200 mg = _____ g

**9.** 0.2 mg = _____ $\mu$g

**10.** 0.65 mg = _____ $\mu$g

## Table of Common Metric Solid Equivalents

Most practicing nurses know certain common equivalents in the metric system. Study Table 4-1 to familiarize yourself with them.

**TABLE 4-1   Common Metric Weight Equivalents**

| Weight | Equivalent |
| --- | --- |
| 1000 mg | 1 g |
| 600 mg | 0.6 g |
| 500 mg | 0.5 g |
| 300 mg | 0.3 g |
| 200 mg | 0.2 g |
| 100 mg | 0.1 g |
| 60 mg | 0.06 g |
| 30 mg | 0.03 g |
| 15 mg | 0.015 g |
| 10 mg | 0.01 g |
| 1 mg | 1000 $\mu$g |
| 0.6 mg | 600 $\mu$g |
| 0.4 mg | 400 $\mu$g |
| 0.3 mg | 300 $\mu$g |
| 0.1 mg | 100 $\mu$g |

**SELF TEST 6   Common Equivalents**

*Fill in the blanks to convert mg to g or to $\mu$g.*

1. 1000 mg = _____ g

2. 600 mg = _____ g

3. 500 mg = _____ g

4. 300 mg = _____ g

5. 200 mg = _____ g

6. 100 mg = _____ g

7. 60 mg = _____ g

8. 30 mg = _____ g

9. 15 mg = _____ g

10. 10 mg = _____ g

11. 0.6 mg = _____ $\mu$g

12. 0.4 mg = _____ $\mu$g

13. 0.3 mg = _____ $\mu$g

14. 0.25 mg = _____ $\mu$g

**SELF TEST 7** | Review of Grams to Milligrams

1. What is the short rule for converting grams to milligrams? _____

_____

2. 1 g = _____ mg        9. 0.3 g = _____ mg

3. 0.01 g = _____ mg     10. 0.2 g = _____ mg

4. 0.2 g = _____ mg      11. 0.1 g = _____ mg

5. 0.12 g = _____ mg     12. 0.06 g = _____ mg

6. 1 g = _____ mg        13. 0.03 g = _____ mg

7. 0.6 g = _____ mg      14. 0.015 g = _____ mg

8. 0.5 g = _____ mg      15. 0.01 g = _____ mg

## ▶ Apothecary System

The apothecary system was used in the past to write prescriptions. It has gradually been replaced by the metric system; today it is rare to see medication orders in apothecary notation. Here is a brief overview of the apothecary system.

### Roman Numerals

In the apothecary system, roman numerals are used to designate amounts. Table 4-2 has the equivalents:

### ▍TABLE 4-2  Apothecary System

| Arabic Number | Roman Number | Arabic Number | Roman Number |
|---|---|---|---|
| ½ | śś | 6 | vi |
| 1 | i | 7 | vii |
| 1½ | iśś | 7½ | viiśś |
| 2 | ii | 8 | viii |
| 3 | iii | 9 | ix |
| 4 | iv | 10 | x |
| 5 | v | 20 | xx |
| | | 30 | xxx |

## TABLE 4-3   Apothecary Abbreviations

| Apothecary Abbreviation | Meaning | Learning Aid |
|---|---|---|
| ʒ | Dram | This is a liquid measure. It is slightly less than a household teaspoon. (One dram equals 4 milliliters; ʒi = 4 mL [see below]) |
| ℥ | Ounce | This is a liquid measure. It is slightly more than a household ounce. (One ounce equals 32 milliliters; ℥ i = 32 mL) |
| gr | Grain | Latin, *granum.* This solid measure was based on the weight of a grain of wheat in ancient times. There is no commonly used equivalent to the grain in the metric system. |
| gtt | Drop | Latin, *guttae.* This liquid measure was based on a drop of water. (One drop equals 1 minim) |
| m ($M$, $M_x$) | Minim | Latin, *minim.* (One minim equals one drop: 1 m = 1 gtt) |
| śś | One-half | Latin, *semis* |
| i | One | ***Example:*** gr i = grains 1; ʒi = 4 mL |
| i śś | One-and-a-half | ***Example:*** gr i śś = grains 1½ |
| ii | Two | ***Example:*** gr ii = grains 2 |
| iii | Three | ***Example:*** gr iii = grains 3 |
| iv | Four | ***Example:*** gr iv = grains 4 ʒiv = drams 4 |
| v | Five | ***Example:*** gr v = grains 5 m v = minims 5 |
| vii | Seven | ***Example:*** gr vii = grains 7 |
| vii śś | Seven-and-a-half | ***Example:*** gr vii śś = grains 7½ |
| x | Ten | ***Example:*** gr x = grains 10 m x = minims 10 |
| xv | Fifteen | ***Example:*** gr xv = grains 15 m xv = minims 15 |

## Apothecary Abbreviations

The apothecary system has specific abbreviations. Table 4-3 has the common apothecary abbreviations.

## Solid Apothecary Measure—The Grain

The only solid dosage measure in the apothecary system is the grain (abbreviated gr) followed by a Roman number, ex. gr v. Arabic numbers have been used, ex. gr 5; 5 gr. Do not confuse the apothecary gr with the metric gram (g, gm).

## Solid Equivalents—Apothecary and Metric

Equivalents between the metric and apothecary systems are not exact (see Table 4-4):

| TABLE 4-4 | Metric and Apothecary Equivalents | | |
|---|---|---|---|
| **Grain** | **Milligram** | **Gram\*** | **Microgram** |
| gr xv | 1000 mg | 1 g | |
| gr x | (650)† 600 mg | 0.6 g | |
| gr vii śś | 500 mg | 0.5 g | |
| gr v | (325)† 300 mg | 0.3 g | |
| gr iii | 200 mg | 0.2 g | |
| gr i śś | 100 mg | 0.1 g | |
| gr i | (65)† 60 mg | 0.06 g | |
| gr śś or gr ½ | 30 mg | 0.03 g | |
| gr ¼ | 15 mg | 0.015 g | |
| gr ⅙ | 10 mg | 0.01 g | |
| gr ¹⁄₁₀₀ | 0.6 mg | | 600 μg |
| gr ¹⁄₁₅₀ | 0.4 mg | | 400 μg |
| gr ¹⁄₂₀₀ | 0.3 mg | | 300 μg |

\* g = gram; μg = microgram or mcg.
† Alternative values.

Three equivalents require explanation:

gr x = 0.6 g = 600 mg or 650 mg

gr v = 0.3 g = 300 mg or 325 mg

gr i = 0.06 g = 60 mg or 65 mg

Note that 15 grains = 1000 mg; 1 grain = 60 mg. If you multiply 15 × 60 the answer should be 1000 mg, but the answer is 900 mg. To remedy this discrepancy some drug companies manufacture 1 grain to equal 65 mg; aspirin and acetaminophen are made this way (5 grains = 325 mg; 10 grains = 650 mg.) In solving dosage problems when the order is written in one system and the stock comes in another system or conversion, use whichever equivalent is closer.

---

**SELF TEST 8** | **Converting Grains to mg**

*Fill in the blanks to convert gr to mg.*

1. gr iss _____   4. gr 15 _____

2. gr v _____   5. gr 4 _____

3. gr ¹⁄₁₅₀ _____

*Convert mg or g to gr.*

6. 3 g _____   9. .5 mg _____

7. 325 mg _____   10. 9 g _____

8. 15 mg _____

# ▶ Household System

## Household Measures

Household measures are used in preparing doses when a standard medication receptacle is used. Household measures are

teaspoon: abbreviated tsp

tablespoon: abbreviated tbsp

ounce: abbreviated oz (or fl oz = fluid ounce)

pint: abbreviated pt

quart: abbreviated qt

pound: abbreviated lb

Household equivalents are

1 tsp = 5 mL   ✳

1 tbsp = 15 mL ✳

1 oz = 30 mL ✳

1 pt = 500 mL ✳

1 qt = 1 L = 1000 mL ✳

2.2 lbs = 1 kg ✳

## Metric Liquid Measures

Liquid measures in the metric system are

Liter: abbreviated L

Milliliter: abbreviated mL (may be seen as ml)

Cubic centimeter: abbreviated cc

Liquid equivalents in the metric system are

1 mL = 1 cc (acceptable in dosage)

1 L = 1000 mL or 1000 cc

## Liquid Apothecary Measures

In the apothecary system, the liquid measures are

Minim: abbreviated M or M̶ or m

Dram: abbreviated ʒ or dr

Ounce: abbreviated ʒ or oz

Drop: abbreviated gtt

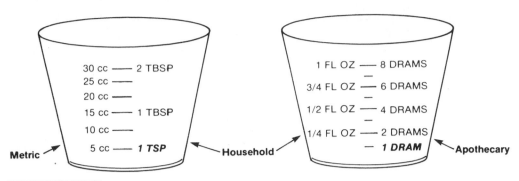

**FIGURE 4-1**

A medicine cup with metric, apothecary, and household equivalents.

An ounce is larger than a dram; hence the symbol for an ounce has two loops.
Liquid equivalents in the apothecary system are

| | |
|---|---|
| 1 m = 1 gtt | 1 minim = 1 drop |
| 1 dr = 4 mL | 1 dram = 4 mL |
| 8 dr = 1 oz | 8 drams = 1 ounce |

## Conversions Among Liquid Measures

Figure 4-1 shows a medicine cup with metric, apothecary, and household equivalents.
Note that

5 cc = 1 tsp

15 cc = 1 tbsp = ½ oz = 4 drams

30 cc = 2 tbsp = 1 oz = 8 drams

Figure 4-2 shows a 3-cc syringe.
Note that 1 cc = 16 minims.

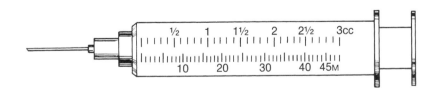

**FIGURE 4-2**

A 3-cc (mL) syringe with metric and apothecary measures.

Table 4-5 combines the common liquid equivalents among the three systems. Remember that equivalents are approximate, not exact. Learn this information, then test your knowledge by completing the exercises that follow. Use the proficiency examination at the end of this chapter to validate your learning.

### TABLE 4-5  Liquid Equivalents Among Metric, Apothecary, and Household Measures

| Metric | | Apothecary | | Household |
|---|---|---|---|---|
| | | 1 minim = 1 gtt | | |
| 1 mL = 1 cc | = | 16 minims | | |
| 4 mL | = | 1 dram | | |
| 5 mL | = | → | | 1 tsp |
| 15 mL | = | 4 drams | = | 1 tbsp |
| 30 mL | = | 8 drams | = | 1 oz = 2 tbsp |
| 500 mL | = | → | | 1 pint |
| 1000 mL = 1 L | = | → | | 1 quart = 2 pints |

---

## SELF TEST 9    Liquid Equivalents

*Practice exercises in liquid equivalents. Answers may be found at the end of the chapter.*

**1.** 1 oz = _____ dr

**2.** 1 tbsp = _____ dr

**3.** ½ oz = _____ cc

**4.** 2 dr = _____ mL

**5.** 1 mL = _____ minims

**6.** 4 dr = _____ oz

**7.** 1 tsp = _____ mL

**8.** 1 oz = _____ tbsp

**9.** 1 oz = _____ mL

**10.** 1 L = _____ mL

---

## SELF TEST 10    Liquid Measures

*Express the liquid measure requested.*

**1.** 4 mL = _____ dram

**2.** 1 tbsp = _____ mL

**3.** 1½ oz = _____ mL

**4.** 5 mL = _____ tsp

**5.** 30 mL = _____ oz

**6.** 30 mL = _____ dr

**7.** 1 minim = _____ gtt

**8.** 1 pt = _____ cc

**9.** 1 qt = _____ mL

**10.** 1 cc = _____ mL

**SELF TEST 11** **Mixed Conversions**

*Fill in the measure requested.*

**1.** 1 dram = _____ cc

**2.** 1 qt = _____ L

**3.** 15 mL = _____ tbsp

**4.** 8 drams = _____ oz

**5.** 2 tbsp = _____ oz

**6.** 16 minims = _____ mL

**7.** 1 L = _____ mL

**8.** 2 drams = _____ cc

**9.** 500 mL = _____ pt

**10.** 1 kg = _____ lb

**PROFICIENCY TEST 1** Solid and Liquid Equivalents

*Name:* _____

*Aim for 90% accuracy or better on this test. There are 40 items each worth 2.5 points. If you have any difficulty, reread and study Chapter 4, which explains this information. Answers will be found on page 329.*

**1.** 100 mg = _____ gm

**2.** 1 oz = _____ cc

**3.** 1 L = _____ mL

**4.** 1 tsp = _____ cc

**5.** 0.015 g = _____ mg

**6.** 10 mg = _____ gm

**7.** 1 cc = _____ mL

**8.** 0.2 gm = _____ mg

**9.** 30 mg = _____ g

**10.** 500 mg = _____ g

**11.** 1 oz = _____ mL

**12.** 1 mL = _____ minims

**13.** 1 tbsp = _____ cc

**14.** 1 kg = _____ lbs

**15.** 1 g = _____ mg

**16.** 60 mg = _____ g

**17.** 30 mL = _____ oz

**18.** 1 minim = _____ gtt

**19.** 2 drams = _____ mL

**20.** 1000 mg = _____ gm

**21.** 0.1 gm = _____ mg

**22.** 4 cc = _____ dr

**23.** 600 mg = _____ gm

**24.** 10 mcg = _____ mg

**25.** 1 L = _____ mL

**26.** 0.5 $\mu$g = _____ mg

**27.** 0.6 mg = _____ g

**28.** 250 mcg = _____ mg

**29.** 1 mg = _____ g

**30.** 0.125 mg = _____ mcg

**31.** 0.01 mg = _____ mcg

**32.** 0.001 mg = _____ $\mu$g

**33.** 1 qt = _____ mL

**34.** gr $\frac{1}{100}$ = _____ mg

**35.** 30 mg = gr _____

**36.** gr ii = _____ mg

**37.** 240 mg = gr _____

**38.** gr $\frac{1}{125}$ = gr _____

**39.** 1 g = gr _____

**40.** gr $\frac{1}{200}$ = gr _____

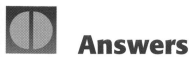

# Answers

**Self-Test 1 Grams to Milligrams**

| | | | |
|---|---|---|---|
| **1.** 300 | **3.** 20 | **5.** 5000 | **7.** 80 |
| **2.** 1 | **4.** 1200 | **6.** 400 | **8.** 275 |

**Self-Test 2 Milligrams to Grams**

| | | | |
|---|---|---|---|
| **1.** 0.004 | **3.** 0.04 | **5.** 0.25 | **7.** 0.05 |
| **2.** 0.12 | **4.** 0.075 | **6.** 0.001 | **8.** 0.6 |

**Self-Test 3 Milligrams to Micrograms**

| | | | |
|---|---|---|---|
| **1.** 300 | **3.** 20 | **5.** 1200 | **7.** 5000 |
| **2.** 1 | **4.** 80 | **6.** 400 | **8.** 700 |

**Self-Test 4 Micrograms to Milligrams**

| | | | |
|---|---|---|---|
| **1.** 0.8 | **3.** 0.014 | **5.** 0.001 | **7.** 0.05 |
| **2.** 0.004 | **4.** 0.025 | **6.** 0.2 | **8.** 0.75 |

**Self-Test 5 Mixed Conversions**

| | | | |
|---|---|---|---|
| **1.** 0.0003 | **4.** 100 | **7.** 14 | **9.** 200 |
| **2.** 30 | **5.** 0.1 | **8.** 0.2 | **10.** 650 |
| **3.** 0.015 | **6.** 0.05 | | |

**Self-Test 6 Common Equivalents**

| | | | |
|---|---|---|---|
| **1.** 1 | **5.** 0.2 | **9.** 0.015 | **12.** 400 |
| **2.** 0.6 | **6.** 0.1 | **10.** 0.01 | **13.** 300 |
| **3.** 0.5 | **7.** 0.06 | **11.** 600 | **14.** 250 |
| **4.** 0.3 | **8.** 0.03 | | |

**Self-Test 7 Review of Grams to Milligrams**

| | |
|---|---|
| **1.** Multiply grams by 1000, or move decimal point three places to the right, or use an arrow with the open part toward gram to show movement of decimal point three places. | **7.** 600 |
| | **8.** 500 |
| | **9.** 300 |
| | **10.** 200 |
| **2.** 1000 | **11.** 100 |
| **3.** 10 | **12.** 60 |
| **4.** 200 | **13.** 30 |
| **5.** 120 | **14.** 15 |
| **6.** 1000 | **15.** 10 |

## Self-Test 8 Converting Grains to mg

| | | | |
|---|---|---|---|
| **1.** 100 mg | **4.** 900 or 1000 mg | **7.** gr 5 | **9.** gr $\frac{1}{120}$ |
| **2.** 300 mg | **5.** 240 mg | **8.** gr ¼ | **10.** gr 135 |
| **3.** .4 mg | **6.** gr 50 | | |

## Self-Test 9 Liquid Equivalents

| | | | |
|---|---|---|---|
| **1.** 8 | **4.** 8 | **7.** 5 | **9.** 30 |
| **2.** 4 | **5.** 16 | **8.** 2 | **10.** 1000 |
| **3.** 15 | **6.** ½ | | |

## Self-Test 10 Liquid Measure

| | | | |
|---|---|---|---|
| **1.** 1 | **4.** 1 | **7.** 1 | **9.** 1000 |
| **2.** 15 | **5.** 1 | **8.** 500 | **10.** 1 |
| **3.** 45 | **6.** 8 | | |

## Self-Test 11 Mixed Conversions

| | | | |
|---|---|---|---|
| **1.** 4 | **4.** 1 | **7.** 1000 | **9.** 1 |
| **2.** 1 | **5.** 1 | **8.** 8 | **10.** 2.2 |
| **3.** 1 | **6.** 1 | | |

# Drug Preparations and Equipment to Measure Doses

Drugs are manufactured in different forms for oral, parenteral, and topical administration. This chapter focuses on the more common drug preparations used in the clinical area and on the equipment that nurses use to prepare accurate doses.

## ▶ Drug Preparations

### Oral Route

Oral drug forms are generally the easiest for the patient to take and the most convenient for the nurse to administer.

*Tablets* are powdered drugs that are compressed or molded into solid shapes. Tables may contain ingredients that bind the powder or aid in its gastrointestinal absorption (Fig. 5-1A). Plain tablets for oral administration may be crushed if a patient has difficulty swallowing.

There are several types of pill or tablet crushers available.

*Scored tablets* have a line down the center so that the tablet can be broken into halves. Unscored tablets should not be broken because there is no certainty that the drug is evenly distributed (see Fig. 5-1B). When in doubt, check with the pharmacist.

*Coated tablets* or film-coated tablets are smooth and easy to swallow because of their coating. If necessary, some tablets may be crushed.

*Enteric-coated tablets* dissolve in the more alkaline secretions of the intestine rather than in the highly acidic stomach juices. The enteric coating protects the drug from being inactivated in the stomach and reduces the chance that the drug will irritate the gastric mucosa. Enteric-coated tablets should *not* be crushed.

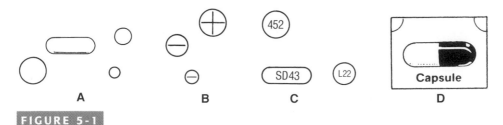

**FIGURE 5-1**

(*A*) Tablets that can be crushed. (*B*) Scored tablets that can be broken. (*C*) Coded tablets—identification of the drug may be by number, letters, or shape. (*D*) Capsule.

*Prolonged-release or extended-release tablets* disintegrate more slowly and have a longer duration of action. The use of these preparations decreases the number of doses needed to only one or two tablets each day. Prolonged-release tablets should not be crushed.

*Sublingual tablets* dissolve quickly under the tongue. Medication is absorbed through the capillaries and reaches the circulation without passing through the gastrointestinal tract.

*Coded tablets* have a number or letters, or both, that make them easily identifiable (see Fig. 5-1*C*).

*Capsules* are gelatin containers that hold a drug in solid or liquid form. Nurses should avoid opening capsules; the drug is encased in the capsule for a reason—possibly because contact with gastric juices will decrease drug potency or because drug could irritate the stomach lining. Occasionally, however, if a patient has difficulty swallowing, the nurse may open a capsule and combine the contents with a semisolid such as applesauce or custard. Before doing this, always check with the pharmacist to find out if the drug is available as a liquid or if there is an alternative (Fig. 5-1*D*).

Some capsules are enteric-coated. Others (called *spansule, timespan, time-release, or sustained-release*) contain particles of the drug that are coated to dissolve at different times. These capsules are long acting and should not be opened.

*Syrups* are solutions of sugar in water that disguise the medication's unpleasant taste. Because they contain sugar syrups may be contraindicated in patients with diabetes mellitus.

*Elixirs* are clear, hydroalcoholic liquids that are sweetened. Elixirs may be contraindicated in patients with a history of alcoholism.

*Fluidextracts* and *tinctures* are alcoholic, liquid concentrations of a drug: they are potent and, consequently, are ordered in small amounts. Tinctures are ordered in drops. The average dose of a fluidextract is 2 teaspoons or less. Fluidextracts are the most concentrated of all liquids.

*Solutions* are clear liquids that contain a drug dissolved in water.

*Suspensions* are solid particles of a drug dispersed in a liquid. The particles settle to the bottom of the container upon standing and must be resuspended to obtain an accurate dose; therefore, oral preparations must be shaken before being poured.

*Magmas* contain large bulky particles, for example, milk of magnesia.

*Gels* have small particles, for example, magnesium hydroxide gel.

*Emulsions* are creamy, white suspensions of fats or oils in an agent that reduces surface tension and makes the oil easier to swallow, for example, emulsified castor oil.

*Powders* are dry, finely ground drugs that are reconstituted according to directions. Oral antibiotics are frequently supplied as powders. In liquid form these preparations become oral suspensions. Powders must be dissolved according to the manufacturer. When the nurse reconstitutes a powder, three facts should be written on the label: the date, the nurse's initials, and the solution made.

## Parenteral Route

The drug forms for parenteral administration include solutions, suspensions, and powders (see definitions above). The term "parenteral" does not indicate a specific route; it is a general term that means *by injection.* Four common parenteral routes are intramuscular (IM), subcutaneous (SC), intravenous (IV), and intravenous piggyback (IVPB). Drug forms for parenteral use are sterile, and sterile technique is used to prepare and administer them.

## Topical Route

Commonly ordered preparations include aerosol powders or liquids, creams, ointments, pastes, suppositories, and transdermal medications. The physician's orders will indicate application to the skin, eye, ear, nose, vagina, or rectum.

*Aerosol powders and liquids* are combined with a propellant and used for sprays on the skin or in nebulizers and inhalers to reach the mucous membranes of the lower respiratory tract.

*Powders* may be applied to the skin in dry form.

*Creams* are semisolid drug preparations applied externally to the skin or mucous membranes. Vaginal creams require a special applicator for insertion.

*Ointments* are semisolid preparations in a petroleum or lanolin base for topical use. Ointments used for the eye must be labeled "ophthalmic."

*Pastes* are thick ointments used to protect the skin. They absorb secretions and soften the skin.

*Suppositories* contain medication molded with a firm base, such as cocoa butter, that melts at body temperature. Suppositories are shaped for insertion into the rectum, vagina, and, less commonly, the urethra.

*Transdermal medications* are drug molecules contained in a unique polymer patch that is applied to the skin as one would an ordinary plastic bandage. The medication is easy to apply and is effective for hours or days at a time as it is slowly released and absorbed through the skin.

*Match Column A with the letters in Column B to identify the meaning of the terms used for drug preparations. Answers can be found at the end of the chapter.*

Column A

1. _____ Scored tablet
2. _____ Enteric-coated
3. _____ Spansule
4. _____ Sublingual tablet
5. _____ Capsule
6. _____ Syrup
7. _____ Elixir
8. _____ Fluidextract
9. _____ Tincture
10. _____ Magma
11. _____ Gel
12. _____ Topical
13. _____ Suppository

Column B

a. Coated drug particles dissolve at different times
b. The most concentrated of all liquids
c. Hydroalcoholic liquid ordered in drops
d. Large particles suspended in a liquid
e. A solid that can be broken in half
f. Route applied to skin or mucous membrane
g. Small particles suspended in a liquid
h. Medication dissolves under the tongue
i. Gelatin containers for solid or liquid drug
j. Molded solid inserted into the rectum
k. Drug dissolves in the more alkaline secretions of the intestine
l. Sweetened, hydroalcoholic liquid
m. Solution of sugar in water to improve the taste of a drug

## ▶ Equipment to Measure Doses

Nurses do not use a scale to weigh oral solid doses such as the gram and the grain. Solids for oral administration come in tablets and capsules. The nurse calculates the number to give and pours the amount needed into a paper cup, a small container that is discarded once the medication has been given.

Liquids may be prepared as unit doses ready to administer or in stock bottles which require calculation and measurement. Liquids must be measured accurately. Two practices will aid in achieving this goal:

1. *Pour liquids to a line.* Never estimate a dose between two lines.

2. *Pour liquids at eye level* (Fig. 5-2). The surface of a liquid has a natural curve called the *meniscus.* At eye level the center of the curve should be on the measurement line. The fluid at the sides of the container will appear to be above the line (Fig. 5-3).

The equipment used most often by nurses to measure liquids are the medicine cup and syringes.

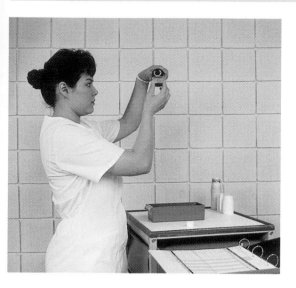

FIGURE 5-2

Liquids are poured at eye level.

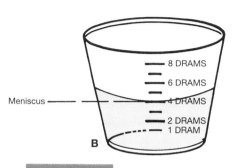

FIGURE 5-3

When viewing the liquid from eye level, the meniscus (lower curve of the fluid) should be on the line.

## Medicine Cup

The medicine cup is a plastic disposable container that has equivalent measures for metric doses in cubic centimeters, for apothecary doses in drams, and for household doses in tablespoons and teaspoons (Fig. 5-4).

The following exercise will help you apply your knowledge of liquid equivalents.

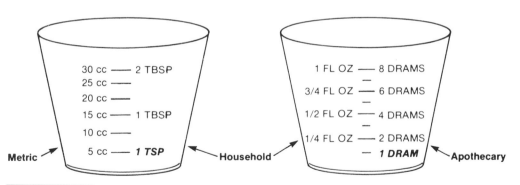

FIGURE 5-4

A medicine cup for measurement of metric, apothecary, or household dose units.

*Look at the medicine cup in Figure 5-4. Two sides are shown. Fill in answers related to this measuring device. Check your answers at the end of the chapter.*

1. Find 30 cc. What other measures are equivalent to this?

   _____    _____    _____    _____

2. Find 5 cc. Hold the page of this book up so that the 5 cc line is at eye level. Is a dram equal to 5 cc? _____

3. If an order reads dram i, what line would you use to pour the dose? _____

4. Find 15 cc. What other equivalents equal this?

   _____    _____    _____    _____

5. Consider the following answers to oral liquid dosage problems. What measurement line would you use?

   **a.** 8 cc    Pour _____

   **b.** 4 tsp    Pour _____

   **c.** ½ oz    Pour _____

6. Suppose an answer to an oral liquid problem is 2 mL. Could you pour this dose into a medicine cup?

   Explain what you would do. _____

   _____

   _____

## Syringes

There are several types of syringes used by nurses to prepare routine parenteral doses. Each is different from the others. Understanding these differences will help you to prepare doses (Figure 5-5).

The 3-mL syringe, 1-mL syringe, and insulin 100 unit and insulin 50 unit syringes will be presented. (Note: these are not drawn to scale.)

*3-mL SYRINGE.* The syringe shown in Figure 5-6 is routinely used for injections. It has a 22-gauge needle, 1½ inches long. The term "gauge" indicates the diameter (width) of the needle.

Note the following on the 3-mL syringe:

- The markings on one side are in cc (mL) to the nearest tenth. Each line indicates 0.1 mL.

- The markings on the opposite side are in minims. Each line indicates 1 minim.

- When preparing a dose, hold the syringe with the needle up, draw down the medication into the barrel. Suppose a dose were calculated to be 1.1 cc or 18 minims. Look at Figure 5-6 and count the lines to reach the dose.

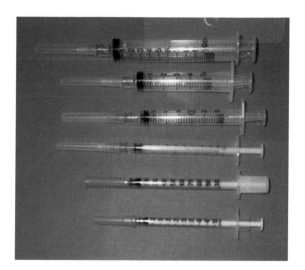

### FIGURE 5-5

(*Top to bottom*) 10-mL syringe, 5-mL syringe, 3-mL syringe, 1-mL syringe (often called a tuberculin syringe), insulin 100-unit syringe, and insulin 50-unit syringe.

### FIGURE 5-6

A 3-mL (cc) syringe with metric and apothecary measures.

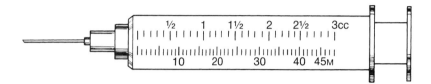

---

**SELF TEST 3 | 3-mL Syringe Amounts**

*Use an arrow to indicate these amounts on the 3-mL syringe in Figure 5-6. Check your answers at the end of this chapter.*

0.3 mL

25 m

1.2 cc

4 m

2.7 mL

---

The 3-mL syringe has markings for 0.7 mL and 0.8 mL. What would you do if a dosage answer were 0.75 mL? Nurses do not approximate doses between lines. There are two ways to handle this problem:

1. Round off 0.75 mL to the nearest tenth. The answer would be 0.8 mL, which can be drawn up onto a line. (Rounding off numbers was discussed in Chapter 1 and is discussed again in this chapter.)

2. Use a different syringe with markings to the nearest hundredth. There is a precision syringe that has markings to the nearest hundredth.

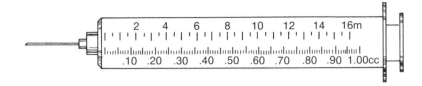

**FIGURE 5-7**

A 1-mL (cc) precision syringe with metric and apothecary measures.

*1-mL PRECISION SYRINGE.* The 1-mL (cc) precision syringe with a 25-gauge, ⅝-inch needle is the most accurate of the syringes nurses use. It is sometimes called a tuberculin syringe. This syringe is marked in hundredths of a milliliter (cubic centimeter) and in half minims (Fig. 5-7).

Note the following on the 1-mL precision syringe:

- The markings on one side are in minims. There is a short line between each half minim and a long line for a whole minim.

- The markings on the other side are in milliliters (mL; cc). There are nine lines before 0.10. Each line is 0.01 mL.

- To prepare an injection, hold the syringe with the needle up then draw down the medication into the barrel. Suppose a dose was calculated to be 0.13 mL or 2 minims. Look at Figure 5-7 and count the lines to reach the dose.

---

**SELF TEST 4** | **1-mL Syringe Amounts**

*Use arrows to mark the following doses on the 1-mL (cc) precision syringe in Figure 5-7. Check your answers at the end of this chapter.*

3 minims

6½ minims

0.61 mL

0.95 mL

## Rounding Off Numbers in Liquid Dosage Answers

For solving liquid injection problems, answers are in milliliters, cubic centimeters, or minims. The answer may not be an even number and the nurse must decide the degree of accuracy to be obtained. *The degree of accuracy depends on the syringe chosen to give the dose.*

**RULE**  **ROUNDING OFF NUMBERS**

1. **When the last number is 5 or more, add 1 to the previous number.**
2. **When the number is 4 or less, drop the number.** ∎

**Example**

0.864 becomes 0.86    4.562 becomes 4.56

1.55 becomes 1.6      2.38 becomes 2.4

0.33 becomes 0.3      0.25 becomes 0.3

With the *3-mL syringe,* carry out decimals two places and round off to the *nearest tenth for milliliters.* Carry out answers in *minims* to the nearest tenth and *round off to the nearest whole number.*

With the *1-mL precision syringe,* carry out decimals three places and round off to the *nearest 100th* for milliliters. Carry out answers in *minims* to the nearest 100th and *round off to the nearest tenth.*

---

**SELF TEST 5** | **3-mL Syringe-Rounding Answers**

*The following are possible answers to dosage problems that require use of a 3-mL syringe. Put a check (√) next to the answer if it is acceptable. If not acceptable, change the answer to a correct form. Check your answers at the end of this chapter.*

**a.** 0.1 mL _____    **e.** 0.2 mL _____    **i.** 0.4 cc _____

**b.** 1½ cc _____    **f.** 8½ minims _____    **j.** 0.65 mL _____

**c.** 0.83 cc _____    **g.** 1.7 ml _____    **k.** 3 minims _____

**d.** 0.98 minims _____    **h.** ½ mL _____    **l.** 5.5 minims _____

---

**SELF TEST 6** | **1-mL Syringe-Rounding Answers**

*The following are possible answers to dosage problems that require the use of a 1-mL precision syringe. Put a check (√) next to the answer if it is acceptable. If not acceptable, change the answer to a correct form. Check your answers at the end of this chapter.*

**a.** 0.65 mL _____    **d.** 12.8 m _____    **g.** 0.758 ml _____

**b.** 12.5 minims _____    **e.** 0.346 mL _____    **h.** 5 minims _____

**c.** 0.04 mL _____    **f.** 0.290 mL _____

---

*1-cc INSULIN SYRINGE.* The 1-cc insulin syringe (for Unit 100 insulin) is marked in units rather than in milliliters or minims. It is used to prepare only U 100 insulins. The physician orders the type of insulin, the strength of insulin, and the number of units (Fig. 5-8).

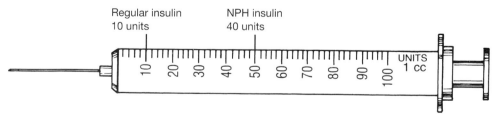

**FIGURE 5-8**

A 1-mL (cc) insulin syringe (for U 100 insulin).

| **Example** | Order: 20 units NPH (U 100) insulin qd SC. |

Look at Figure 5-8. Note that there are four short lines between 10 units and 20 units. This indicates that each line is equal to 2 units on this syringe. Always check the markings on a syringe to be certain you understand what each line equals.

---

**SELF TEST 7    1-mL Insulin Syringe**

*Use arrows on the insulin syringe in Figure 5-8 to indicate the following amounts. Check your answers at the end of this chapter.*

6 units

34 units

50 units

---

Odd-numbered insulin doses should not be drawn up with the syringe in Figure 5.8. Another insulin syringe should be used to prepare these doses. Doses should be exact, not approximate.

*LOW-DOSE INSULIN SYRINGE.* The low-dose unit 100 insulin syringe with a 28-gauge, ½-inch needle (Fig. 5-9) has four short lines between 10 and 15. This indicates that each line is equal to 1 unit. The syringe is marked for 50 units, so any dose of insulin (U 100) up to 50 units can be drawn up with this syringe.

---

**SELF TEST 8    .5-mL Insulin Syringe**

*Use arrows on the insulin syringe in Figure 5-9 to indicate the following amounts. Answers may be found at the end of this chapter.*

Units 33

Units 7

Units 40

---

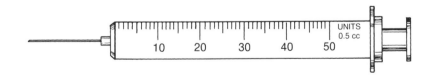

**FIGURE 5-9**

Low-dose insulin syringe for U 100 insulin.

## Needles for Intramuscular and Subcutaneous Injections

Each of the four syringes discussed has a different injection needle.

| Syringe | Gauge | Length (inches) |
| --- | --- | --- |
| 3 mL | 22 g | 1½–3 |
| 1 mL | 25 g | ⅝–⅞ |
| U 100 insulin | 25–26 g | ½–⅝ |
| U 100 low-dose insulin | 25–28 g | ½–⅝ |

*Gauge* (g) indicates the diameter or width of the needle. *The higher the gauge number, the finer the needle.* In the gauges just given, the low-dose insulin syringe has the needle with the smallest diameter (28-gauge) and, hence, is the finest needle in this group. A 15-gauge needle would be very wide and would have a wide opening. It is used to transfuse blood cells.

The *length* of the needle used depends on the route of injection. For deep intramuscular injections, a long needle is necessary. A short needle is used for subcutaneous injections.

The nurse determines what types of needle to use for adults and children depending on the route of administration, the size and condition of the patient, and the amount of adipose tissue present at the site. (Figure 5-10)

You have looked at medication orders, types of drug preparations, labels, systems of dosage, and measurement equipment. The next chapters will concentrate on solving dosage problems for oral and parenteral routes.

Needles usually used for **intradermal** injections are ⅜" to ⅝" (1 to 1.5 cm) long and are 25G. Such needles usually have short bevels.

Needles for **subcutaneous** injections are ⅝" to ⅞" (1.5 to 2 cm) long, have medium bevels, and are 25G to 23G.

Needles for **intramuscular** use are 1" to 3" (2.5 to 7.5 cm) long, have medium bevels, and are 23G to 18G.

Needles for **intravenous** use are 1" to 3" long, have long bevels, and are 25G to 14G.

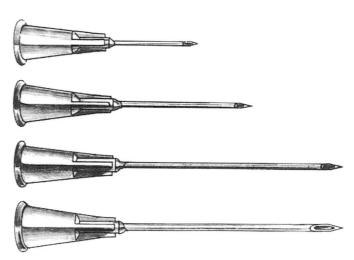

**FIGURE 5-10**

When choosing a needle, the nurse must consider the needle gauge, bevel, and length. Gauge refers to the inside diameter of the needle; the smaller the gauge, the larger the diameter. Bevel refers to the angle at which the needle tip is opened, and length is the distance from the tip to the hub of the needle.

*Name:* _____

*Complete these statements. Answers will be found on page 330.*

1. Elixirs may be contraindicated for patients with a history of _____
   or _____

2. The average dose of a fluidextract is _____ .

3. In giving medications parenterally, four common routes are _____ ,
   _____ , _____ , and _____

4. When a powder is reconstituted, what three facts must the nurse write on the label?
   a. _____
   b. _____
   c. _____

5. What route(s) require(s) sterile technique in preparing and administering drugs?
   _____

6. An example of a drug listed as a magma is _____

7. What action must always be carried out before pouring an oral suspension?
   _____

8. List six drug preparations that can be administered topically.

   _____     _____

   _____     _____

   _____     _____

9. List two advantages in using transdermal medications.

   _____

   _____

10. Define an ointment. _____

    _____

11. List two practices that aid in pouring oral liquids accurately.
    a. _____
    b. _____

12. Define the following:
    a. Meniscus _____

    _____

    b. Needle gauge _____

    _____

*(continued)*

**13.** What factors determine the needle length chosen for an injection?

_____

_____

_____

**14.** List two rules for rounding off numbers.

a. _____

_____

b. _____

_____

**15.** What determines how dosage answers are rounded off?

_____

_____

_____

# Answers

## Self-Test 1 Terms

**1.** e        **4.** h        **6.** m        **8.** b        **10.** d        **12.** f
**2.** k        **5.** i        **7.** l        **9.** c        **11.** g        **13.** j
**3.** a

## Self-Test 2 Medicine Cup Measurements

**1.** Other equivalents are 2 tbsp, 1 oz, 8 drams, 30 mL.
(Remember 1 mL = 1 cc.)
**2.** No, a dram is slightly less than 5 mL (5 cc).
**3.** Use the 1-dram line!
**4.** 15 cc is equal to 1 tbsp, ½ oz, 4 drams, and 15 mL.

**5. a.** Pour 2 drams.
   **b.** 4 tsp × 5 mL = 20 mL; use the 20-cc line
   **c.** ½ oz. Use the liner for ½ oz.
**6.** No, there is no line for 2 mL. Use a syringe to obtain the 2 mL and then pour the amount into a medicine cup.

## Self-Test 3 3-mL Syringe Amounts

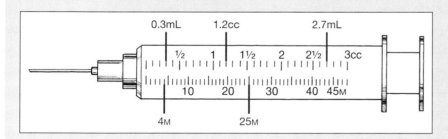

## Self-Test 4 1-mL Syringe Amounts

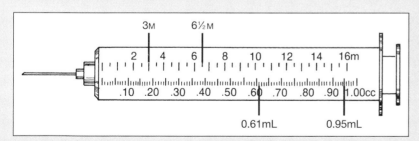

## Self Test 5 3-mL Syringe-Rounding Answers

**a.** 0.1 mL    ✓
**b.** 1½ cc    ✓
**c.** 0.83 cc    0.8 cc
**d.** 0.98 m    1 minim

**e.** 0.2 mL    ✓
**f.** 8½ m    9 m
**g.** 1.7 mL    ✓
**h.** ½ mL    ✓

**i.** 0.4 cc    ✓
**j.** 0.65 mL    0.7 mL
**k.** 3 minims    ✓
**l.** 5.5 minims    6 minims

## Self Test 6 1-mL Syringe-Rounding Answers

**a.** 0.65 mL _____√_____     **d.** 12.8 m ____13 minims____     **g.** 0.758 mL ____0.76 mL____
**b.** 12.5 m _____√_____     **e.** 0.346 mL ____0.35 mL____     **h.** 5 minims _____√_____
**c.** 0.04 mL _____√_____     **f.** 0.290 mL ____0.29 mL____

## Self Test 7 1-mL Insulin Syringe

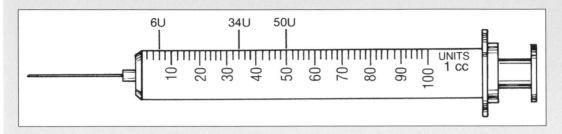

## Self Test 8 .5-mL Insulin Syringe

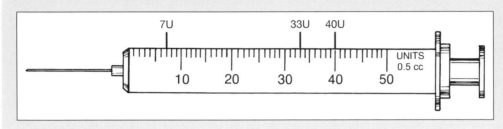

# Calculation of Oral Medications—Solids and Liquids

Drugs for oral administration are prepared by pharmaceutical companies as solids (tablets, capsules) and liquids. When the dose ordered by the physician differs from the stock, the nurse calculates the amount to be given. The problems are solved using a rule derived from ratio and proportion. All measurements need to be in the same system and the same unit or size (use smallest numbers).

A proportion can be used to solve dosage problems. In dosage, three pieces of information are given:

| | |
|---|---|
| The doctor's order: | D = doctor's order or desired dose |
| The quantity or strength of drug on hand | H = on hand or have |
| The solid or liquid form of stock drug (in which the drug comes) | S = stock form |
| The unknown is the amount of drug to administer, usually designated as X or x. It can also be abbreviated as: | A = answer or amount of stock to give |

## ▶ Proportion Expressed As Two Fractions

Using fractions, set up proportions so that like units are across from each other (the units and the numerator match and the units and denominators match). The 1st fraction is the known equivalent.

Example: 1 tablet is equal to 50 mg would be written: $\dfrac{1\ tablet}{50\ mg}$

The 2nd fraction is the unknown and the desired amount. Example: x tablets is equal to 100 mg, and

is written: $\dfrac{x\ tablets}{100\ mg}$

The completed proportion looks like:

$$\frac{S}{H} = \frac{x}{D} \quad \text{or} \quad \frac{S}{H} = \frac{A}{D}$$

**Learning Aid**

You can use the letter X or the letter A to denote the unknown amount. In this text, the letter X will be used with ratio/proportion problems and the letter A will be used when problems are solved using the formula method.

In the example above, it would look like: $\frac{1 \text{ tablet}}{50 \text{ mg}} = \frac{x \text{ tablets}}{100 \text{ mg}}$ or $\frac{1 \text{ tablet}}{50 \text{ mg}} = \frac{A \text{ tablets}}{100 \text{ mg}}$

To solve for x:

1. Cross multiply.

1. $\dfrac{S}{H} = \dfrac{x}{D}$

   $\dfrac{S}{H} \diagup\!\!\!\!\diagdown \dfrac{x}{D}$

   $SD = xH$

2. Clear x by dividing both sides by H.

2. $\dfrac{SD}{H} = \dfrac{xH}{H}$

3. Solve for x.

3. $\dfrac{SD}{H} = \dfrac{x\cancel{H}}{\cancel{H}}$

   $\dfrac{SD}{H} = x$

In our example, it would look like this:

1. $\dfrac{1 \text{ tablet}}{50 \text{ mg}} = \dfrac{x \text{ tablets}}{100 \text{ mg}}$

   $\dfrac{1 \text{ tablet}}{50 \text{ mg}} \diagup\!\!\!\!\diagdown \dfrac{x \text{ tablets}}{100 \text{ mg}}$

   $100 \times 1 = 50x$

2. $\dfrac{100 \times 1}{50} = \dfrac{50x}{50}$

3. $\dfrac{100}{50} = \dfrac{5\cancel{0}x}{5\cancel{0}}$

   $\dfrac{100}{50} = x$

**Learning Aid**

Always divide by the number that is multiplied by x.

Answer: 2 tablets = x.

# ▶ Proportion Expressed As Two Ratios

A ratio using colons can be set up. Double colons separate the two ratios. The 1st ratio is the known equivalent; 2nd ratio is desired amount and the unknown; ratio must always follow the same sequence.

1. Multiply the means (inner two numbers) and the extremes (outer two numbers)
2. Clear x by dividing both sides by H.
3. Solve for x.

1. $S : H :: X : D$      1 tablet: 50 mg = x: 100 mg

   $SD = xH$        $1 \times 100 = 50x$

2. $\dfrac{SD}{H} = \dfrac{xH}{H}$     $\dfrac{1 \times 100}{50} = \dfrac{50x}{50}$

   $\dfrac{SD}{H} = \dfrac{x\cancel{H}}{\cancel{H}}$     $\dfrac{100}{50} = \dfrac{\cancel{50}x}{\cancel{50}}$

3. $\dfrac{SD}{H} = x$     $\dfrac{100}{50} = x$

Both of these methods can be simplified by using the formula method. This is the formula derived from step 3:

$\dfrac{D}{H} \times S = A$      $\dfrac{\text{Desire}}{\text{Have}} \times \text{Stock} = \text{Amount}$

The formula method eliminates the need to cross-multiply, which can be a possible source of error in calculation.

For the purpose of this book, the formula method and the ratio proportion method will be shown side-by-side. (A proportion expressed as two fractions will be shown.) The most important thing is for a nurse to thoroughly understand and use whichever method makes sense to him/her.

Another method used in dosage calculations is the dimensional analysis method. This is briefly discussed in Appendix A.

# ▶ Oral Solids

## Application of the Rule for Oral Solids

| RULE | *Formula Method* |
| --- | --- |

$\dfrac{\text{Desire}}{\text{Have}} \times \text{Stock} = \text{Amount}$

*Ratio Proportion Method*

$\dfrac{\text{Stock}}{\text{Have}} = \dfrac{\text{x or Amount}}{\text{Desire}}$

**Learning Aid**

Abbreviate the rule:

$\dfrac{D}{H} \times S = A$      $\dfrac{S}{H} = \dfrac{x}{D}$

**Example**

Order: alprazolam 0.5 mg po bid

Stock: Read the label.

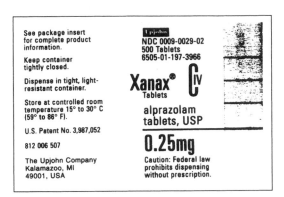

*Desire:* The desire is the physician's order. In the example, desired is 0.5 mg.

*Have:* Have is the strength of the drug supplied in the container. In the example, the label indicates that each tablet contains 0.25 mg.

*Stock:* The stock is the unit form in which the drug comes. Alprazolam comes in tablet form. Because tablets and capsules are single entities, the stock for oral solid drugs is always one.

*Amount:* The amount is how much stock to give. For oral solids the answer will be the number of tablets or capsules to administer.

To solve any problem, first check that the order and the stock are in the same weight measure. If they are not, you must convert one or the other amount to its equivalent. In this example no equivalent is needed; both the order and the stock are in mg.

**Example**

*Formula Method*

Order: alprazolam 0.5 mg

Stock: tablets of 0.25 mg

Rule: $\dfrac{D}{H} \times S = A$

$$\frac{\overset{2}{0.50 \text{ mg}}}{\underset{1}{0.25 \text{ mg}}} \times 1 \text{ tab} = 2 \text{ tabs}$$

*Ratio Proportion Method*

$$\frac{1 \text{ tab}}{0.25 \text{ mg}} = \frac{x}{0.50 \text{ mg}}$$

$$\frac{0.50}{0.25} = x$$

$$2 \text{ tabs} = x$$

## *Clearing Decimals*

When the numerator and denominator in $\dfrac{D}{H}$ are decimals, add zeros to make the number of decimal places the same. Then drop the decimal points. This is a short arithmetic operation to replace long division:

$$\frac{\overset{\text{added}}{\overset{\downarrow}{0.50}} \text{ mg}}{0.25 \text{ mg}} \quad \frac{\text{numerator}}{\text{denominator or divisor}}$$

In division the denominator is the divisor and must be cleared of decimal points before the arithmetic is carried out. The decimal point in the numerator is moved the same number of places. Refer to Chapter 1 for further help in division of decimals.

---

**Example**

Order: digoxin 0.125 mg po qd

Stock: scored tablets labeled 0.25 mg

No equivalent is needed. Both are in mg.

$$\frac{0.125 \text{ mg}^{1}}{0.250 \text{ mg}_{2}} \times 1 \text{ tab} = \frac{1}{2} \text{ tab}$$

---

### Learning Aid

Long division

$$0.25\overline{)0.125} = \frac{0.5}{10} = \frac{5}{10} = \frac{1}{2} \text{ tab}$$

Short way

$$\frac{0.125}{0.250} = \frac{1}{2} \text{ tab}$$

Note that a zero was added. In short arithmetic when the number of decimal places is the same in the numerator and denominator, the decimal is dropped.

---

**Example**

Order: Amoxicillin 1 g po q 6h

Stock: 1 capsule equals 500 mg.

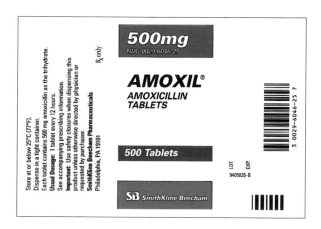

(Courtesy of GlaxoSmithKline.)

Equivalent: 1 g = 1000 mg

**Formula Method**

$$\frac{D}{H} \times S = A$$

$$\frac{\overset{2}{\cancel{1000\ mg}}}{\underset{1}{\cancel{500\ mg}}} \times 1\ cap = 2\ caps$$

**Ratio Proportion Method**

$$\frac{1}{500\ mg} = \frac{x}{1000\ mg}$$

$$\frac{1000}{500} = x$$

2 caps = x

**Example**

Order: penicillin VK 800,000 units po
q 4 h × 10 days

Stock: 1 tablet equals 400,000 units

**Formula Method**

$$\frac{D}{H} \times S = A$$

$$\frac{\overset{2}{\cancel{800,000\ units}}}{\underset{1}{\cancel{400,000\ units}}} \times 1\ tab = 2\ tabs$$

**Ratio Proportion Method**

$$\frac{1\ tab}{400,000\ units} = \frac{x}{800,000\ units}$$

$$\frac{800,000}{400,000} = x$$

2 tabs = x

**Example**

Order: Synthroid 100 mcg po qd

Stock: Read the label.

| NDC 0053 | See full prescribing information for dosage and administration |
|---|---|
| **Levothyroxine Sodium Tablets** | |
| | Dispense in a tight, light-resistant container. Store at controlled room temperature 15-30°C. |
| **100 mcg (0.1 mg)** | |
| 100 tablets | |

Note that the label gives the equivalent measure: 100 mcg = 0.1 mg

Because the order and the stock are in the same weight measure, no calculation is necessary.

Give 1 tablet.

**Example**

Order: Myambutol 1.2 g po qd

Stock: 1 tablet equals 400 mg

Equivalent: 1.2 g = 1200 mg

**Learning Aid**

Reminder 1 g = 1000 mg. Equivalents are in Chapter 4.

The quick rule for converting states that you write the equivalent you wish to change first. Then write the conversion you want. The open arrow faces the larger measure.

1.2 g = _____ mg

1.2 g > mg

The arrow tells you to move the gram number three places to the right:

1.2 g = 1200 mg

*Formula Method*

Rule: $\dfrac{D}{H} \times S = A$

$$\dfrac{\overset{3}{\cancel{1200}\text{ mg}}}{\underset{1}{\cancel{400}\text{ mg}}} \times 1 \text{ tab} = 3 \text{ tabs}$$

*Ratio Proportion Method*

$$\dfrac{1 \text{ tablet}}{400 \text{ mg}} = \dfrac{x}{1200 \text{ mg}}$$

$$\dfrac{1200}{400} = x$$

$$3 \text{ tablets} = x$$

**Example**

Order: levothyroxine sodium 37.5 μg po qd

Stock: scored tablets of 0.025 mg

Equivalent 0.025 mg = 25 μg

**Learning Aid**

Remember 1 mg = 1000 μg. The quick rule for converting states that you write the equivalent you want to change first. Then write the conversion you want. Change the mg to μg. To find the equivalent, the open arrow faces the larger measure.

mg > μg

The arrow tells you to move mg three places to the right.

0.025 mg = 25 μg

**Formula Method**

Rule: $\dfrac{D}{H} \times S = A$

**Ratio Proportion Method**

$\dfrac{1 \text{ tablet}}{25 \ \mu g} = \dfrac{x}{37.5 \ \mu g}$

$\dfrac{37.5 \ \mu g}{25 \ \mu g} \times 1 = A$

$\dfrac{37.5}{25} = x$

$1.5 \text{ tablets} = x$

Use the quick way to clear the decimal point.

$\dfrac{\overset{3}{\cancel{37.5}}}{\underset{2}{\cancel{25.0}}} \times 1 \text{ tab} = \dfrac{3}{2}$

(Divided by 125)

$\dfrac{3}{2} = 1\tfrac{1}{2} \text{ tabs}$

You can administer $1\tfrac{1}{2}$ tablets because the stock is scored.

**Example**

EXAMPLE 1:

Order: pentobarbital 0.1 g po hs prn

Stock: capsules labeled 100 mg

Equivalent 0.1 g = 100 mg

**Formula Method**

Rule: $\dfrac{D}{H} \times S = A$

**Ratio Proportion Method**

$\dfrac{1 \text{ capsule}}{100 \text{ mg}} = \dfrac{x}{100 \text{ mg}}$

$\dfrac{\overset{1}{\cancel{100 \text{ mg}}}}{\underset{1}{\cancel{100 \text{ mg}}}} \times 1 \text{ cap} = 1 \text{ cap}$

$\dfrac{100}{100} = x$

$1 \text{ cap} = x$

EXAMPLE 2:

Order: Mycostatin 1 million units po tid

Stock: scored tablets labeled 500,000 units

No equivalent needed.

**Formula Method**

Rule: $\dfrac{D}{H} \times S = A$

**Ratio Proportion Method**

$\dfrac{1 \text{ tablet}}{500,000 \text{ units}} = \dfrac{x}{1,000,000 \text{ units}}$

$\dfrac{\overset{2}{\cancel{1,000,000 \text{ units}}}}{\underset{1}{\cancel{500,000 \text{ units}}}} \times 1 \text{ tab} = 2 \text{ tabs}$

$\dfrac{1,000,000}{500,000} = x$

$2 \text{ tabs} = x$

*Solve these practice problems. Answers may be found at the end of the chapter. Remember the*

**Formula Method**

$$\frac{D}{H} \times S = A$$

**Ratio Proportion Method**

$$\frac{S}{H} \times \frac{x}{D}$$

1. Order: Decadron 1.5 mg po bid
   Stock: tablets labeled 0.75 mg

2. Order: digoxin 0.25 mg po qd
   Stock: scored tablets labeled 0.5 mg

3. Order: ampicillin 0.5 Gm po q6h
   Stock: capsules labeled 250 mg

4. Order: prednisone 10 mg po tid
   Stock: tablets labeled 2.5 mg

5. Order: aspirin 650 mg po stat
   Stock: tablets labeled 325 mg

6. Order: digitoxin 200 mcg po qd
   Stock: scored tablets labeled 0.1 mg

7. Order: Equanil 0.2 g po q4h
   Stock: scored tablets labeled 400 mg

8. Order: penicillin G potassium 200,000 units po q8h
   Stock: scored tablets labeled 400,000 units

9. Order: digoxin 0.5 mg po qd
   Stock: scored tablets labeled 0.25 mg

10. Order: Lasix 60 mg po qd
    Stock: scored tablets labeled 40 mg

## Special Types of Oral Solid Orders

Drugs that contain a number of active ingredients are ordered by the number to be administered and do not require calculation. These include over-the-counter (OTC) preparations and multivitamins.

**Example**    Multivitamin tabs i po qd

Gelusil tabs i po q4h prn

Physicians occasionally specify the weight measure of the drug and the number of tablets to be given. These orders do not require calculation.

**Example**

*EXAMPLE 1:*

Darvon 65 mg caps ii po hs prn

This is interpreted: Give two capsules of Darvon 65 mg by mouth at the hour of sleep if needed.

*EXAMPLE 2:*

aspirin 325 mg ii po stat

This is interpreted: Give two tablets of aspirin 325 mg by mouth immediately.

# ▶ Oral Liquids

## *Application of the Rule for Oral Liquids*

**RULE**   *Formula Method*

$$\frac{\text{Desire}}{\text{Have}} \times \text{Stock} = \text{Amount}$$

*Ratio Proportion Method*

$$\frac{\text{Stock}}{\text{Have}} = \frac{\text{x or Amount}}{\text{Desire}}$$

**Learning Aid**

Abbreviate the rule:

$$\frac{D}{H} \times S = A \qquad \frac{S}{H} = \frac{x}{D}$$

**Example**

Order: azithromycin oral susp 400 mg po qd × 4 days

Stock: Read the label below.

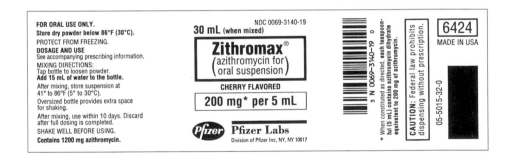

*Formula Method*

$$\frac{D}{H} \times S = A$$

$$\frac{\overset{2}{\cancel{400 \text{ mg}}}}{\underset{1}{\cancel{200 \text{ mg}}}} \times 5 \text{ mL} = 10 \text{ mL}$$

*Ratio Proportion Method*

$$\frac{5 \text{ mL}}{200 \text{ mg}} = \frac{x}{400 \text{ mg}}$$

$$\frac{2000}{200} = x$$

$$10 \text{ mL} = x$$

Before solving each problem, check to be certain that the order and your supply are in the same measure. If they are not, you must convert one or the other to its equivalent. Convert whichever one is easier for you to solve.

**Example**    Order: cloxacillin sodium 0.25 g

Stock: 125 mg per 5 mL

Equivalent: 0.25 g = 250 mg

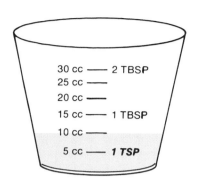

**Learning Aid**

There are several ways to solve the math.

$$\dfrac{\overset{10}{\cancel{\overset{250}{\cancel{250}}}}}{\underset{1}{\cancel{\underset{25}{\cancel{125}}}}} \times \overset{1}{\cancel{5}} = 10 \text{ mL}$$

$$250 \times 5 = \dfrac{\overset{10}{\cancel{1250}}}{\underset{1}{\cancel{125}}} = 10 \text{ mL}$$

***Formula Method***

Rule: $\dfrac{D}{H} \times S = A$

$$\dfrac{\overset{2}{\cancel{250}} \text{ mg}}{\underset{1}{\cancel{125}} \text{ mg}} \times 5 \text{ mL} = 10 \text{ mL}$$

***Ratio Proportion Method***

$$\dfrac{5 \text{ mL}}{125 \text{ mg}} = \dfrac{x}{250 \text{ mg}}$$

$$\dfrac{\overset{2}{\cancel{250}} \times 5}{\underset{1}{\cancel{125}}} = x$$

$$10 \text{ mL} = x$$

**Example**    Order: furosemide 34 mg po qd.

Stock: Read the label below.

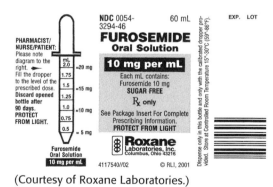

(Courtesy of Roxane Laboratories.)

**Learning Aid**

Because the drug comes with a calibrated dropper, you are alerted that your answer will be a small amount. See Figure 11-2 for equipment used to measure small amounts of liquid doses.

*Formula Method*
No equivalent is needed

*Ratio Proportion Method*

$$\frac{D}{H} \times S = A$$

$$\frac{1 \text{ mL}}{10 \text{ mg}} = \frac{x}{34 \text{ mg}}$$

$$\frac{34 \text{ mg}}{10 \text{ mg}} \times 1 \text{ mL} = \frac{34}{10} \quad 10\overline{)34.0}^{\phantom{0}3.4}$$

$$\frac{34}{10} = x$$

Give 3.4 mL

3.4 mL = x

| Example | Order: penicillin VK 0.4 g po q 6 h |

Stock: 250 mg Penicillin V per 5 mL

Equivalent: 0.4 g = 400 mg

*Formula Method*

$$\frac{D}{H} \times S = A$$

*Ratio Proportion Method*

$$\frac{5 \text{ mL}}{250 \text{ mg}} = \frac{x}{400 \text{ mg}}$$

$$\frac{\overset{8}{400 \text{ mg}}}{\underset{1}{\underset{5}{250 \text{ mg}}}} \times \overset{1}{5} = 8 \text{ mL}$$

$$\frac{2000}{250} = x$$

$$8 \text{ mL} = x$$

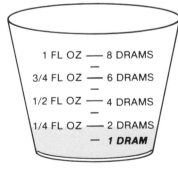

**Example**

Order: Amoxicillin oral suspension 500 mg po q 8h

Stock: Read the label below

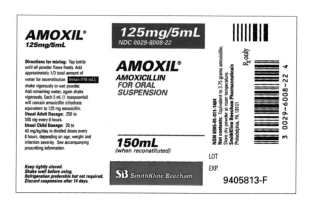

(Courtesy of GlaxoSmithKline.)

*Formula Method*

$$\frac{D}{H} \times S = A$$

$$\frac{\overset{4}{\cancel{500\ mg}}}{\underset{1}{\cancel{125\ mg}}} \times 5\ mL = 20\ mL$$

*Ratio Proportion Method*

$$\frac{5\ mL}{125\ mg} = \frac{x}{500\ mg}$$

$$\frac{2500}{125} = x$$

$$20\ mL = x$$

---

**SELF TEST 2** | **Oral Liquids**

*Solve these oral liquid problems. Answers may be found at the end of the chapter.*

1. Order: erythromycin susp. 0.75 g po qid
   Stock: liquid labeled 250 mg/5 mL

   $\frac{5}{250}\ \frac{x}{150}$   $\frac{50x}{50} = \frac{750}{50} = 50\overline{)750}$   $15\ mL$

2. Order: ampicillin susp. 500 mg po q8h
   Stock: liquid labeled 250 mg/5 mL

   $\frac{5}{250}\ \frac{x}{500}$   $\frac{50x}{50} = \frac{500}{50}$   $10\ mL$

3. Order: Cephalex in oral suspension 0.35 Gm po q6h
   Stock: liquid labeled 125 mg/5 mL

   $\frac{5}{125}\ \frac{x}{350}$   $\frac{25x}{25} = \frac{350}{25}$   $14\ mL$

4. Order: cyclosporine 150 mg po stat and qd
   Stock: liquid labeled 100 mg/mL in a bottle with a calibrated dropper

   $\frac{1}{100}\ \frac{x}{150}$   $\frac{100x}{100} = \frac{150}{100}$   $1.5\ mL$

5. Order: sulfasoxizole susp. 300 mg po qid
   Stock: liquid labeled 250 mg/5 mL

   $\frac{5}{250} = \frac{x}{300}$   $\frac{50x}{50} = \frac{300}{50}$   $6\ mL$

6. Order: digoxin 0.02 mg po qd
   Stock: pediatric elixir 0.05 mg/mL in a bottle with a dropper marked in tenths of a milliliter

   $\frac{1}{0.05} = \frac{x}{0.02}$   $\frac{0.05x}{0.05} = \frac{0.02}{0.05}$   $0.4\ mL$

   *(continued)*

**7.** Order: potassium chloride 30 mEq po qd
Stock: liquid labeled 20 mEq/15 mL

**8.** Order: elixir digoxin 0.25 mg via nasogastric tube qd
Stock: liquid labeled 0.5 mg/10 mL

**9.** Order: hydrocortisone cypionate oral susp. 30 mg po q6h
Stock: liquid labeled 10 mg/5 mL

**10.** Order: promethazine HCl syrup 12.5 mg po tid
Stock: liquid labeled 6.25 mg/5 mL

## Special Types of Oral Liquid Orders

Some liquids, including OTC preparations and multivitamins, are ordered in the amount to be poured and administered. No calculation is required.

**Example**

*EXAMPLE 1:*

Order: terpin hydrate elixir 2 tsp q 4 h prn po

Stock: liquid labeled terpin hydrate elixir

No calculation is needed. Pour 2 teaspoons every 4 hours by mouth if necessary.

*EXAMPLE 2:*

Order: milk of magnesia 30 cc hs tonight po

Stock: liquid labeled milk of magnesia

No calculation is required. Pour 30 cc of milk of magnesia and give tonight by mouth.

## ▶ Mental Drill for Oral Solid and Liquid Problems

As you develop proficiency in solving problems, you will be able to calculate many answers without written work. This drill combines your knowledge of equivalents and dosage.

## SELF TEST 3 | Mental Drill Oral Solids

*Solve the problems mentally and write only the amount to be given. Answers will be found at the end of the chapter. Keep the rule in mind as you solve each problem.*

| Order | Stock (Scored Tablets) | Answer |
|---|---|---|
| **1.** 20 mg | 10 mg | 2 tablets |
| **2.** 0.125 mg | 0.25 mg | 1/2 tablet |
| **3.** 0.25 mg | 0.125 mg | 2 tablets |
| **4.** 200,000 units | 100,000 units | 2 tablets |
| **5.** 0.5 mg | 0.25 mg | 2 tablets |
| **6.** 0.2 Gm | 400 mg | 1/2 tablet |
| **7.** 1 Gm | 1000 mg | 1 tablet |
| **8.** 0.1 Gm | 100 mg | 1 tablet |
| **9.** 0.01 Gm | 20 mg | 1/2 tablet |
| **10.** 650 mg | 325 mg | 2 tablets |
| **11.** 500 mg | 250 mg | 2 tablets |
| **12.** gr i | 60 mg | 1 tablet |
| **13.** 50 mg | 0.1 Gm | 1/2 tablet |
| **14.** 4 mg | 2 mg | 2 tablets |

## SELF TEST 4 | Mental Drill Oral Liquids

| Order | Stock | Answer |
|---|---|---|
| **1.** 20 mg | 10 mg per 5 mL | 2x = 20  = 10 mL |
| **2.** 10 mg | 2 mg/5 cc | |
| **3.** 0.5 Gm | 250 mg/5 mL | |
| **4.** 0.1 Gm | 200 mg per 10 mL | |
| **5.** 250 mg | 0.1 g per 6 mL | |
| **6.** 100 mg | 50 mg/10 cc | |
| **7.** 12 mg | 4 mg/5 mL | |
| **8.** 15 mg | 30 mg/10 mL | |
| **9.** 15 mg | 10 mg per 4 mL | |
| **10.** 0.25 mg | 0.5 mg/5 mL | |

**PROFICIENCY TEST 1** Calculation of Oral Doses

*Name:* _____

*For liquid answers, draw a line on the medicine cup indicating the amount you would pour. Answers will be found on page 330.*

**1.** Order:     KCl elixir 20 mEq po bid
     Stock:     liquid labeled 30 mEq/15 mL

     Answer ____10 mL____

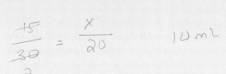

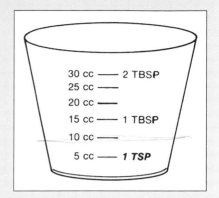

**2.** Order:     Dilantin susp 150 mg po tid
     Stock:     liquid labeled 75 mg/7.5 mL

     Answer ____15 mL____

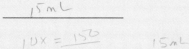

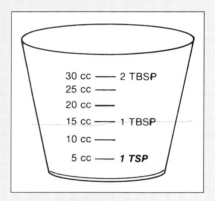

**3.** Order:     elixir digoxin 0.125 mg po qd
     Stock:     liquid labeled 0.25 mg/10 mL

     Answer ____5 mL____

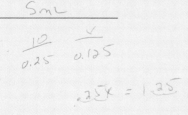

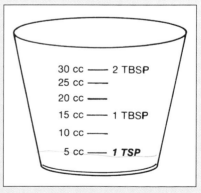

*(continued)*

**4.** Order:    Dilantin oral suspension 150
              mg po tid

Stock:    liquid labeled 75 mg/6 mL

Answer _____

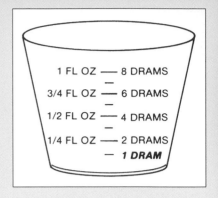

**5.** Order:    Proximyl 10 mg po bid

Stock:    liquid labeled 2 mg/5 mL

Answer _____

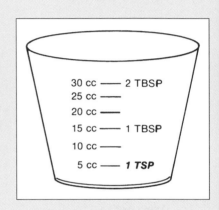

**6.** Order:    digoxin 0.5 mg po qd

Stock:    tablets labeled 0.25 mg

Answer _____

**7.** Order:    Lanoxin 10 μg qd po

Stock:    0.02 mg scored tablets

Answer _____

**8.** Order:    Zyloprim 250 mg po qd

Stock:    scored tablets 100 mg

Answer _____

**9.** Order:    ampicillin 0.5 g po q6h

Stock:    capsules labeled 250 mg

Answer _____

**10.** Order:    Synthroid 0.3 mg po qd

Stock:    tablets labeled 300 μg scored

Answer _____

**PROFICIENCY TEST 2 | Calculation of Oral Doses (Test 2)**

*Name:* _____

*For liquid answers, draw a line on the medicine cup indicating the amount you would pour. Answers will be found on page 332.*

**1.** Order:     ibuprofen 0.8 gm po tid
     Stock:     tablets labeled 400 mg

     Answer    _____

**2.** Order:     isoniazid 0.3 Gm po qd
     Stock:     tablets labeled 300 mg

     Answer    _____

**3.** Order:     ethambutol HCl 600 mg po qd
     Stock:     tablets scored and labeled 400 mg

     Answer    _____

**4.** Order:     acetaminophen 0.65 Gm po q4h
     Stock:     tablets labeled 325 mg

     Answer    _____

**5.** Order:     ascorbic acid 250 mg po bid
     Stock:     tablets scored and labeled 500 mg

     Answer    _____

**6.** Order:     colistin sulfate oral suspension
     80 mg po tid
     Stock:     liquid labeled 25 mg/tsp

     Answer    _____

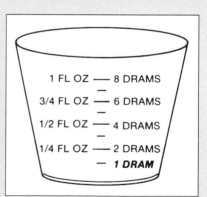

**7.** Order:     oxacillin sodium 0.75 Gm po q6h
     Stock:     liquid labeled 250 mg/5 mL

     Answer    _____

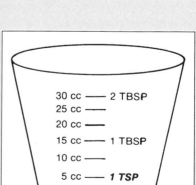

*(continued)*

**8.** Order:     penicillin V potassium 600 mg
                     po q6h
     Stock:     liquid labeled 250 mg/5 mL

     Answer  _____

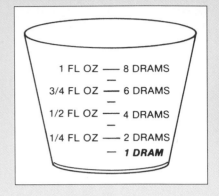

**9.** Order:     Mylanta II 30 ml q4h prn
     Stock:     liquid labeled Mylanta II

     Answer  _____

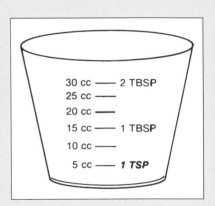

**10.** Order:     Elixophyllin 160 mg po q6h
      Stock:     liquid labeled 80 mg/15 mL

      Answer  _____

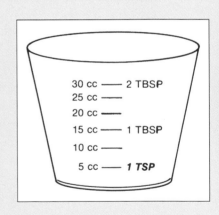

*Name:* _____

*Aim for 90% or better on this test. There are 20 questions, each worth 5 points. Determine the amount to be given. If you have any difficulty, reread Chapter 6, which explains this information. Answers will be found on page 334.*

1. Order: potassium chloride 20 mEq po in juice
   Stock: liquid in a bottle labeled 30 mEq/15 mL

2. Order: syrup of tetracycline hydrochloride 80 mg po q6h
   Stock: liquid in a dropper bottle labeled 125 mg/5 mL

3. Order: propranolol 0.02 g po bid
   Stock: scored tablets labeled 10 mg

4. Order: ampicillin sodium 0.5 g po q6h
   Stock: capsules of 250 mg

5. Order: digoxin 0.5 mg po qd
   Stock: scored tablets of 0.25 mg

6. Order: Levothroid susp. 100 mcg qd po
   Stock: liquid in a bottle labeled 0.2 mg/10 mL

7. Order: hydrochlorothiazide 75 mg po qd
   Stock: scored tablets 50 mg

8. Order: furosemide 40 mg po qd
   Stock: scored tablets of 80 mg

9. Order: digoxin 0.125 mg po
   Stock: liquid in a dropper bottle labeled 500 $\mu$g/10 mL

10. Order: Dilantin Susp 75 mg po tid
    Stock: liquid in a bottle labeled 50 mg/10 mL

11. Order: diazepam 5 mg po q4h prn
    Stock: scored tablets 2 mg

12. Order: Synthroid 0.15 mg po qd
    Stock: scored tablets 300 $\mu$g

13. Order: Antabuse 375 mg po today
    Stock: scored tablets 250 mg

14. Order: ibuprofen 0.6 g po q4h prn
    Stock: Film-coated tablets 300 mg

15. Order: chlorpheniramine maleate syr 1.5 mg po bid
    Stock: liquid in a bottle 1 mg/8 mL

*(continued)*

16. Order:   diphenhydramine maleate syrup 25 mg po q4h while awake
    Stock:   liquid labeled 12.5 mg/5 mL

17. Order:   simethicone liq 60 mg po in ½ glass H$_2$O
    Stock:   liquid in a dropper bottle labeled 40 mg/0.6 mL

18. Order:   chlorothiazide oral susp 0.5 g via NGT po qd
    Stock:   liquid labeled 250 mg/5 mL

19. Order:   meperidine HCl syrup 15 mg po q4h prn
    Stock:   liquid labeled 50 mg/5 mL

20. Order:   hydroxyzine syrup 7.5 mg po q6h
    Stock:   liquid labeled 10 mg/5 mL

# Answers

## Self-Test 1 Oral Solids

**1.**

*Formula Method*

Rule: $\dfrac{D}{H} \times S = A$.

No equivalent needed

$$\dfrac{\overset{2}{\cancel{1.50\ \text{mg}}}}{\underset{1}{\cancel{0.75\ \text{mg}}}} \times 1\ \text{tab} = 2\ \text{tablets}$$

*Ratio Proportion Method*

$$\dfrac{S}{H} = \dfrac{x}{D}$$

$$\dfrac{1\ \text{tab}}{0.75\ \text{mg}} = \dfrac{x}{1.5\ \text{mg}}$$

$$\dfrac{1.50}{0.75} = x$$

$$2\ \text{tablets} = x$$

*Learning Aid*

$$\begin{array}{r} 2. \\ 0.75\,\overline{)1.50} \\ \underline{1\ 50} \\ 0 \end{array}$$

**2.** No equivalent necessary

*Formula Method*

$$\dfrac{\overset{1}{\cancel{0.25\ \text{mg}}}}{\underset{2}{\cancel{0.50\ \text{mg}}}} \times 1\ \text{tab} = \dfrac{1}{2}\ \text{tablet}$$

*Ratio Proportion Method*

$$\dfrac{1\ \text{tablet}}{0.5\ \text{mg}} = \dfrac{x}{0.25\ \text{mg}}$$

$$\dfrac{0.25}{0.50} = x$$

$.5$ tablet $= x$

*Learning Aid*

$$\begin{array}{r} 0.5 \\ 0.5\,\overline{)0.2.5} \\ \underline{25} \\ 0 \end{array} \text{ or } \dfrac{1}{2}$$

**3.** Equivalent 0.5 Gm = 500 mg

*Formula Method*

$$\dfrac{\overset{2}{\cancel{500\ \text{mg}}}}{\underset{1}{\cancel{250\ \text{mg}}}} \times 1\ \text{tab} = 2\ \text{tablets}$$

*Ratio Proportion Method*

$$\dfrac{1\ \text{tablet}}{250\ \text{mg}} = \dfrac{x}{500\ \text{mg}}$$

$$\dfrac{500}{250} = x$$

$2$ tablets $= x$

*Learning Aid*

$$\begin{array}{r} 2. \\ 250\,\overline{)500.} \\ \underline{500} \\ 0 \end{array}$$

**4.** No equivalent necessary

**Formula Method**

$$\frac{\overset{4}{\cancel{10.0}} \text{ mg}}{\underset{1}{\cancel{2.5}} \text{ mg}} \times 1 \text{ tab} = 4 \text{ tablets}$$

**Ratio Proportion Method**

$$\frac{1 \text{ tablet}}{2.5 \text{ mg}} = \frac{x}{10}$$

$$\frac{10}{2.5} = x$$

$$4 \text{ tablets} = x$$

**Learning Aid**

$$2.5\overline{)10.0}\;\overset{4.}{}$$

**5.** No equivalent necessary

**Formula Method**

$$\frac{\overset{2}{\cancel{650}} \text{ mg}}{\underset{1}{\cancel{325}} \text{ mg}} \times 1 \text{ tab} = 2 \text{ tablets}$$

**Ratio Proportion Method**

$$\frac{1 \text{ tablet}}{325 \text{ mg}} = \frac{x}{650 \text{ mg}}$$

$$\frac{650}{325} = x$$

$$2 \text{ tablets} = x$$

**Learning Aid**

$$325\overline{)650.}\;\overset{2.}{}$$
$$\phantom{325)}\underline{650}$$
$$\phantom{325)}0$$

**6.** Equivalent 1 mg = 1000 mcg

mg > mcg

0.1 mg = 100 mcg

**Formula Method**

$$\frac{\overset{2}{\cancel{200}} \text{ mcg}}{\underset{1}{\cancel{100}} \text{ mcg}} \times 1 \text{ tab} = 2 \text{ tablets}$$

**Ratio Proportion Method**

$$\frac{1 \text{ tablet}}{100 \text{ mcg}} = \frac{x}{200 \text{ mcg}}$$

$$\frac{200}{100} = x$$

$$2 \text{ tablets} = x$$

**Learning Aid**

Move decimal three places to the right.

0.100 = 100 mcg

**7.** Equivalent 0.2 g = 200 mg

$g > mg$

*Formula Method*

$$\frac{\overset{1}{\cancel{200\text{ mg}}}}{\underset{2}{\cancel{400\text{ mg}}}} \times 1\text{ tab} = \frac{1}{2}\text{ tablet}$$

*Ratio Proportion Method*

$$\frac{1\text{ tablet}}{400\text{ mg}} = \frac{x}{200\text{ mg}}$$

$$\frac{200}{400} = x$$

.5 tablet = x

**Learning Aid**

Move decimal point three places to the right.

0.200 = 200 mg

Important! Do not invert the numbers in the answer. The answer is

$\frac{1}{2}$ tablet, not 2 tablets.

**8.** No equivalent necessary

*Formula Method*

$$\frac{\overset{1}{\cancel{200{,}000\text{ units}}}}{\underset{2}{\cancel{400{,}000\text{ units}}}} = \frac{1}{2}\text{ tablet}$$

*Ratio Proportion Method*

$$\frac{1\text{ tablet}}{400{,}000\text{ units}} = \frac{x}{200{,}000}$$

$$\frac{200{,}000}{400{,}000} = x$$

.5 tablet = x

**9.** No equivalent necessary

*Formula Method*

$$\frac{\overset{2}{\cancel{0.50\text{ mg}}}}{\underset{1}{\cancel{0.25\text{ mg}}}} \times 1\text{ tab} = 2\text{ tablets}$$

*Ratio Proportion Method*

$$\frac{1\text{ tablet}}{0.25\text{ mg}} = \frac{x}{0.50\text{ mg}}$$

$$\frac{0.50}{0.25} = x$$

2 tablets = x

**Learning Aid**

$$0.25\overline{)0.50}$$
$$\underline{50}$$
$$0$$

(answer 2.)

**10.** No equivalent necessary

*Formula Method*

$$\frac{\overset{3}{\cancel{60\text{ mg}}}}{\underset{2}{\cancel{40\text{ mg}}}} \times 1\text{ tab} = 1\tfrac{1}{2}\text{ tablets}$$

*Ratio Proportion Method*

$$\frac{1\text{ tablet}}{40\text{ mg}} = \frac{x}{60\text{ mg}}$$

$$\frac{60}{40} = x$$

1.5 tablets = x

**Learning Aid**

$$40\overline{)60.0}$$
$$\underline{40}$$
$$200$$
$$\underline{200}$$
$$0$$

(answer 1.5)

## Self Test 2 Oral Liquids

**1.**

*Formula Method*

Rule: $\dfrac{D}{H} \times S = A$

Equivalent 0.75 g = 750 mg

$\dfrac{\overset{3}{\cancel{750 \text{ mg}}}}{\underset{1}{\cancel{250 \text{ mg}}}} \times 5 \text{ mL} = 15 \text{ mL}$

*Ratio Proportion Method*

$\dfrac{S}{H} = \dfrac{x}{D}$

$\dfrac{5 \text{ mL}}{250 \text{ mg}} = \dfrac{x}{750 \text{ mg}}$

$\dfrac{5 \times \overset{3}{\cancel{750}}}{\underset{1}{\cancel{250}}} = x$

$15 \text{ mL} = x$

**Learning Aid**

Calculations may be done in different ways. Answers should be the same regardless of the method chosen to solve the problem.

**2.** No equivalent necessary

*Formula Method*

$\dfrac{\overset{2}{\cancel{500 \text{ mg}}}}{\underset{1}{\cancel{250 \text{ mg}}}} \times 5 \text{ mL} = 10 \text{ mL}$

*Ratio Proportion Method*

$\dfrac{5 \text{ mL}}{250 \text{ mg}} = \dfrac{x}{500}$

$\dfrac{2500}{250} = x$

$10 \text{ mL} = x$

**Learning Aid**

Alternate arithmetic

$500 \times 5 = 2500$

$\begin{array}{r} 10. \\ 250 \overline{)2500.} \\ 250 \phantom{0000} \\ \hline 0 \end{array}$

**3.** Equivalent 0.35 Gm = 350 mg

*Formula Method*

$\dfrac{\overset{\overset{\overset{14}{\cancel{70}}}{\cancel{350 \text{ mg}}}}{\underset{\underset{\underset{1}{\cancel{5}}}{\cancel{25}}}{\cancel{125 \text{ mg}}}} \times 5 \text{ mL} = 14 \text{ mL}$

*Ratio Proportion Method*

$\dfrac{5 \text{ mL}}{125 \text{ mg}} = \dfrac{x}{350 \text{ mg}}$

$\dfrac{5 \times 350}{125} = x$

$\dfrac{1750}{125} = x$

$14 \text{ mL} = x$

**Learning Aid**

Alternate arithmetic

$350 \times 5 = 1750$

$\begin{array}{r} 14. \\ 125 \overline{)1750.} \\ 125 \phantom{00} \\ \hline 500 \\ 500 \\ \hline 0 \end{array}$

**4.** No equivalent necessary

*Formula Method*

$$\frac{\overset{3}{\cancel{150}\ \text{mg}}}{\underset{2}{\cancel{100}\ \text{mg}}} \times 1\ \text{mL} = \frac{3}{2} = 1.5\ \text{mL}$$

*Ratio Proportion Method*

$$\frac{1\ \text{mL}}{100\ \text{mg}} = \frac{x}{150\ \text{mg}}$$

$$\frac{150}{100} = x$$

$$1.5\ \text{mL} = x$$

**Learning Aid**

Alternate arithmetic

```
        1.5
100 )150.0
     100
     500
     500
       0
```

**5.** No equivalent necessary

*Formula Method*

$$\frac{\overset{6}{\cancel{300}\ \text{mg}}}{\underset{5}{\cancel{250}\ \text{mg}}} \times \frac{1}{\cancel{5}}\ \text{mL} = 6\ \text{mL}$$

*Ratio Proportion Method*

$$\frac{5\ \text{mL}}{250\ \text{mg}} = \frac{x}{300\ \text{mg}}$$

$$\frac{1500}{250} = x$$

$$6\ \text{mL} = x$$

**Learning Aid**

Alternate arithmetic

$$300 \times 5 = 1500$$

```
        6.
250 )1500.
     1500
        0
```

**6.** No equivalent necessary

*Formula Method*

$$\frac{0.02\ \text{mg}}{0.05\ \text{mg}} \times 1\ \text{mL} = \frac{2}{5} = 0.4\ \text{mL}$$

*Ratio Proportion Method*

$$\frac{1\ \text{mL}}{0.05\ \text{mg}} = \frac{x}{0.02}$$

$$\frac{0.02}{0.05} = x$$

$$.4\ \text{mL} = x$$

**Learning Aid**

```
           0.4
0.05 )0.02 0
           20
            0
```

**7.** No equivalent necessary

*Formula Method*

$$\frac{\cancel{3}\ \text{mEq}}{\cancel{2}\ \text{mEq}} \times 15\ \text{mL} = \frac{45}{2)45.0}\ \frac{22.5}{} = 22.5\ \text{mL}$$

*Ratio Proportion Method*

$$\frac{15\ \text{mL}}{20\ \text{mEq}} = \frac{x}{30\ \text{mEq}}$$

$$\frac{450}{20} = x$$

$$22.5\ \text{mL} = x$$

**8.** No equivalent necessary

*Formula Method*

$$\dfrac{\overset{1}{\cancel{0.25}}\text{ mg}}{\underset{2}{\cancel{0.50}}\text{ mg}} \times \overset{5}{\cancel{10}} \text{ mL} = 5 \text{ mL}$$

*Ratio Proportion Method*

$$\dfrac{10 \text{ mL}}{0.5 \text{ mg}} = \dfrac{x}{0.25 \text{ mg}}$$

$$\dfrac{10 \times .25}{.5} = x$$

$$\dfrac{2.5}{.5} = x$$

$$5 \text{ mL} = x$$

---

**Learning Aid**

$0.25 \times 10 = 2.5$

$$0.5\,\overline{)2.5}\;\;^{5.}$$
$$\underline{25}$$

---

**9.** No equivalent necessary

*Formula Method*

$$\dfrac{\cancel{3}\text{ mg}}{\cancel{1}\text{ mg}} \times 5 \text{ mL} = 15 \text{ mL}$$

*Ratio Proportion Method*

$$\dfrac{5 \text{ mL}}{10 \text{ mg}} = \dfrac{x}{30 \text{ mg}}$$

$$\dfrac{150}{10} = x$$

$$15 \text{ mL} = x$$

---

**Learning Aid**

Alternate arithmetic

$30 \times 5 = 150$

$$10\,\overline{)150.}\;\;^{15.}$$
$$\underline{10}$$
$$50$$
$$\underline{50}$$

---

**10.** No equivalent necessary

*Formula Method*

$$\dfrac{\overset{10}{\cancel{12.5}}\text{ mg}}{\underset{1.25}{\cancel{6.25}}\text{ mg}} \times \overset{1}{\cancel{5}} \text{ mL} = 10 \text{ mL}$$

*Ratio Proportion Method*

$$\dfrac{5 \text{ mL}}{6.25 \text{ mg}} = \dfrac{x}{12.5}$$

$$\dfrac{62.5}{6.25} = x$$

$$10 \text{ mL} = x$$

---

**Learning Aid**

Alternate arithmetic

$12.5 \times 5 = 62.5$

$$6.25\,\overline{)62.50}\;\;^{10.}$$
$$\underline{625}$$
$$0$$

---

## Self-Test 3 Mental Drill Oral Solids

| | | | | |
|---|---|---|---|---|
| **1.** 2 tablets | **4.** 2 tablets | **7.** 1 tablet | **10.** 2 tablets | **13.** ½ tablet |
| **2.** ½ tablet | **5.** 2 tablets | **8.** 1 tablet | **11.** 2 tablets | **14.** 2 tablets |
| **3.** 2 tablets | **6.** ½ tablet | **9.** ½ tablet | **12.** 1 tablet | |

## Self-Test 4 Mental Drill Oral Liquids

| | | | | |
|---|---|---|---|---|
| **1.** 10 mL | **3.** 10 mL | **5.** 15 mL | **7.** 15 mL | **9.** 6 mL |
| **2.** 25 cc | **4.** 5 mL | **6.** 20 cc | **8.** 5 mL | **10.** 2.5 mL |

# Liquids for Injection

**CONTENT TO MASTER**

▶ The rule for solving injection-from-liquid problems is

$$\frac{\text{Desire}}{\text{Have}} \times \text{Stock} = \text{Amount}$$

▶ The marks on the syringe determine the accuracy of calculations:

   3 cc syringe—nearest tenth

   1 cc precision syringe—nearest hundredth

   insulin syringes— units

▶ Mixing two insulins requires special technique

▶ Liquids for injection may be labeled solutions of g or mg per mL

   as ratio

   as percent

Liquid drugs for injection are prepared by pharmaceutical companies as sterile solutions or suspensions. Sterile techniques are used to prepare and administer them. As with oral medications, the nurse may be required to calculate the correct dosage.

**RULE**  **CALCULATING LIQUID INJECTIONS**

**The rule used to solve liquid injection problems is the same as that for oral solids and liquids.** ■

$$\frac{\text{Desire}}{\text{Have}} \times \text{Stock} = \text{Amount} \qquad \frac{\text{Stock}}{\text{Have}} = \frac{\text{x}}{\text{Desire}}$$

**Example**  Order: Stelazine 1.5 mg IM q 6 h prn

Label:

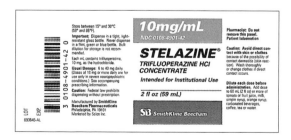

(Courtesy of GlaxoSmithKline.)

*Desire* is the order: 1.5 mg

*Have* is the strength of the drug supplied: 10 mg

*Stock* is the unit form of the drug: 1 mL

*Answer* is how much liquid to give by injection in mL

# ▶ Calculating Injection Problems

## *3-cc Syringe*

The degree of accuracy in calculating injection answers depends on the syringe used. Figure 7-1 shows a 3-cc (3-mL) syringe marked in milliliters to the nearest tenth and in minims to the nearest whole number. *To calculate milliliter answers for this 3-mL syringe, the arithmetic is carried out to the hundredth place and the answer is rounded off to the nearest tenth.*

1.25 mL becomes 1.3 mL

*To calculate minims on the 3-mL syringe, the arithmetic is carried out to the tenth place and the answer is rounded off to the nearest whole number.*

19.7 minims becomes 20 minims

## *1-cc Precision Syringe*

Figure 7-2 shows a 1-cc (1-mL) precision syringe marked in milliliters to the nearest hundredth and in minims to the nearest half-minim. *To calculate milliliters when the 1-mL syringe is used, the arithmetic is carried out to the thousandth place and the answer is rounded off to the nearest hundredth.*

0.978 mL becomes 0.98 mL

*To calculate minims for the 1-mL syringe, the arithmetic is carried out to the nearest hundredth and the answer is reported as the closest half minim.*

> **Learning Aid**
>
> Rules for round-off numbers can be reviewed in Chapter 1.

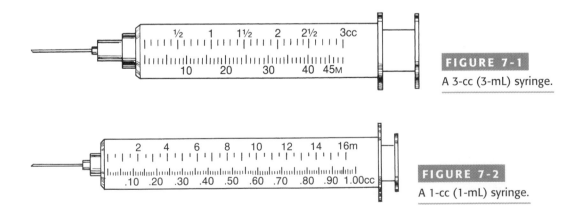

**FIGURE 7-1**

A 3-cc (3-mL) syringe.

**FIGURE 7-2**

A 1-cc (1-mL) syringe.

**Example**   14.28 minims becomes 14 minims. (The answer 14.28 rounds off to 14.3. Because 0.3 is less than 0.5, it is dropped.)

A syringe is provided for each of the examples that follow. Calculate milliliters to the degree of accuracy required by the syringe markings. **Calculation of minims is not provided because this is an apothecary measure. Draw a line on the syringe indicating the answer for milliliters only.**

**Example**   Order: Demerol HCl 75 mg IM q4h prn

Label:

**Learning Aid**

Calculate answers in milliliters (mL). Avoid minims, an apothecary measure.

⊐ 1 mL    NDC 0074-1179-31
                        LD-83
**10 Carpuject®**
sterile cartridge units
**with Luer Lock**   (C II

DETECTO-SEAL® PAK Tamper Detection Package
**Demerol®**
meperidine
hydrochloride
injection, USP
Warning: May be habit forming.
**50 mg/mL**

*Formula Method*

Rule: $\dfrac{D}{H} \times S = A$

$\dfrac{\overset{3}{\cancel{75\ mg}}}{\underset{2}{\cancel{50\ mg}}} \times 1\ mL = \dfrac{3}{2} = 1.5\ mL$

Give 1.5 mL IM.

*Ratio Proportion Method*

$\dfrac{1\ mL}{50\ mg} = \dfrac{x}{75\ mg}$

$\dfrac{75}{50} = x$

1.5 mL = x

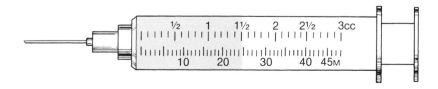

**Example**

Order: heparin sodium 1500 units SC bid

Label:

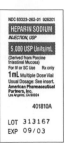

NDC 63323-262-01 926201
**HEPARIN SODIUM**
*INJECTION, USP*
**5,000 USP Units/mL**
(Derived from Porcine Intestinal Mucosa)
For IV or SC Use    Rx only
**1 mL** Multiple Dose Vial
Usual Dosage: See insert.
**American Pharmaceutical Partners, Inc.**
Los Angeles, CA 90024

401810A

LOT 313167
EXP 09/03

(Courtesy of American Pharmaceutical Partners, Inc.)

*Formula Method*

Rule: $\dfrac{D}{H} \times S = A$

$$\dfrac{\overset{3}{\cancel{1500 \text{ units}}}}{\underset{10}{\cancel{5000 \text{ units}}}} \times 1 \text{ mL} = \dfrac{3}{10} = 0.3 \text{ mL}$$

Give 0.3 mL.

*Ratio Proportion Method*

$$\dfrac{1 \text{ mL}}{5000 \text{ units}} = \dfrac{x}{1500 \text{ units}}$$

$$\dfrac{1500}{5000} = x$$

$$0.3 \text{ mL} = x$$

**Learning Aid**

$$\dfrac{3}{10 \overline{)3.0}} \quad \dfrac{.3}{}$$

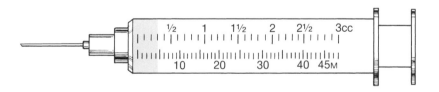

**Example**

Order: Lanoxin 120 mcg IM qd

Label:

**Learning Aid**

Since you are using a 1-mL precision syringe, you can draw the medication up to the nearest 100th.

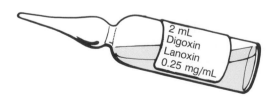

2 mL
Digoxin
Lanoxin
0.25 mg/mL

*Formula Method*

Rule: $\dfrac{D}{H} \times S = A$

Equivalent: 0.25 mg = 250 mcg

$\dfrac{\cancel{120\ mcg}}{\cancel{250\ mcg}} \times 1\ mL = \begin{array}{r} .48 \\ 25\overline{)12.00} \\ \underline{100} \\ 200 \\ \underline{200} \end{array}$

*Ratio Proportion Method*

$\dfrac{1\ mL}{250\ mcg} = \dfrac{x}{120\ mcg}$

$\dfrac{120}{250} = x$

0.48 mL = x

Give 0.48 mL IM.

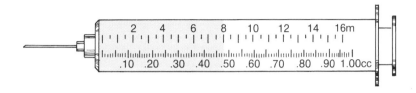

---

**Example**  Order: Gantrisin 400 mg IM q12h

Label: vial labeled 2 g/5 mL.

Logic: You have milligrams in the order and grams in the stock. Use an equivalent (2 g = 2000 mg).

*Formula Method*

Rule: $\dfrac{D}{H} \times S = A$

$\dfrac{\overset{1}{\cancel{400\ mg}}}{\underset{\underset{1}{5}}{\cancel{2000\ mg}}} \times 5\ mL = 1\ mL$

Give: 1 mL IM.

*Ratio Proportion Method*

$\dfrac{5\ mL}{2000\ mg} = \dfrac{x}{400\ mg}$

$\dfrac{2000}{2000} = x$

1 mL = x

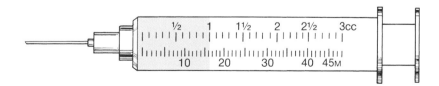

| SELF TEST 1 | Calculation of Liquids for Injections |
|---|---|

*Practice calculations of injections from a liquid. Report your answer in milliliters; mark the syringe in milliliters. Answers may be found at the end of the chapter.*

**1.** Order: Cleocin 0.3 Gm IM q6h
  Stock: liquid in a vial labeled 300 mg/2 mL

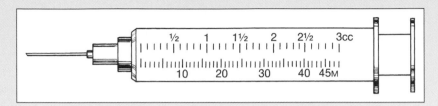

**2.** Order: morphine $SO_4$ 12 mg SC stat
  Stock: vial of liquid labeled 15 mg/mL

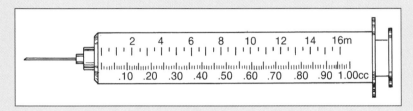

**3.** Order: vitamin $B_{12}$ 1 mg IM qd
  Stock: vial of liquid labeled 1000 $\mu$g/mL

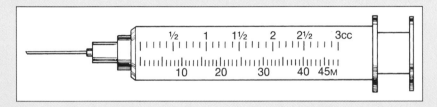

**4.** Order: gentamicin 9 mg IM q8h
  Stock: pediatric ampule labeled 20 mg/2 mL

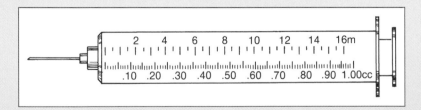

**5.** Order: digoxin 0.5 mg IM qd
  Stock: vial labeled 0.25 mg/mL

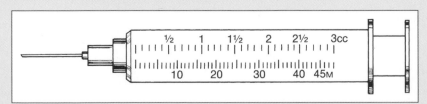

*(continued)*

**6.** Order:   gentamicin 50 mg IM q8h
   Stock:   vial labeled 40 mg/mL

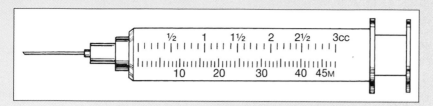

**7.** Order:   phenobarbital 100 mg IM stat
   Stock:   ampule labeled 130 mg/mL

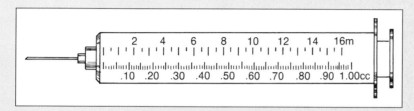

**8.** Order:   Lanoxin 0.25 mg IM stat
   Stock:   ampule labeled 0.5 mg/2 mL

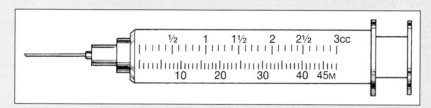

**9.** Order:   heparin 6000 units SC q4h
   Stock:   vial labeled 10,000 U/cc

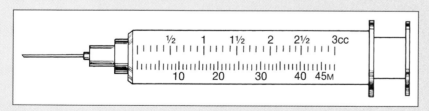

**10.** Order:   tobramycin 70 mg IM q8h
   Stock:   ampule labeled 80 mg/2 mL

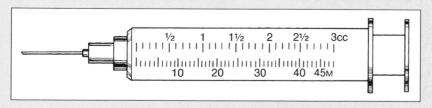

# ▶ Special Types of Problems in Injections From a Liquid

## When Stock Is a Ratio

Labels may state the strength of a drug as a ratio.

**Example**     Adrenalin 1:1000

*Ratios are always interpreted in the metric system as grams per milliliters.* In the example given, 1:1000 means 1 g in 1000 mL. Ratios may be stated in three ways:

1 g per 1000 mL

1 g = 1000 mL

1 g/1000 mL

**SELF TEST 2   Ratios**

*Write the following ratios in three ways. Answers may be found at the end of the chapter.*

**1.** 1:20 _____     _____     _____

**2.** 2:15 _____     _____     _____

**3.** 1:500 _____     _____     _____

Some nurses have difficulty understanding the meaning of ratio in relation to drugs. A deductive line of reasoning may help to make this clear.

Figure 7-3 shows an ampule of epinephrine that is labeled 2 mL and is a 1:1000 solution. You know that 1:1000 means 1 g in 1000 mL. You also know that 1 g is equivalent to 1000 mg. Therefore, the solution can be interpreted as 1000 mg = 1000 mL. Logic tells you that if there are 1000 mg in 1000 mL, then there is 1 mg in 1 mL.

$$\frac{\cancel{1000} \text{ mg}}{\cancel{1000} \text{ mL}} = \frac{1 \text{ mg}}{1 \text{ mL}}$$

Because the ampule contains 2 mL, the ampule contains 2 mg of the drug. Be careful reading and writing milligram (mg) and milliliter (mL). Milligram is the solid measure; milliliter is the liquid measure.

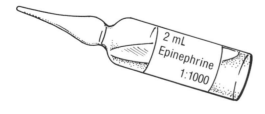

**FIGURE 7-3**
A 2-mL ampule of epinephrine 1:1000.

**Example**

*EXAMPLE 1:*

Order: epinephrine 1 mg SC stat

Label: ampule labeled 1:1000

Equivalent: 1:1000 means
    1 g in 1000 mL
    1 g = 1000 mg, therefore
    stock is 1000 mg = 1000 mL

| **Formula Method** | ***Ratio Proportion Method*** |
|---|---|
| Rule: $\dfrac{D}{H} \times S = A$ | $\dfrac{1000 \text{ mL}}{1000 \text{ mg}} = \dfrac{x}{1 \text{ mg}}$ |
| $\dfrac{1 \text{ mg}}{1000 \text{ mg}} \times \dfrac{1}{1000} \text{ mL} = 1 \text{ mL}$ | $\dfrac{1000}{1000} = x$ |
| Give: 1 mL SC. | $1 \text{ mL} = x$ |

*EXAMPLE 2:*

Order: isoproterenol HCl 0.2 mg IM stat

Label: ampule labeled 1:5000

Equivalents: 1:5000 means
    1 g in 5000 mL
    1 g = 1000 mg

Therefore, the solution is 1000 mg/5000 mL.

| **Formula Method** | ***Ratio Proportion Method*** |
|---|---|
| Rule: $\dfrac{D}{H} \times S = A$ | $\dfrac{5000 \text{ mL}}{1000 \text{ mg}} = \dfrac{x}{.2 \text{ mg}}$ |
| $\dfrac{0.2 \text{ mg}}{1000 \text{ mg}} \times \dfrac{5}{5000} \text{ mL} = \dfrac{5 \times 0.2}{1.0} \text{ mL}$ | $\dfrac{1000}{1000} = x$ |
| Give: 1 mL IM. | $1 \text{ mL} = x$ |

**SELF TEST 3** | **Using Ratios with Liquids for Injection**

*Solve these problems involving ratios. Answers may be found at the end of the chapter.*

1. Order: neostigmine 0.5 mg SC
   Stock: ampule labeled 1:2000

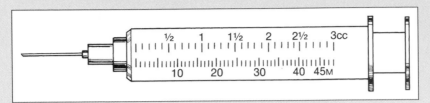

2. Order: Isuprel 1 mg: add to IV
   Stock: vial labeled 1:5000
   A 10-mL syringe is available.

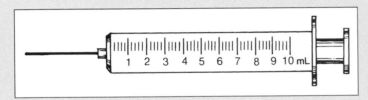

3. Order: neostigmine methylsulfate 0.75 mg SC
   Stock: ampule labeled 1:1000

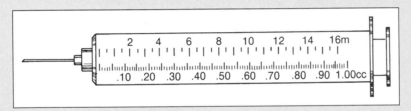

4. Order: ponthaline 50 mg IM
   Stock: ampule labeled 1:20

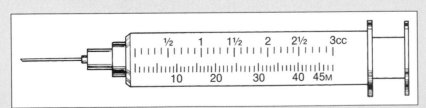

5. Order: neostigmine methylsulfate 1.5 mg IM tid
   Stock: 1:2000

## When Stock Is a Percent

Labels may state the strength of a drug as a percent. Percent means parts per hundred. *Percentages are always interpreted in the metric system as grams per 100 mL.*

**Example**    Lidocaine 2% (2 g in 100 mL)

Percents may be stated in three ways:

2 g per 100 mL

2 g = 100 mL

2 g/100 mL

---

### SELF TEST 4  Percentages

*Write the following percentages in three ways. Answers may be found at the end of the chapter.*

**1.** 0.9% _____    _____    _____

**2.** 10% _____    _____    _____

**3.** 0.45% _____    _____    _____

---

Percent problems can be solved by applying the meaning of ratio.

**Example**    *EXAMPLE 1:*

Order: lidocaine 30 mg for injection before suturing wound

Stock: ampule labeled 2%

Equivalents: 2% means

   2 g in 100 mL
   1 g = 1000 mg
   2 g = 2000 mg

Stock is 2000 mg in 100 mL.

| *Formula Method* | *Ratio Proportion Method* |
|---|---|
| Rule: $\dfrac{D}{H}$ S = A | $\dfrac{100 \text{ mL}}{2000 \text{ mg}} = \dfrac{x}{30 \text{ mg}}$ |

$$\frac{30 \text{ mg}}{2000 \text{ mg}} \times \frac{1}{100 \text{ mL}} = \frac{3}{2} \quad \frac{1.5}{2\overline{)3.0}} \qquad \frac{3000}{2000} = x$$

Prepare 1.5 mL for physician.    1.5 mL = x

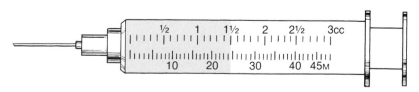

*EXAMPLE 2:*

Order: calcium gluconate 1 g; add to IV stat

Stock: vial of liquid labeled 10%

Equivalents: 10% means 10 g in 100 mL

| *Formula Method* | *Ratio Proportion Method* |
|---|---|
| Rule: $\dfrac{D}{H} \times S = A$ | $\dfrac{100 \text{ mL}}{10 \text{ g}} = \dfrac{x}{1 \text{ g}}$ |
| $\dfrac{1 \cancel{g}}{\underset{1}{\cancel{10 g}}} \times \underset{10}{\cancel{100}} \text{ mL} = 10 \text{ mL}$ | $\dfrac{100}{10} = x$ |
| | $10 \text{ mL} = x$ |

Add: 10 mL to IV. (Amount is correct. The route is IV, not IM.)

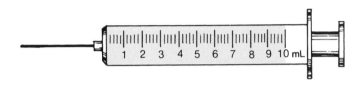

---

**SELF TEST 5** | **Using Percentages with Liquids for Injection**

*Solve these problems involving percentages. Answers may be found at the end of the chapter. Answeres in milliliters (mL).*

**1.** Order:   epinephrine 5 mg SC stat
   Stock:   ampule labeled 1%

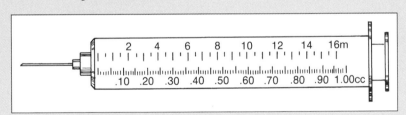

**2.** Order:   Mesterin 2.5 mg IM
   Stock:   ampule labeled 0.5%

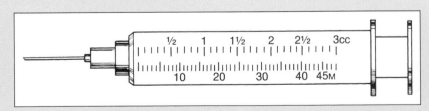

*(continued)*

**3.** Order: phenylephrine HCl 3 mg SC stat
Stock: ampule labeled 1%

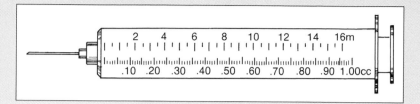

**4.** Order: Prepare for IV use calcium gluconate 0.3 g
Stock: ampule labeled 10%

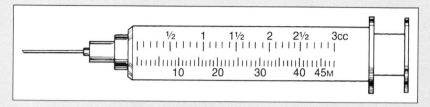

**5.** Order: Prepare for IV use sodium tetradecyl sulfate 0.015 g
Stock: ampule labeled 3%

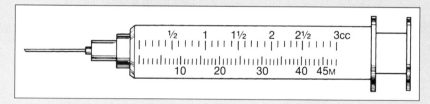

# ❱ Insulin Injections

## *Types of Insulin*

Insulin is a hormone that regulates glucose metabolism. It is measured in units and is administered by injection. Insulin is supplied in 10-mL vials containing 100 units per milliliter. There are many types of insulin currently available. Insulins may be prepared from animal tissue or semisynthetically from human recombinant DNA. Insulins are classified as rapid, intermediate, or long acting. Because onset of action, time of peak activity, and duration of action vary, *nurses must be careful to choose the correct insulin.* Table 7-1 summarizes the onset, peak, and duration of various insulins.

| TABLE 7-1 | Onset, Peak, and Duration of Different Types of Insulin | | |
|---|---|---|---|
| **Type** | **Onset** | **Peak** | **Duration** |
| Regular | 1 hour | 2–4 hours | 5–7 hours |
| Humalog | 5 minutes | 1 hour | 2–4 hours |
| NPH or Lente | 1–2.5 hours | 6–12 hours | 18–24 hours |
| Ultralente | 4–8 hours | 12–20 hours | 24–48 hours |
| Mixed insulins | 30–60 minutes then 1–2 hours | 2–4 hours then 6–12 hours | 6–8 hours then 18–24 hours |

*RAPID-ACTING INSULINS.* These begin acting within 1 hour and peak in 2 to 4 hours; actions may last 5 to 7 hours. Insulins are administered subcutaneously except for regular insulin, which can be given IV.

Note the large "R" on the label for quick identification as regular insulin. Most insulin used clinically is human insulin, "Humulin", which is synthesized in the laboratory using recombinant DNA technology. Pork insulin, made from the porcine pancreas, is occasionally used for patients.

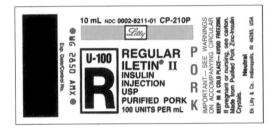
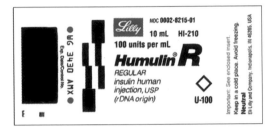

*HUMALOG—A UNIQUE, RAPID-ACTING INSULIN.* Humalog (lispro) is the newest human insulin product made by recombinant DNA technology. Like regular insulin it lowers blood sugar but much more rapidly. Humalog starts acting 5 minutes after injection, peaks in 1 hour, and lasts 2 to 4 hours.

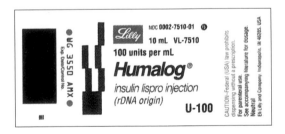

*INTERMEDIATE-ACTING INSULINS.* These begin action in 1 to 3 hours, peak around 6 to 12 hours, and may last 24 hours. The letters "N" or "L" or the term "isophane" indicate that regular insulin has been modified with the addition of zinc and protamine to delay absorption and prolong the time of action. These intermediate insulins can be prepared from pork or Humulin R. The letters NPH also are used to denote an intermediate action. These letters mean the following: N = the solution is neutral pH; P = the protamine content; H = Hagedorn, the laboratory which first prepared this type of insulin.

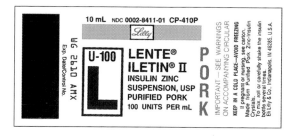

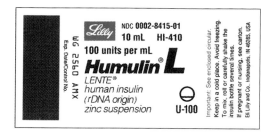

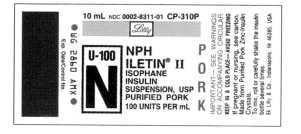

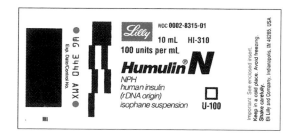

*LONG-ACTING INSULINS.* These have also been modified with the addition of zinc and protamine, a basic protein. These insulins take 4 to 8 hours to act, peak in 12 to 20 hours; duration of action can last as long as 36 hours.

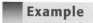
**Example**

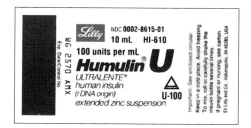

*MIXED INSULINS.* An order may require that two insulins be mixed in one syringe and administered together. Mixed insulins combine rapid and intermediate insulin. They save nursing time in preparation and are more convenient for the patient, who must learn to draw up and self-administer an injection.

**Example**

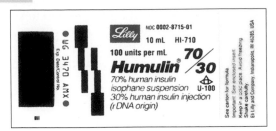 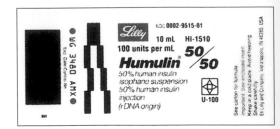

*HIGH-POTENCY INSULINS.* These are manufactured for some patients who require large doses and for emergency situations. To protect against error these insulins should be carefully stored away from the usual Units-100/mL insulins.

**Example**

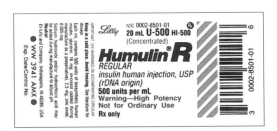

Regular insulin should appear clear and colorless; it is the only insulin that may be given IV. Other insulins appear cloudy. Insulin vials should be gently rotated between the hands to resuspend the particles. *Never shake insulin vials.* This may result in the formation of bubbles or froth and interfere with accurate measurement of the dose ordered.

### Types of Insulin Syringes

Insulin doses are administered subcutaneously with an insulin syringe. Two standard syringes are available to measure U 100 insulin. The first measures doses up to 100 units (Fig. 7-4). The second, called a low-dose insulin syringe, can be used when the dose is 50 units or less (Fig. 7-5).

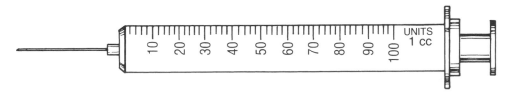

**FIGURE 7-4**

1-cc insulin syringe marked in units. Each line equals 2 units.

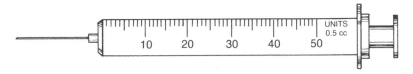

**FIGURE 7-5**

½ cc low-dose insulin syringe. Each line equals 1 unit.

## Preparing an Injection Using an Insulin Syringe

No calculation is required to prepare an insulin dose. The physician's order is in units; the stock comes in 100 units/mL. Both syringes are calibrated (lined) for 100 units/mL.

**Example**

*EXAMPLE 1:*

Order: Units 60 NPH SC qd

Label:

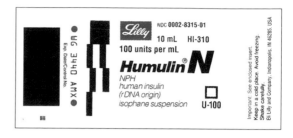

Ask yourself three questions:

1. What is the order? NPH Units 60

2. What is the stock? NPH U 100/mL

3. Is a U 100 insulin syringe available? Yes.

Using sterile technique, draw up the amount required into the syringe.

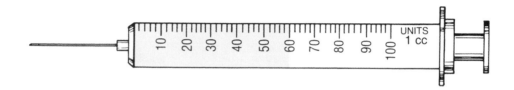

*EXAMPLE 2:*

Order: U 35 Regular Insulin SC stat

Label:

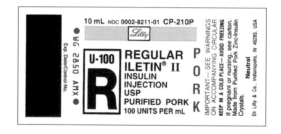

Ask yourself three questions:

1. What is the order? Regular Insulin U 35

2. What is the stock? U 100/mL Regular Insulin

3. What syringe should be used? Low-dose insulin syringe

Using sterile technique, draw up the amount required into the syringe.

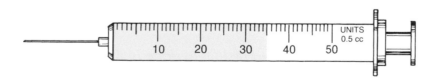

## Mixing Two Insulins in One Syringe

Sometimes the physician will order regular insulin to be mixed with another insulin and injected together at the same site. The method of preparing two medications in one syringe is handled later in this book. For now, remember two facts:

1. The regular insulin is always drawn up first into the syringe.

2. The total number of units in the syringe will be the addition of the two insulin orders.

Regular insulin is often ordered with NPH insulin. Regular insulin is clear and NPH insulin is cloudy. The mnemonic "clear to cloudy" may be helpful to remember which insulin is drawn up first. (note: when drawing up medication, air is injected into the vial equal to the amount of medication to be drawn up. When using this method with regular and NPH insulin, air is injected first into the NPH vial equal to the amount of medication; then air is injected into the regular insulin vial equal to the amount of medication; the regular insulin is withdrawn, then the NPH insulin is withdrawn.)

**Example**    Order: Regular Humulin Insulin Units 15⎫
               NPH Humulin Insulin Units 10⎬ qd SC

Label: Regular Humulin Insulin U 100/mL
NPH Humulin insulin U 100/mL

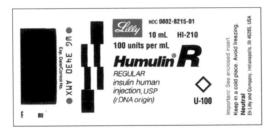   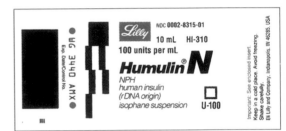

1. What are the orders? Regular (Humulin) Insulin Units 15; NPH Insulin Units 10 (Humulin)

2. What is the stock? Regular (Humulin) Insulin Units 100/mL. NPH (Humulini) Insulin Units 100/mL

3. Is there an insulin syringe? Yes.

4. What will be the total units in the syringe? 25 units

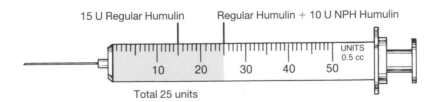

## Preparing an Insulin Injection When No Insulin Syringe is Available

When an insulin syringe is not available, it is possible to calculate and administer an insulin dose. Handle the order as an injection from a liquid and use a 1-mL precision syringe.

**Example**  Order: Lente Insulin Units 40 SC qd

Label: Lente Insulin U 100/mL

No insulin syringe is available.

*Formula Method*

Rule: $\dfrac{D}{H} \times S = A$

$\dfrac{\overset{2}{\cancel{40 \text{ Units}}}}{\underset{5}{\cancel{100 \text{ Units}}}} \times 1 \text{ mL} \quad 5\overline{\smash{)}\,2.0}\ \ \dfrac{2}{}\ 0.4$

Give: 0.4 mL SC

*Ratio Proportion Method*

$\dfrac{1 \text{ mL}}{100 \text{ units}} = \dfrac{x}{40}$

$\dfrac{40}{100} = x$

$0.4 \text{ mL} = x$

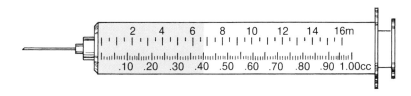

**Example**  Order: Regular Insulin Units 25 SC if Blood Glucose >250

Label: Regular Insulin U 100/mL

No insulin syringe available

*Formula Method*

$\dfrac{\overset{1}{\cancel{25 \text{ Units}}}}{\underset{4}{\cancel{100 \text{ Units}}}} \times 1 \text{ mL} \quad 4\overline{\smash{)}\,1.00}\ \ \dfrac{1}{}\ 0.25$

Give 0.25 mL SC.

*Ratio Proportion Method*

$\dfrac{1 \text{ mL}}{100 \text{ units}} = \dfrac{x}{25}$

$\dfrac{25}{100} = x$

$0.25 \text{ mL} = x$

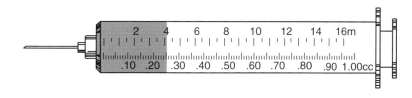

**SELF TEST 6** | **Insulin Calculations**

*Solve these insulin problems. Draw a line on the syringe to indicate the dose you would prepare. Answers may be found at the end of the chapter.*

1. Order: NPH Insulin 56 Units SC qd
   Stock: vial of NPH Iletin Isophane Insulin Suspension U 100/mL

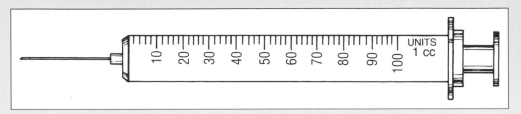

2. Order: 7 Units Regular Insulin U 100 and 20 Units NPH Insulin
   U 100 SC qd 7 AM
   Stock: vial of Regular Insulin U 100/mL (pork) and NPH Iletin I
   Isophane Insulin Suspension U 100/mL

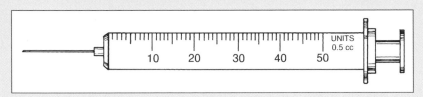

3. Order: Regular Humulin Insulin 4 Units SC stat
   Stock: vial of Novolin R Regular Insulin U 100/mL

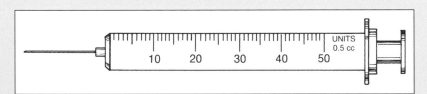

4. Order: Semilente Insulin Units 28 SC
   Stock: Semilente Insulin Prompt Insulin Zinc Suspension U 100/mL

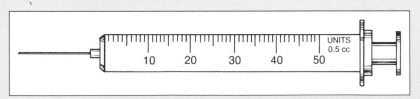

*(continued)*

**5.** Order: 20 Units of NPH 100 SC qd
  Stock: vial of NPH Iletin I Isophane Insulin Suspension U 100/mL

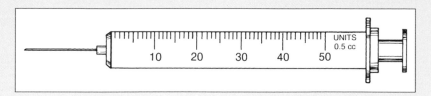

**6.** Order: Regular Insulin 16 Units with NPH Insulin Units 64 SC qd
  Stock: vial of Regular Insulin U 100/mL and vial of NPH Iletin I Isophane Insulin Suspension U 100/mL

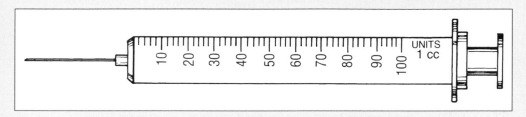

**7.** Order: Regular Insulin 3 Units SC stat
  Stock: vial of Regular Insulin U 100/mL

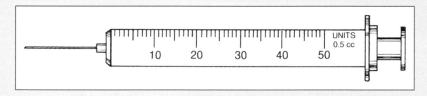

**8.** Order: Semilente Insulin Units 30 SC qd
  Stock: vial of Semilente Insulin Prompt Insulin Zinc Suspension U 100/mL

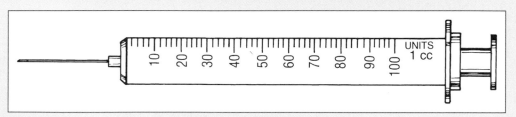

*(continued)*

**SELF TEST 6** | **Insulin Calculations (Continued)**

9. Order: Regular Insulin 10 Units with NPH Insulin 40 Units SC qd

   Stock: vial of Regular Insulin U 100/mL vial of NPH Iletin I Isophane Insulin Suspension U 100/mL

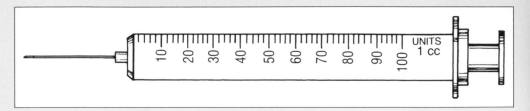

10. Order: Regular Humulin Insulin 13 Units SC stat

    Stock: vial of Novolin R Regular Insulin U 100/mL

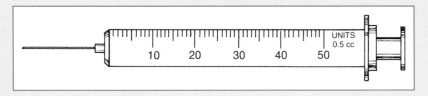

## TEST YOUR CLINICAL SAVVY

You are a nursing student about to graduate from one of the most prestigious nursing schools in Ame On your last day of clinical, you are to give insulin to the last patient in your nursing school career. Unfortunately, the hospital has run out of insulin syringes. This chapter discusses how to prepare an i injection when no insulin syringe is available (pg. 144). Ideally a 1-cc syringe is used, but the hospita also run out of these. Your instructor is going to check your insulin before you administer it.

A. Could you use a 3-mL syringe to draw up insulin? If so, how is this done and what would be the precautions?

B. Could a 5-mL syringe be used to draw up insulin?

C. What would be the danger in using either of these syringes?

D. What amount of insulin would be safe to draw up in either a 3-mL or 5-mL syringe (or neither)?

E. Even if a 1-mL syringe were available, what would be the precautions in using a non-insulin syring

**PROFICIENCY TEST 1** | **Calculations of Liquid Injections (Test 1)**

Name: _____

*Solve these injection problems. Draw a line on the syringe indicating the amount you would prepare in milliliters (mL). Aim for 100% accuracy! Answers will be found on page 338.*

**1.** Order:  sodium amytal 0.1 Gm IM at 7 AM
    Stock:  ampule of liquid labeled 200 mg/3 mL

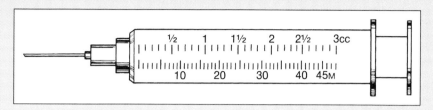

**2.** Order:  morphine sulfate 5 mg SC stat
    Stock:  vial of liquid labeled 15 mg/mL

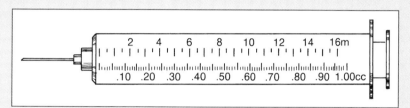

**3.** Order:  Benadryl 25 mg IM q4h prn
    Stock:  ampule of liquid labeled 50 mg (2-cc size)

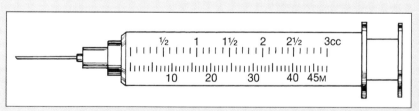

**4.** Order:  NPH Insulin 15 units and Humulin Insulin 5 units SC qd 7 AM
    Stock:  vials of NPH Insulin U 100 and Humulin Insulin U 100

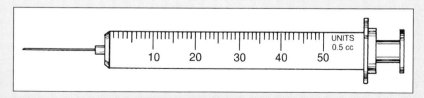

**5.** Order:  add 20 mEq potassium chloride to IV stat
    Stock:  vial of liquid labeled 40 mEq (3 g) per 20 mL

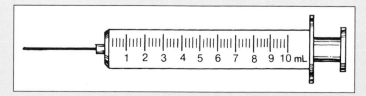

*(continued)*

**6.** Order: scopolamine 0.6 mg SC stat
Stock: vial labeled 0.4 mg/mL

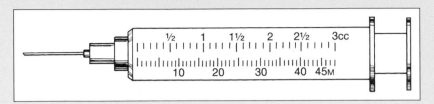

**7.** Order: atropine sulfate 0.8 mg IM at 7 AM
Stock: vial labeled 0.4 mg/mL

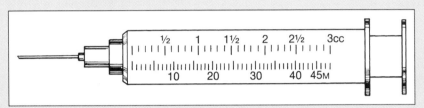

**8.** Order: add 0.5 Gm dextrose 25% to IV stat
Stock: vial of liquid labeled Infant 25% Dextrose Injection 250 mg/mL

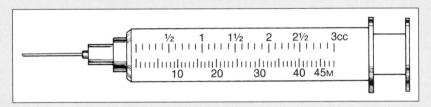

**9.** Order: ascorbic acid 200 mg IM bid
Stock: ampule labeled 500 mg/2 mL

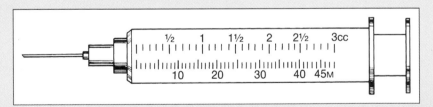

**10.** Order: epinephrine 7.5 mg SC stat
Stock: ampule labeled 1:100

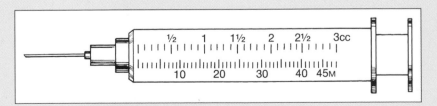

**PROFICIENCY TEST 2** | Calculations of Liquid Injections (Test 2)

*Name:* _____

*Solve these problems for injections from a liquid. Draw a line on the syringe indicating the amount you would prepare in milliliters (mL). Aim for 100% accuracy! Answers will be found on page 341.*

**1.** Order:  morphine sulfate 10 mg SC stat
    Stock:  vial labeled 15 mg/mL

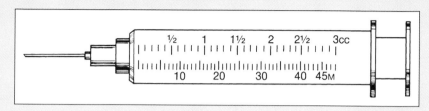

**2.** Order:  Demerol 25 mg IM stat
    Stock:  vial of liquid labeled 100 mg in 1 mL

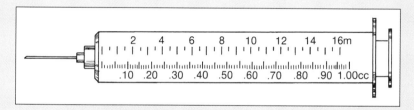

**3.** Order:  phenobarbital 0.1 g IM q6h
    Stock:  ampule of liquid labeled 200 mg/3 mL

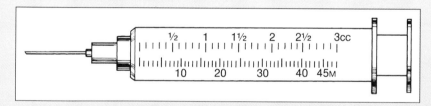

**4.** Order:  vitamin B$_{12}$ 1000 $\mu$g IM qd
    Stock:  vial labeled 5000 $\mu$g/mL

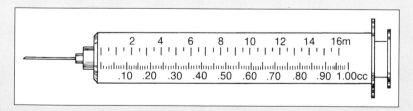

**5.** Order:  prepare 25 mg lidocaine for physician to use
    Stock:  vial of liquid labeled 1%

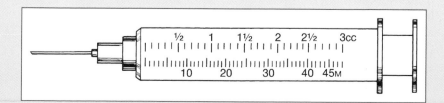

*(continued)*

6. Order:   scopolamine 0.5 mg SC stat
   Stock:   vial labeled 0.4 mg/mL

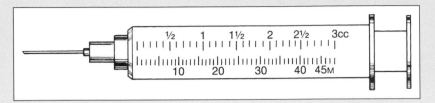

7. Order:   NPH Insulin 10 units and Humulin Insulin 3 units SC qd 7 AM
   Stock:   vials of NPH Insulin U 100 and Humulin Insulin U 100

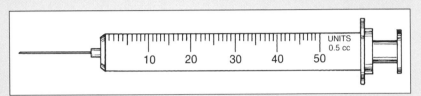

8. Order:   add sodium bicarbonate 1.2 mEq to IV stat
   Stock:   vial labeled Infant 4.2% Sodium Bicarbonate 5 mEq (0.5 mEq/mL)

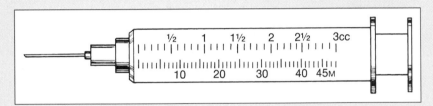

9. Order:   dromostanolone proprionate 75 mg IM tiw
   Stock:   vial labeled 50 mg/mL

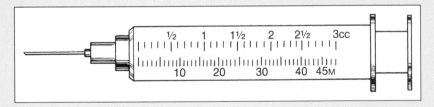

10. Order:   adrenalin 500 μg SC stat
    Stock:   ampule of liquid labeled 1:1000

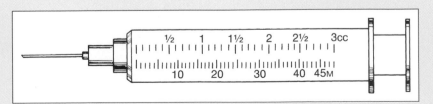

**PROFICIENCY TEST 3** | Calculations of Liquid Injections (Test 3)

*Name:* _____

*Aim for 90% or better on this test. There are 20 questions, each worth 5 points. If you have any difficulty, reread and study Chapter 7, which explains this information. Assume you have only a 3-cc syringe. Answers will be found on page 345.*

1. Order:   Lanoxin 0.25 mg IM qd
   Stock:   ampule labeled 0.5 mg/2 mL

2. Order:   diphenhydramine hydrochloride 40 mg IM stat
   Stock:   ampule labeled 50 mg (2-cc size)

3. Order:   morphine sulfate 8 mg SC q4h prn
   Stock:   vial labeled 15 mg/mL

4. Order:   Demerol Hydrochloride 25 mg IM q4h prn
   Stock:   vial labeled 100 mg/mL

5. Order:   ascorbic acid 200 mg IM qd
   Stock:   ampule labeled 500 mg/2 mL

6. Order:   vitamin $B_{12}$ 1500 $\mu$g qd IM
   Stock:   vial labeled 5000 $\mu$g/mL

7. Order:   atropine sulfate 0.6 mg SC at 7:30 AM
   Stock:   vial labeled 0.4 mg/mL

8. Order:   Sodium Amytal 0.1 gm IM stat
   Stock:   ampule 200 mg/3 mL

9. Order:   hydromorphone HCl 1.5 mg IM q4h prn
   Stock:   vial labeled 2 mg/mL

10. Order:   penicillin G procaine 600,000 units IM q12h
    Stock:   vial labeled 500,000 USP units/mL

11. Order:   add nitroglycerin 200 $\mu$g to IV stat
    Stock:   vial labeled 0.8 mg/mL

12. Order:   neostigmine methylsulfate 500 mcg SC
    Stock:   ampule labeled 1:4000

13. Order:   levorphanol tartrate 3 mg SC
    Stock:   vial labeled 2 mg/mL

14. Order:   epinephrine 0.4 mg SC stat
    Stock:   ampule labeled 1:1000 (2-mL size)

15. Order:   magnesium sulfate 500 mg IM
    Stock:   ampule labeled 50% (2-mL size)

16. Order:   oxymorphone HCl 0.75 mg SC
    Stock:   vial labeled 1.5 mg/mL

*(continued)*

**PROFICIENCY TEST 3** | Calculations of Liquid Injections (Test 3) (Continued)

17. Order:  add lidocaine 100 mg to IV stat
    Stock:  ampule labeled 20%

18. Order:  Lanoxin 0.125 mg IM 10 AM
    Stock:  ampule labeled 0.25 mg/2 mL

19. Order:  nalbuphine HCl 12 mg IM
    Stock:  vial 10 mg/mL

20. Order:  add 10 mEq KCl to IV
    Stock:  vial 40 mEq/20 mL

## PROFICIENCY TEST 4  Mental Drill in Liquids for Injection Problems

Name: _____

As you develop proficiency in solving problems, you will be able to calculate many answers without written work. This drill combines your knowledge of equivalents and dosages. Solve these problems mentally and write only the amount to give. Keep the rule in mind as you solve each problem. Answers will be found on page 348.

| Order | Stock | Give |
|---|---|---|
| **1.** 0.5 g IM | 250 mg/mL | _____ |
| **2.** 10 mEq IV | 40 mEq/20 mL | _____ |
| **3.** 0.5 mg IM | 0.25 mg/mL | _____ |
| **4.** 100 mg IM | 0.2 Gm per 2 mL | _____ |
| **5.** 50 mg IM | 100 mg = 1 mL | _____ |
| **6.** 0.25 mg IM | 0.5 mg per 2 mL | _____ |
| **7.** 0.3 mg SC | 0.4 mg/mL | _____ |
| **8.** 1 mg SC | 1:1000 solution | _____ |
| **9.** 1 g IV | 5% solution | _____ |
| **10.** 0.1 g IM | 200 mg/5 mL | _____ |
| **11.** 400,000 units IM | 500,000 U/mL | _____ |
| **12.** 0.5 mg IM | 0.5 mg per 2 mL | _____ |
| **13.** 1 g IV | 50% solution | _____ |
| **14.** 75 mg IM | 100 mg per 2 mL | _____ |
| **15.** 15 mg IM | 1:100 solution | _____ |
| **16.** 35 mg IM | 100 mg/mL | _____ |
| **17.** 0.6 mg SC | 0.4 mg per mL | _____ |
| **18.** 0.15 g IM | 0.2 g/2 mL | _____ |

# Answers

### Self Test 1 Calculation of Liquids for Injection

**1.** Equivalent 0.3 Gm = 300 mg

*Formula Method*

$$\frac{\overset{1}{\cancel{300\ mg}}}{\underset{1}{\cancel{300\ mg}}} \times 2\ mL = 2\ mL$$

Give 2 mL IM.

*Ratio Proportion Method*

$$\frac{2\ mL}{300\ mg} = \frac{x}{300\ mg}$$

$$\frac{600}{300} = x$$

$$2\ mL = x$$

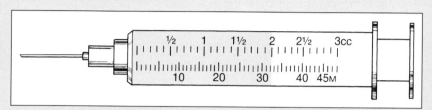

*Formula Method*

**2.** $\dfrac{\overset{4}{\cancel{12\ mg}}}{\underset{5}{\cancel{15\ mg}}} \times 1\ mL = \dfrac{4}{5} \overset{.8}{\overline{)4.0}}$

Give 0.8 mL SC.

*Ratio Proportion Method*

$$\frac{1\ mL}{15\ mg} = \frac{x}{12\ mg}$$

$$\frac{12}{15} = x$$

$$0.8\ mL = x$$

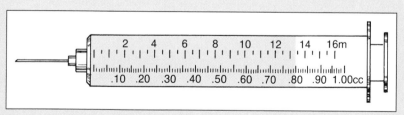

**3.** Equivalent 1 mg = 1000 $\mu$g

*Formula Method*

$$\frac{\overset{1}{\cancel{1000\ \mu g}}}{\underset{1}{\cancel{1000\ \mu g}}} \times 1\ mL = 1\ mL$$

Give 1 mL IM.

*Ratio Proportion Method*

$$\frac{1\ mL}{1000\ mcg} = \frac{x}{1000\ mcg}$$

$$\frac{1000}{1000} = x$$

$$1\ mL = x$$

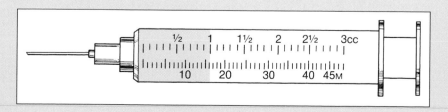

*Formula Method*

**4.** $\dfrac{9\ \text{mg}}{20\ \text{mg}} \times 2\ \text{mL} = \dfrac{18}{20} \overset{.9}{)\overline{18.0}}$
$\phantom{\dfrac{9\ \text{mg}}{20\ \text{mg}} \times 2\ \text{mL} = \dfrac{18}{20}}\underline{18.0}$

Give 0.9 mL IM. You are using a 1-mL precision syringe.

*Ratio Proportion Method*

$\dfrac{2\ \text{mL}}{20\ \text{mg}} = \dfrac{x}{9\ \text{mg}}$

$\dfrac{18}{20} = x$

0.9 mL = x

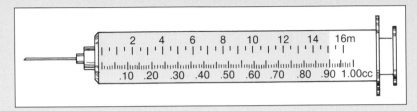

*Formula Method*

**5.** $\dfrac{\overset{2}{\cancel{0.50}}\ \text{mg}}{\underset{1}{\cancel{0.25}}\ \text{mg}} \times 1\ \text{mL} = 2\ \text{mL}$

Give 2 mL IM.

*Ratio Proportion Method*

$\dfrac{1\ \text{mL}}{0.25\ \text{mg}} = \dfrac{x}{0.5\ \text{mg}}$

$\dfrac{0.5}{0.25} = x$

2 mL = x

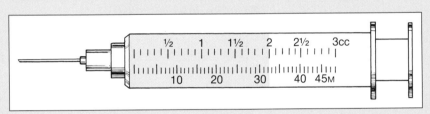

*Formula Method*

**6.** $\dfrac{50\ \text{mg}}{40\ \text{mg}} \times 1\ \text{mL} = \dfrac{5}{4} \overset{1.25}{)\overline{5.00}}$
$\phantom{xxxxxxxxxxxxxxxxx}\underline{4}$
$\phantom{xxxxxxxxxxxxxxxxxx}1\ 0$
$\phantom{xxxxxxxxxxxxxxxxxxx}\underline{8}$
$\phantom{xxxxxxxxxxxxxxxxxxx}20$
$\phantom{xxxxxxxxxxxxxxxxxxx}\underline{20}$

Give 1.3 mL IM.

*Ratio Proportion Method*

$\dfrac{1\ \text{mL}}{40\ \text{mg}} = \dfrac{x}{50\ \text{mg}}$

$\dfrac{50}{40} = x$

1.25 mL = x

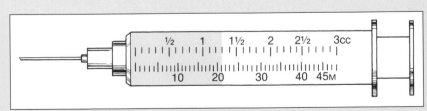

*Formula Method*

7. $\dfrac{100 \text{ mg}}{130 \text{ mg}} \times 1 \text{ mL} = \dfrac{10}{13}$

$$13\overline{)10.000} \quad .769$$
$$\phantom{13)}\underline{9\,1}$$
$$\phantom{13)1}9\,0$$
$$\phantom{13)1}\underline{7\,8}$$
$$\phantom{13)1}1\,20$$
$$\phantom{13)1}\underline{1\,17}$$
$$\phantom{13)1}\phantom{1}3$$

*Ratio Proportion Method*

$$\dfrac{1 \text{ mL}}{130 \text{ mg}} = \dfrac{x}{100 \text{ mg}}$$

$$\dfrac{100}{130} = x$$

$.769$ or $.77$ mL $= x$

Give 0.77 mL IM. You are using a 1-mL precision syringe, hence, milliliters to the nearest hundredth.

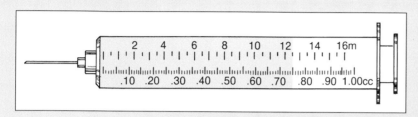

*Formula Method*

8. $\dfrac{\overset{1}{\cancel{0.25}} \text{ mg}}{\underset{2}{\cancel{0.50}} \text{ mg}} \times \overset{1}{\cancel{2}} \text{ mL} = 1 \text{ mL}$

$\phantom{8.}\dfrac{\phantom{0}}{1}$

Give 1 mL IM.

*Ratio Proportion Method*

$$\dfrac{2 \text{ mL}}{0.5 \text{ mg}} = \dfrac{x}{0.25 \text{ mg}}$$

$$\dfrac{0.5}{0.5} = x$$

$1$ mL $= x$

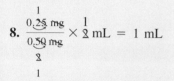

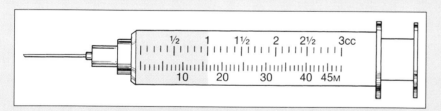

*Formula Method*

9. $\dfrac{6000 \text{ units}}{10000 \text{ units}} \times 1 \text{ cc} = \dfrac{6}{10} = 0.6$

Give 0.6 mL SC.

*Ratio Proportion Method*

$$\dfrac{1 \text{ cc}}{10,000 \text{ u}} = \dfrac{x}{6000 \text{ u}}$$

$$\dfrac{6000}{10000} = x$$

$0.6$ mL $= x$

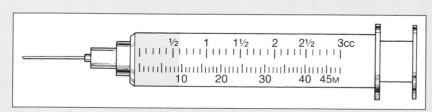

*Formula Method*

**10.** $\dfrac{\cancel{70} \text{ mg}}{\cancel{80} \text{ mg}} \times \dfrac{1}{\cancel{2}} \text{ mL} = \dfrac{7}{4}$

$$
\begin{array}{r}
1.75 \\
4\overline{)7.00} \\
\underline{4\phantom{.00}} \\
3\;0\phantom{0} \\
\underline{2\;8}\phantom{0} \\
20 \\
\underline{20}
\end{array}
$$

40

Give 1.8 mL IM.

*Ratio Proportion Method*

$$\frac{2 \text{ mL}}{80 \text{ mg}} = \frac{\text{x}}{70 \text{ mg}}$$

$$\frac{140}{80} = \text{x}$$

1.75 or 1.8 mL = x

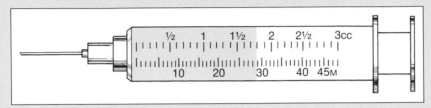

## Self Test 2 Ratios

1. 1 g per 20 mL; 1 g = 20 mL; 1 g/20 mL
2. 2 g per 15 mL; 2 g = 15 mL; 2 g/15 mL
3. 1 g per 500 mL; 1 g = 500 mL; 1 g/500 mL

## Self Test 3 Using Ratios with Liquids for Injection

1. Equivalent 1:2000 means
   1 g in 2000 mL
   1 g = 1000 mg

Hence, the solution is 1000 mg/2000 mL.

*Formula Method*

$$\frac{\text{D}}{\text{H}} \times \text{S} = \text{A}$$

$$\frac{0.5 \text{ mg}}{\cancel{1000} \text{ mg}} \times \overset{2}{\cancel{2000}} \text{ mL} = \begin{array}{r} 0.5 \\ \underline{\times\;2} \\ 1.0 \end{array}$$

Give 1 mL SC.

*Ratio Proportion Method*

$$\frac{2000 \text{ mL}}{1000 \text{ mg}} = \frac{\text{x}}{0.5 \text{ mg}}$$

$$\frac{1000}{1000} = \text{x}$$

1 mL = x

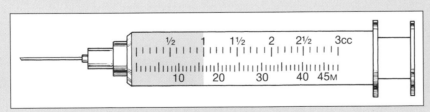

**2.** Equivalent 1:5000 means

1 g in 5000 mL

1 g = 1000 mg

Hence, the solution is 1000 mg/5000 mL.

*Formula Method*

$$\frac{D}{H} \times S = A$$

$$\frac{1 \text{ mg}}{1000 \text{ mg}} \times 5000 \text{ mL} = 5 \text{ mL}$$

Add 5 mL to IV. (This is correct because route is IV, not IM.)

*Ratio Proportion Method*

$$\frac{5000 \text{ mL}}{1000 \text{ mg}} = \frac{x}{1 \text{ mg}}$$

$$\frac{5000}{1000} = x$$

$$5 \text{ mL} = x$$

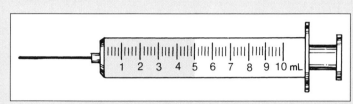

**3.** Equivalent 1:1000 means

1 g in 1000 mL and 1 g = 1000 mg,

Hence, the solution is 1000 mg/1000 mL or 1 mg/mL.

*Formula Method*

$$\frac{D}{H} \times S = A$$

$$\frac{0.75 \text{ mg}}{1 \text{ mg}} \times 1 \text{ mL} = 0.75 \text{ mL}$$

You have a 1-cc syringe marked in hundredths. Draw up 0.75 mL. Do not round off.

*Ratio Proportion Method*

$$\frac{1 \text{ mL}}{1 \text{ mg}} = \frac{x}{0.75 \text{ mg}}$$

$$\frac{0.75}{1} = x$$

$$0.75 \text{ mL} = x$$

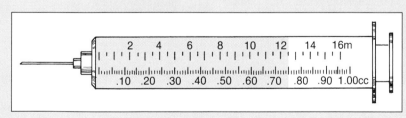

**4.** Equivalent 1:20 means
   1 g in 20 ml
   1 g = 1000 mg

Hence, the solution is 1000 mg/20 mL.

*Formula Method*

$$\dfrac{\overset{1}{\cancel{50 \text{ mg}}}}{\underset{20}{\cancel{1000 \text{ mg}}}} \times \overset{1}{\cancel{20}} \text{ mL} = 1 \text{ mL}$$

Give 1 mL IM.

*Ratio Proportion Method*

$$\dfrac{20 \text{ mL}}{1000 \text{ mg}} = \dfrac{\text{x}}{50 \text{ mg}}$$

$$\dfrac{1000}{1000} = \text{x}$$

$$1 \text{ mL} = \text{x}$$

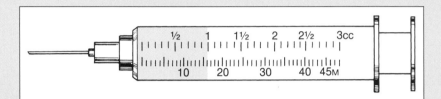

**5.** Equivalent 1:2000 = 1000 mg/2000 mL or 1 mg per 2 mL

*Formula Method*

$$\dfrac{\text{D}}{\text{H}} \times \text{S} = \text{A} \qquad \dfrac{1.5 \text{ mg}}{1 \text{ mg}} \times 2 \text{ mL} = \begin{array}{r} 1.5 \\ \times 2 \\ \hline 3.0 \text{ mL} \end{array}$$

*Ratio Proportion Method*

$$\dfrac{2 \text{ mL}}{1 \text{ mg}} = \dfrac{\text{x}}{1.5 \text{ mg}}$$

$$\dfrac{3.0}{1} = \text{x}$$

$$3.0 \text{ mL} = \text{x}$$

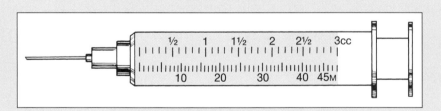

## Self Test 4 Percentages

**1.** 0.9 g per 100 mL; 0.9 g = 100 mL; 0.9 g/100 mL
**2.** 10 g per 100 mL; 10 g = 100 mL; 10 g/100 mL
**3.** 0.45 g per 100 mL; 0.45 g = 100 mL; 0.45 g/100 mL

## Self Test 5 Using Percentages with Liquids for Injection

**1.** Equivalent 1%  1 g in 100 mL

$$1 \text{ g} = 1000 \text{ mg}$$

Hence, the solution is 1000 mg/100 mL.

*Formula Method*

$$\frac{\overset{1}{\cancel{5 \text{ mg}}}}{\underset{\underset{2}{\cancel{10}}}{\cancel{1000 \text{ mg}}}} \times \overset{1}{\cancel{100}} \text{ mL} = \frac{1}{2} \text{ mL or } 0.5$$

Give 0.5 mL SC.

*Ratio Proportion Method*

$$\frac{100 \text{ mL}}{1000 \text{ mg}} = \frac{x}{5 \text{ mg}}$$

$$\frac{500}{1000} = x$$

$$0.5 \text{ mL} = x$$

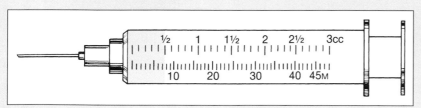

**2.** Equivalent 0.5%  0.5 g in 100 mL

$$0.5 \text{ g} = 500 \text{ mg}$$

Hence, the solution is 500 mg/100 mL.

*Formula Method*

$$\frac{2.5 \text{ mg}}{\underset{5}{\cancel{500 \text{ mg}}}} \times \overset{1}{\cancel{100}} \text{ mL} = \frac{2.5}{5} \quad 5\overline{)2.5}^{\,0.5}$$

Give 0.5 mL IM.

*Ratio Proportion Method*

$$\frac{100 \text{ mL}}{500 \text{ mg}} = \frac{x}{2.5}$$

$$\frac{2500}{500} = x$$

$$0.5 \text{ mL} = x$$

**3.** Equivalent 1%  1 g in 100 mL

$$1 \text{ g} = 1000 \text{ mg}$$

Hence, the solution is 1000 mg per 100 mL.

**Formula Method**

$$\frac{\overset{3}{\cancel{3 \text{ mg}}}}{\underset{10}{\cancel{1000 \text{ mg}}}} \times \overset{1}{\cancel{100}} \text{ mL} = \frac{3}{10} = 0.3 \text{ mL}$$

Give 0.3 mL SC.

**Ratio Proportion Method**

$$\frac{100 \text{ mL}}{1000 \text{ mg}} = \frac{x}{3 \text{ mg}}$$

$$\frac{300}{1000} = x$$

$$0.3 \text{ mL} = x$$

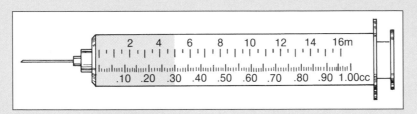

**4.** Equivalent 10% means 10 g in 100 mL or 1 g in 10 mL

**Formula Method**

$$\frac{D}{H} \times S = A \qquad \frac{0.3 \cancel{g}}{1 \cancel{g}} \times 10 \text{ mL} \qquad \begin{array}{r} 10 \\ \times\ 0.3 \\ \hline 3.0 \text{ mL} \end{array}$$

Prepare the syringe with 3 mL for IV use.

**Ratio Proportion Method**

$$\frac{10 \text{ mL}}{1 \text{ g}} = \frac{x}{0.3 \text{ g}}$$

$$\frac{3}{1} = x$$

$$3.0 \text{ mL} = x$$

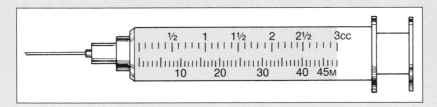

**5.** Equivalent 3% means 3 g in 100 mL or 3000 mg in 100 ML.

This can be reduced $\dfrac{3000 \text{ mg}}{100 \text{ mL}} = 30 \text{ mg/mL}$

Equivalent 0.015 g = 15 mg

<table>
<tr><td>

***Formula Method***

$$\dfrac{D}{H} \times S = A \qquad \dfrac{\overset{1}{\cancel{15 \text{ mg}}}}{\underset{2}{\cancel{30 \text{ mg}}}} \times 1 \text{ mL} = \dfrac{1}{2} \text{ mL}$$

Prepare 0.5 mL (½ mL) for IV use.

</td><td>

***Ratio Proportion Method***

$$\dfrac{1 \text{ mL}}{30 \text{ mg}} = \dfrac{\text{x}}{15 \text{ mg}}$$

$$\dfrac{15}{30} = \text{x}$$

$$0.5 \text{ mL} = \text{x}$$

</td></tr>
</table>

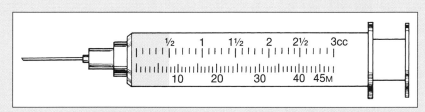

## Self Test 6 Insulin Calculations

**1.**

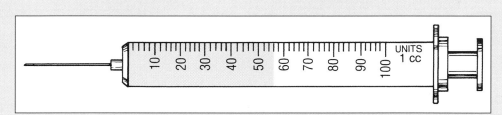

**2.**

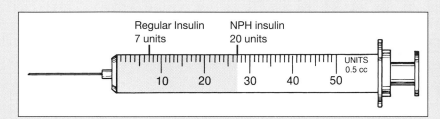

Regular Insulin
7 units

NPH insulin
20 units

**3.**

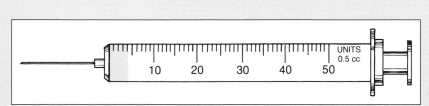

**4.**

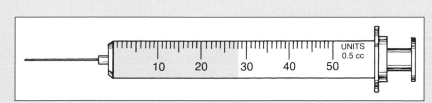

**5.**

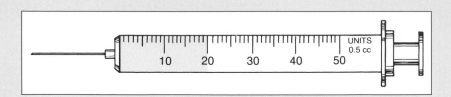

**6.**

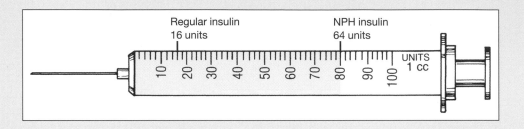

**7.**

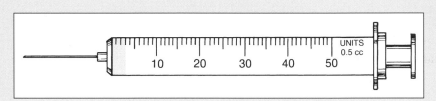

**8.**

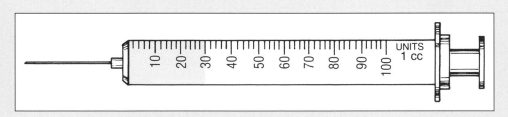

**9.**

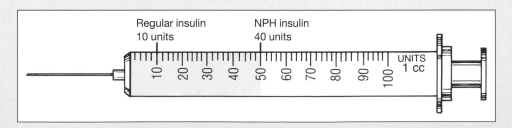

**10.**

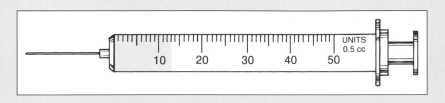

# Injections From Powders

CONTENT TO MASTER

▶ Principles for reconstituting drugs from powder form

▶ Reading and understanding drug manufacturer's label and package insert directions when
dissolving powders accurately; storing reconstituted drugs safely; labeling reconstituted drugs

▶ Acceptable fluids for diluting powders for injection

▶ Terms used when reconstituting powders:
displacement, dilution, sterile technique, concentration, new stock, diluting fluids

Some medications are prepared in a dry form, powder, or crystal. As liquids they are unstable and lose potency over time. The drug must be reconstituted according to the manufacturer's directions, which will give the type and amount of diluent to use.

## ▶ Injections From Powders

The rule used to solve injection from powder problems is the same as that for oral medications and for injection from a liquid, because the powdered drug *becomes a liquid* once the powder is dissolved.

### Application of the Rule for Injections From Powders

**RULE**

*Formula Method*

$$\frac{Desire}{Have} \times Stock = Amount$$

*Ratio Proportion Method*

$$\frac{Stock}{Have} = \frac{x}{Desire}$$

**Example**

Order: cefonicid sodium 0.65 g IM qd.

Label:

*Label directions:* Add 2.5 mL Sterile Water for Injection. Shake well. Provides an approximate volume of 3.1 mL (325 mg/mL). Stable 24 hours at room temperature or 72 hours if refrigerated (5°C).

*Desire:* The order in the example is 0.65 g.

*Have:* The strength of the drug supplied. The example is 1 gram as a dry powder; when reconstituted, it is 325 mg/mL. Remember that the manufacturer gives the strength of the solution; the nurse does not have to determine it.

*Stock:* The fluid portion of the solution made. In this example it is 1 mL = 325 mg.

*Answer:* How much liquid to give, stated as mL or cc.

Equivalent 0.65 g = 650 mg

**Formula Method**

$$\frac{D}{H} \times S = A \quad \frac{\overset{2}{\cancel{650\ mg}}}{\underset{1}{\cancel{325\ mg}}} \times 1\ mL = 2\ mL$$

**Ratio Proportion Method**

$$\frac{1\ mL}{325\ mg} = \frac{x}{650\ mg}$$

$$\frac{650}{325} = x$$

$$2\ mL = x$$

Give 2 mL. The remaining solution is stored in the refrigerator. The vial is labeled with the date, the solution made (325 mg/mL), and the initials of the nurse who dissolved the powder.

## ▶ Distinctive Features of Injections From Powders

Sterile technique is used to prepare and administer the medication, which is given parenterally (usually IM, IV, or IVPB). The dry drug is supplied in vials of powder or crystals and may come in different strengths. Because powders deteriorate in solution, choose the strength closest to the amount ordered.

The powder is usually diluted with one of the following:

Sterile water for injection

Bacteriostatic water for injection with a preservative added

Normal saline for injection (0.9% sodium chloride)

Directions will state which fluids may be used. Read this information carefully because some fluids may be incompatible (i.e., unsuitable) as diluents. When the powder goes into solution, *displacement* occurs. This means that the *volume* added to the vial is *increased* by the powder as it dissolves. There is no uniformity in the way powders go into solution.

Refer to the label in Figure 8-1 again. The manufacturer tells the nurse to add 2.5 mL of sterile water to provide an approximate volume of 3.1 mL. In this example 0.6 mL is the displacement volume. *Injections from powder problems are solved by using the solution made, not the displacement volume.* The manufacturer will give the solution.

**Example**  The package insert information concerning the dilution of cefoperazone sodium (Cefobid) injection is reproduced in Figure 8-2. Examine the directions with the intention of solving the following problem, then read the explanation:

Order: cefoperazone 0.5 g IM q 12 h

Stock powder: 1 gram vial of powder

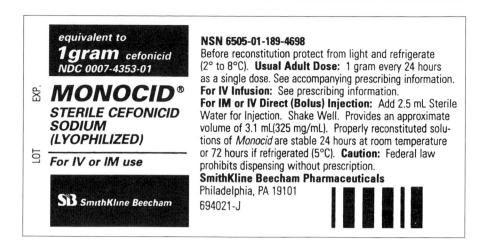

**FIGURE 8-1**

Label of cefonicid sodium (Monocid). (Courtesy of SmithKline Beecham Pharmaceuticals.)

Search the directions for three pieces of information to dissolve your stock, which is 1 gram:

- Type of fluid needed to dissolve the powder
- Amount of fluid to add
- Solution made

## Explanation

1. Figure 8-2 gives *Solutions for Initial Reconstitution:* sterile water for injection, bacteriostatic water for injection, and 0.9% sodium chloride injection. Choose one.

2. The heading *Preparation for Intramuscular Injection* states that when a concentration of 250 mg or more is to be administered, a 2% lidocaine solution should be used together with sterile water for injection in a two-step dilution.

3. Two tables are given. The upper table has the two-step dilution, the lower one does not. Because the order requires two steps, use the directions in the top table.

4. Two strengths of powder are listed in the upper table. Look at the extreme left. They are 1-g vial and 2-g vial. Our supply is a 1-g vial. Follow directions for 1 g.

5. The next heading is *Final Cefoperazone Concentration.* Two possibilities are given for the dilution: 333 mg/mL and 250 mg/mL. Because the order calls for 0.5 g, choose 250 mg/mL. This concentration makes the arithmetic easy. Do you see that the answer will be 2 mL?

6. To make the solution of 250 mg/mL, the following are added: 2.8 mL of sterile water and 1.0 mL of 2% lidocaine.

7. The last column to the right is headed *Withdrawable Volume* and lists 4 mL. Ignore this column; it does not affect the answer: When you add 2.8 mL and 1.0 mL, you expect to have 3.8 mL. The package insert states you will end up with 4 mL. The manufacturer is giving the displacement.

8. You now have all the information needed to prepare the dose ordered. Your solution is 250 mg/mL. Equivalent 0.5 g = 500 mg.

## RECONSTITUTION

The following solutions may be used for the initial reconstitution of CEFOBID sterile powder:

**Table 1. Solutions for Initial Reconstitution**

5% Dextrose Injection (USP)  
5% Dextrose and 0.9% Sodium Chloride Injection (USP)  
5% Dextrose and 0.2% Sodium Chloride Injection (USP)  
10% Dextrose Injection (USP)  
Bacteriostatic Water for Injection [Benzyl Alcohol or Parabens] (USP)*†

0.9% Sodium Chloride Injection (USP)  
Normosol® M and Dextrose Injection  
Normosol® R  
Sterile Water for Injection*

\* Not to be used as a vehicle for intravenous infusion.  
† Preparation containing Benzyl Alcohol should not be used in neonates.

### Preparation for Intramuscular Injection

Any suitable solution listed above may be used to prepare CEFOBID sterile powder for intramuscular injection. When concentrations of 250 mg/ml or more are to be administered, a lidocaine solution should be used. These solutions should be prepared using a combination of Sterile Water for Injection and 2% Lidocaine Hydrochloride Injection (USP) that approximates a 0.5% Lidocaine Hydrochloride Solution. A two-step dilution process as follows is recommended: First, add the required amount of Sterile Water for Injection and agitate until CEFOBID powder is completely dissolved. Second, add the required amount of 2% lidocaine and mix.

| | Final Cefoperazone Concentration | Step 1 Volume of Sterile Water | Step 2 Volume of 2% Lidocaine | Withdrawable Volume*† |
|---|---|---|---|---|
| 1 g vial | 333 mg/ml | 2.0 ml | 0.6 ml | 3 ml |
| | 250 mg/ml | 2.8 ml | 1.0 ml | 4 ml |
| 2 g vial | 333 mg/ml | 3.8 ml | 1.2 ml | 6 ml |
| | 250 mg/ml | 5.4 ml | 1.8 ml | 8 ml |

When a diluent other than Lidocaine HCl Injection (USP) is used reconstitute as follows:

| | Cefoperazone Concentration | Volume of Diluent to be Added | Withdrawable Volume* |
|---|---|---|---|
| 1 g vial | 333 mg/ml | 2.6 ml | 3 ml |
| | 250 mg/ml | 3.8 ml | 4 ml |
| 2 g vial | 333 mg/ml | 5.0 ml | 6 ml |
| | 250 mg/ml | 7.2 ml | 8 ml |

\* There is sufficient excess present to allow for withdrawal of the stated volume.  
† Final lidocaine concentration will approximate that obtained if a 0.5% Lidocaine Hydrochloride Solution is used as diluent.

### STORAGE AND STABILITY

CEFOBID sterile powder is to be stored at or below 25°C (77°F) and protected from light prior to reconstitution. After reconstitution, protection from light is not necessary.

The following parenteral diluents and approximate concentrations of CEFOBID provide stable solutions under the following conditions for the indicated time periods. (After the indicated time periods, unused portions of solutions should be discarded.)

**Controlled Room Temperature (15ʏ–25ʏC/59ʏ–77ʏF)**

| 24 Hours | Approximate |
|---|---|
| Bacteriostatic Water for Injection [Benzyl Alcohol or Parabens] (USP) | 300 mg/ml |
| 5% Dextrose Injection (USP) | 2 mg to 50 mg/ml |
| 5% Dextrose and Lactated Ringer's Injection | 2 mg to 50 mg/ml |
| 5% Dextrose and 0.9% Sodium Chloride Injection (USP) | 2 mg to 50 mg/ml |
| 5% Dextrose and 0.2% Sodium Chloride Injection (USP) | 2 mg to 50 mg/ml |
| 10% Dextrose Injection (USP) | 2 mg to 50 mg/ml |
| Lactated Ringer's Injection (USP) | 2 mg/ml |
| 0.5% Lidocaine Hydrochloride Injection (USP) | 300 mg/ml |
| 0.9% Sodium Chloride Injection (USP) | 2 mg to 300 mg/ml |
| Normosol® M and 5% Dextrose Injection | 2 mg to 50 mg/ml |
| Normosol® R | 2 mg to 50 mg/ml |
| Sterile Water for Injection | 300 mg/ml |

Reconstituted CEFOBID solutions may be stored in glass or plastic syringes, or in glass or flexible plastic parenteral solution containers.

**Refrigerator Temperature (2ʏ–8ʏC/36ʏ–46ʏF)**

| 5 Days | Approximate Concentrations |
|---|---|
| Bacteriostatic Water for Injection [Benzyl Alcohol or Parabens] (USP) | 300 mg/ml |
| 5% Dextrose Injection (USP) | 2 mg to 50 mg/ml |
| 5% Dextrose and 0.9% Sodium Chloride Injection (USP) | 2 mg to 50 mg/ml |
| 5% Dextrose and 0.2% Sodium Chloride Injection (USP) | 2 mg to 50 mg/ml |
| Lactated Ringer's Injection (USP) | 2 mg/ml |
| 0.5% Lidocaine Hydrochloride Injection (USP) | 300 mg/ml |
| 0.9% Sodium Chloride Injection (USP) | 2 mg to 300 mg/ml |
| Normosol® M and 5% Dextrose Injection | 2 mg to 50 mg/ml |
| Normosol® R | 2 mg to 50 mg/ml |
| Sterile Water for Injection | 300 mg/ml |

Reconstituted CEFOBID solutions may be stored in glass or plastic syringes, or in glass or flexible plastic parenteral solution containers.

**FIGURE 8-2**

Reconstitution directions for cefoperazone sodium (Cefobid). (Courtesy of Pfizer Laboratories.)

---

*Formula Method*

$$\frac{D}{H} \times S = A$$

$$\frac{\overset{2}{\cancel{500 \text{ mg}}}}{\underset{1}{\cancel{250 \text{ mg}}}} \times 1 \text{ mL} = 2 \text{ mL}$$

Give 2 mL IM.

*Ratio Proportion Method*

$$\frac{1 \text{ mL}}{250 \text{ mg}} = \frac{x}{500 \text{ mg}}$$

$$\frac{500}{250} = x$$

2 mL = x

9. Write on the label the solution you made, the date, and your initials.

10. Note the storage directions and stability expiration.

**STEPS FOR RECONSTITUTING POWDERS WITH DIRECTIONS**

1. Read the order.
2. Identify the stock.
3. Dilute the fluid.
4. Identify the solution and new stock.
5. Apply the rule and arithmetic.
6. Obtain the amount to give.
7. Write on label.
8. Store according to directions.

**Example**

Order: cefoperazone 0.5 g IM = 500 mg (Refer to Fig. 8-2.)

Stock powder: 1 g

Diluting fluid and number of milliliters

Step 1. Add 2.8 mL sterile water.

Step 2. Add 1 mL 2% lidocaine.

Solution and new stock: 250 mg/mL

Rule and arithmetic: $\dfrac{D}{H} \times S = A$

*Formula Method*

$$\dfrac{\overset{2}{\cancel{500 \text{ mg}}}}{\underset{1}{\cancel{250 \text{ mg}}}} \times 1 \text{ mL} = 2 \text{ mL}$$

*Ratio Proportion Method*

$$\dfrac{1 \text{ mL}}{250 \text{ mg}} = \dfrac{x}{500 \text{ mg}}$$

$$\dfrac{500}{250} = x$$

$$2 \text{ mL} = x$$

Amount to give: 2 mL IM

Write on label: 250 mg/mL; date; initials.

Store: Refrigerate. Stable for 5 days

## Where to Find Information About Reconstitution of Powders

Information about reconstitution of powders may be found from

- The label on the vial of powder
- The package insert that comes with the vial of powder
- Nursing drug handbooks
- Other references such as the *Physician's Desk Reference (PDR)*

**RECONSTITUTION**

**Preparation of Parenteral Solution**

Parenteral drug products should be SHAKEN WELL when reconstituted, and inspected visually for particulate matter prior to administration. If particulate matter is evident in reconstituted fluids, the drug solutions should be discarded. When reconstituted or diluted according to the instructions below, Ancef (sterile cefazolin sodium, SK&F) is stable for 24 hours at room temperature or for 96 hours if stored under refrigeration. Reconstituted solutions may range in color from pale yellow to yellow without a change in potency.

**Single-Dose Vials**

For I.M. injection, I.V. direct (bolus) injection, or I.V. infusion, reconstitute with Sterile Water for Injection according to the following table. SHAKE WELL.

| Vial Size | Amount of Diluent | Approximate Concentration | Approximate Available Volume |
|---|---|---|---|
| 250 mg. | 2.0 ml. | 125 mg./ml. | 2.0 ml. |
| 500 mg. | 2.0 ml. | 225 mg./ml. | 2.2 ml. |
| 1 gram | 2.5 ml. | 330 mg./ml. | 3.0 ml. |

**FIGURE 8-3**

Reconstitution directions for cefazolin sodium (Ancef). (Courtesy of SmithKline Beecham Pharmaceuticals.)

**Example**

EXAMPLE 1:

Order: cefazolin sodium 0.3 g IM (Fig. 8-3)

Stock powder: 500 mg

Diluting fluid: 2.0 mL sterile water for injection

Solution and new stock: 225 mg/mL

**Formula Method**

Rule and arithmetic: $\dfrac{D}{H} \times S = A$

Equivalent 0.3 g = 300 mg

$$\dfrac{300 \text{ mg}}{225 \text{ mg}} \times 1 \text{ mL} = \dfrac{4}{3} \quad 3\overline{)4.00} = 1.33$$

**Ratio Proportion Method**

$$\dfrac{1 \text{ mL}}{225 \text{ mg}} = \dfrac{x}{300 \text{ mg}}$$

$$\dfrac{300}{225} = x$$

1.33 or 1.3 mL = x

Give 1.3 mL IM.

Write on label: 225 mg/mL, date, initials.

Storage: Refrigerate. Stable for 96 hours

EXAMPLE 2:

Order: penicillin G potassium 1 million units IM q6h (Fig. 8-4)

Stock powder: 5 million unit vial

Diluting fluid and number of milliliters: Use sterile water for injection. Write out the directions for the 5 million unit vial (stock).

```
PENICILLIN G POTASSIUM for injection
Preparation of Solutions
Use sterile water for injection
           RECONSTITUTION
1,000,000 u vial
Diluent                        Desired Concentration
9.6 ml                              100,000 u/ml
4.6 ml                              200,000 u/ml
3.6 ml                              250,000 u/ml
5,000,000 u vial
Diluent                        Desired Concentration
23 ml                               200,000 u/ml
18 ml                               250,000 u/ml
8 ml                                500,000 u/ml
3 ml                              1,000,000 u/ml
Storage
Prepared solutions may be kept in the refrigerator one week.
```

**FIGURE 8-4**

Preparation of solution for the 1,000,000-unit and the 5,000,000-unit vials of penicillin G potassium.

23 mL will provide 200,000 U/mL.

18 mL will provide 250,000 U/mL.

8 mL will provide 500,000 U/mL.

3 mL will provide 1 million U/mL.

Choose 3 mL to dilute the powder.

Solution and new stock: 1 million units/mL

Rule: not needed because

**Formula Method**

$$\frac{D}{H} \times S = A$$

$$\frac{1 \text{ million units}}{1 \text{ million units}} \times 1 \text{ mL} = 1 \text{ mL}$$

**Ratio Proportion Method**

$$\frac{1 \text{ mL}}{1 \text{ million units}} = \frac{x}{1 \text{ million units}}$$

$$\frac{1 \text{ million}}{1 \text{ million}} = x$$

$$1 \text{ mL} = x$$

Give 1 mL IM.

Write on label: 1 million units/mL; date; initials.

Storage: Refrigerate. Stable for 1 week.

Note: This solution (1 million units/mL) may be so concentrated that it is painful when injected. The nurse could decide to dilute the powder with 8 mL to make 500,000 U/mL and give 2 mL to the patient. This more dilute solution may be less painful.

Here are a few tips before you begin Self Test 1.

* When reading the directions for reconstitution, look first at the solutions you can make. Think the problem through mentally and choose one dilution. This provides a focus as you read.

* If your answer is more than 3 mL for an IM injection, consider using two syringes and injecting in two different sites.

- Experience in administering injections will guide you in choosing the solution's concentration. Stronger concentrations, although smaller in volume, may be more painful; a more dilute solution may be more suitable despite its larger volume.

- Each powder problem is unique. Read the directions carefully!

- Choose one diluting fluid—generally sterile water or 0.9% sodium chloride for injection. Do not list all of them in your answer.

- For the following practice problems and self-tests, assume that the doses ordered and the order are correct. Chapter 12 discusses the nurse's responsibilities in drug knowledge. Dosages for infants and children are discussed in Chapter 11.

---

**SELF TEST 1**   Injections from Powders

*Solve the following problems in injections from powders and write your answers using the steps. Answers are found at the end of the chapter.*

1. Order:   ceftazidime 1 g IM q6h (Fig. 8-5)
   Stock:   1 g powder

   **a.** Diluting fluid and number of milliliters:
   **b.** Solution and new stock:
   **c.** Rule and arithmetic:
   **d.** Answer:
   **e.** Write on label:
   **f.** Storage:

2. Order:   ampicillin sodium 250 mg IM q6h (Fig. 8-6)
   Stock:   500-mg vial of powder

   **a.** Diluting fluid and number of milliliters:
   **b.** Solution and new stock:
   **c.** Rule and arithmetic:
   **d.** Answer:
   **e.** Write on label:
   **f.** Storage:

---

**CEFTAZIDIME INJECTION**

Reconstitution
Single dose vials: Reconstitute with sterile water. Shake well.

| Vial Size | Diluent | Approx. Avail. Volume | Approx. Avg. Concentration |
|---|---|---|---|
| IM or IV bolus injection | | | |
| 1 gram | 3.0 mL | 3.6 mL | 280 mg/mL |
| | | | |
| IV infusion | | | |
| 1 gram | 10 mL | 10.6 mL | 95 mg/mL |
| 2 gram | 10 mL | 11.2 mL | 180 mg/mL |

Stable for 18 hours at room temperature or seven days if refrigerated.

**FIGURE 8-5**

Label and reconstitution directions for ceftazidime.

*(continued)*

## SELF TEST 1 Injections from Powders (Continued)

**AMPICILLIN**
**Reconstitution**
Dissolve contents of a vial with the amount of Sterile Water or Bacteriostatic Water.

| Amount Ordered | Recommended Amount of Diluent | Withdraw Volume | Concentration in mg/ml |
|---|---|---|---|
| 500 mg | 1.8 ml | 2.0 ml | 250 mg |
| 1.0 Gram | 3.4 ml | 4.0 ml | 250 mg |
| 2.0 gram | 6.8 ml | 8.0 ml | 250 mg |

**Storage**
Use within one hour of reconstitution.

**FIGURE 8-6**

Reconstitution directions for ampicillin sodium for IM or IV injection.

**3.** Order: Ancef 225 mg IM q6h (Fig. 8-7)
Stock: On the shelf there are three vial sizes of powder: 250 mg, 500 mg, 1 g

**a.** Stock chosen:
**b.** Diluting fluid and number of milliliters:
**c.** Solution and new stock:
**d.** Rule and arithmetic:
**e.** Answer:
**f.** Write on label:
**g.** Storage:

**4.** Order: Fortaz 500 mg IM q 6 h (Fig. 8-8)
Stock: 1 g powder

**a.** Diluting fluid and number of milliliters:
**b.** Solution and new stock:
**c.** Rule and arithmetic:
**d.** Answer:
**e.** Write on label:
**f.** Storage:

RECONSTITUTION
**Preparation of Parenteral Solution**
Parenteral drug products should be SHAKEN WELL when reconstituted, and inspected visually for particulate matter prior to administration. If particulate matter is evident in reconstituted fluids, the drug solutions should be discarded. When reconstituted or diluted according to the instructions below, Ancef (sterile cefazolin sodium, SK&F) is stable for 24 hours at room temperature or for 96 hours if stored under refrigeration. Reconstituted solutions may range in color from pale yellow to yellow without a change in potency.
**Single-Dose Vials**
For I.M. injection, I.V. direct (bolus) injection, or I.V. infusion, reconstitute with Sterile Water for Injection according to the following table. SHAKE WELL.

| Vial Size | Amount of Diluent | Approximate Concentration | Approximate Available Volume |
|---|---|---|---|
| 250 mg. | 2.0 ml. | 125 mg./ml. | 2.0 ml. |
| 500 mg. | 2.0 ml. | 225 mg./ml. | 2.2 ml. |
| 1 gram | 2.5 ml. | 330 mg./ml. | 3.0 ml. |

**FIGURE 8-7**

Reconstitution directions for cefazolin sodium (Ancef). (Courtesy of SmithKline Beecham Laboratories.)

*(continued)*

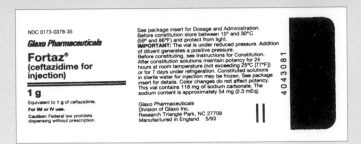

NDC 0173-0378-35

*Glaxo Pharmaceuticals*

**Fortaz®**
(ceftazidime for
injection)

**1 g**

Equivalent to 1 g of ceftazidime.

For IM or IV use.

Caution: Federal law prohibits
dispensing without prescription.

See package insert for Dosage and Administration.
Before constitution store between 15° and 30°C
(59° and 86°F) and protect from light.
IMPORTANT: The vial is under reduced pressure. Addition
of diluent generates a positive pressure.
Before constituting, see Instructions for Constitution.
After constitution solutions maintain potency for 24
hours at room temperature (not exceeding 25°C [77°F])
or for 7 days under refrigeration. Constituted solutions
in sterile water for injection may be frozen. See package
insert for details. Color changes do not affect potency.
This vial contains 118 mg of sodium carbonate. The
sodium content is approximately 54 mg (2.3 mEq).

Glaxo Pharmaceuticals
Division of Glaxo Inc.
Research Triangle Park, NC 27709
Manufactured in England   5/93

4043081

| | Table 5: Preparation of Fortaz Solutions | | |
|---|---|---|---|
| Size | Amount of Diluent to Be Added (mL) | Approximate Available Volume (mL) | Approximate Ceftazidime Concentration (mg/mL) |
| Intramuscular | | | |
| 500-mg vial | 1.5 | 1.8 | 280 |
| 1-gram vial | 3.0 | 3.6 | 280 |
| Intravenous | | | |
| 500-mg vial | 5.0 | 5.3 | 100 |
| 1-gram vial | 10.0 | 10.6 | 100 |
| 2-gram vial | 10.0 | 11.5 | 170 |
| Infusion pack | | | |
| 1-gram vial | 100* | 100 | 10 |
| 2-gram vial | 100* | 100 | 20 |
| Pharmacy bulk package | | | |
| 6-gram vial | 26 | 30 | 200 |

*Note:** Addition should be in two stages (see Instructions for Constitution).

**COMPATIBILITY AND STABILITY:**
**Intramuscular:** Fortaz®, when constituted as directed with sterile water for injection, bacteriostatic water for injection, or 0.5% or 1% lido-caine hydrochloride injection, maintains satisfactory potency for 24 hours at room temperature or for 7 days under refrigeration. Solutions in sterile water for injection that are frozen immediately after constitution in the original container are stable for 3 months when stored at -20°C. Once thawed, solutions should not be refrozen. Thawed solutions may be stored for up to 8 hours at room temperature or for 4 days in a refrigerator.

**FIGURE 8-8**

Preparation of Fortaz solutions. (Reproduced with permission of GlaxoSmithKline.)

5. Order:   cefoxitin sodium 200 mg IM q4h
   Stock:   vial of powder labeled 1 g.
            Refer to Figure 8-9.

   **a.** Diluting fluid and number of milliliters:
   **b.** Solution made and new stock:
   **c.** Rule and arithmetic:
   **d.** Answer:
   **e.** Write on label:
   **f.** Storage:

6. Order:   Mefoxin 0.6 g IM q6h (refer to Fig. 8-9)
            Stock powder: 1 gram

   **a.** Diluting fluid and number of milliliters:
   **b.** Solution made and new stock:
   **c.** Rule and arithmetic:
   **d.** Amount to give:
   **e.** Write on label:
   **f.** Storage:

*(continued)*

| Table 3 — Preparation of Solution | | | |
|---|---|---|---|
| Strength | Amount of Diluent to be Added (mL) + + | Approximate Withdrawable Volume (mL) | Approximate Average Concentration (mg/mL) |
| 1 gram Vial | 2 (Intramuscular) | 2.5 | 400 |
| 2 gram Vial | 4 (Intramuscular) | 5 | 400 |
| 1 gram Vial | 10 (IV) | 10.5 | 95 |
| 2 gram Vial | 10 or 20 (IV) | 11.1 or 21.0 | 180 or 95 |
| 1 gram Infusion Bottle | 50 or 100 (IV) | 50 or 100 | 20 or 10 |
| 2 gram Infusion Bottle | 50 or 100 (IV) | 50 or 100 | 40 or 20 |
| 10 gram Bulk | 43 or 93 (IV) | 49 or 98.5 | 200 or 100 |

+ + Shake to dissolve and let stand until clear.

*Intramuscular*
MEFOXIN, as constituted with Sterile Water for Injection, Bacteriostatic Water for Injection, or 0.5 percent or 1 percent lidocaine hydrochloride solution (without epinephrine), maintains satisfactory potency for 24 hours at room temperature, for one week under refrigeration (below 5°C), and for at least 30 weeks in the frozen state.

## FIGURE 8-9

Directions to reconstitute cefoxitin sodium (Mefoxin). (Courtesy of Merck Sharp & Dohme.)

**7.** Order:     amytal sodium 250 mg IM stat
   Stock:     ampule of crystals labeled 0.5 g
   Directions:   To derive a 20% solution, add 2.5 mL of sterile water for injection.
   *Note:*     You may wish to review Chapter 7, "When Stock Is a Percent."

   **a.** Diluting fluid and number of milliliters:
   **b.** Solution made and new stock:
   **c.** Rule and arithmetic:
   **d.** Amount to give:
   **e.** Write on label:
   **f.** Storage:

**8.** Order:   ceftazidime 0.3 g IV q 8h (refer to Fig. 8-5 for directions)
   Stock powder: 1 gram
   Write the steps.

*As you develop proficiency in solving these problems, you will be able to calculate many answers without written work. Here are two drills to sharpen your skill. The first drill (Set A) should be easy because the specific directions needed are given. In the second exercise (Set B) you must choose the direction you need. Aim for 100%! We will not indicate storage directions. Answers will be shown as follows at the end of the chapter:*

   **a.** Diluting fluid and number of milliliters:
   **b.** Solution made and new stock:
   **c.** Answer:
   **d.** Label:

*(continued)*

| SELF TEST 2 | Mental Drill in Injection From Powder Problems (Continued) |
|---|---|

*Set A*

1. Order:        penicillin G 300,000 units IM
   Stock:        powder labeled 1 million units
   Directions:   Dissolve with 4.6 mL sterile water for injection to make 200,000 units/mL.

2. Order:        hydrocortisone sodium succinate 100 mg IM
   Stock:        vial of powder labeled 100 mg and an ampule of 2 mL diluent
   Directions:   Add diluent to powder. Each 2 mL = 100 mg.

3. Order:        acetazolamide 150 mg IM
   Stock:        vial of powder labeled 500 mg
   Directions:   Reconstitute powder with 5 mL sterile water for injection. Solution will be 100 mg/mL.

4. Order:        colycillin 250 mg IM
   Stock:        vial of powder labeled 1 g
   Directions:   Add 1.5 mL sterile water for injection to prepare a solution of 500 mg/cc.

5. Order:        ampicillin 400 mg IM
   Stock:        vial of powder labeled 500 mg
   Directions:   Add 1.8 mL sterile water for injection to make a solution of 250 mg/mL.

*Set B*

*Directions for these problems are located throughout Chapter 8. Choose the directions you need to give the ordered dose. Aim for 100%.*

1. Order:   ceftazidime sodium 90 mg IM q12h
   Stock:   vial of powder labeled Tazicef 1 gram (refer to Fig. 8-5)

2. Order:   cefazolin sodium 0.45 g IM q12h
   Stock:   vial of powder labeled cefazolin sodium 500 mg (refer to Fig. 8-3)

3. Order:   ampicillin sodium 400 mg IM q 6 h (refer to Fig. 8-6)
             Stock powder: 500 mg

4. Order:   ceftazidime 0.5 g IM q 6 h (refer to Fig. 8-5)
             Stock powder: 1 gram

5. Order:   cefoxitin sodium 0.5 gm IM q12h
   Stock:   vial of powder labeled Mefoxin 1 gram (refer to Fig. 8-9)

# T EST YOUR CLINICAL SAVVY

You are working in a medical-surgical unit of a large city hospital. A patient is to receive 500,000 units of Penicillin G potassium, IV, q 12 hours. Normally a vial containing 1 million units is considered stock drug (reconstituted: 250,000 units = 1 mL). Because of a nationwide shortage, a vial with 5 million units of Penicillin G Potassium is supplied (reconstituted 1,000,000 units = 1 mL).

A. What should you do to ensure no mistakes are made for the initial dosing and for subsequent dosing of Penicillin?
B. What is the danger in administering too much of any drug?
C. What is the danger in administering too much Penicillin and/or potassium?

*Name:* _____

*There are 5 questions, each worth 20 points. Aim for 90% or better on this test. If you have any difficulty doing the problems, review and study Chapter 8. Answers will be found on page 348.*

1. Order:   Fortaz 250 mg IM q 8 hours
   Stock:   vial of powder labeled 1 g powder (refer to Fig. 8-8)

   a. Diluting fluid and number of milliliters:
   b. Solution and new stock:
   c. Rule and arithmetic:
   d. Amount to give:
   e. Write on label:
   f. Storage:

2. Order:   ticarcillin disodium 1 g IM
   Stock:   vial of powder labeled Ticar 1 gram (Fig. 8-10)

   a. Diluting fluid and number of milliliters:
   b. Solution and new stock:
   c. Rule and arithmetic:
   d. Amount to give:
   e. Write on label:
   f. Storage:

3. Order:   ampicillin sodium 300 mg IM q8h
   Stock:   vial of 500 mg powder (refer to Fig. 8-11)

   a. Diluting fluid and number of milliliters:
   b. Solution and new stock:
   c. Rule and arithmetic:
   d. Amount to give:
   e. Write on label:
   f. Storage:

**DIRECTIONS FOR USE**
**—1 Gm, 3 Gm and 6 Gm Standard Vials—**
**INTRAMUSCULAR USE:** (Concentration of approximately 385 mg/ml).
For initial reconstitution use Sterile Water for Injection, USP, Sodium Chloride Injection, USP or 1% Lidocaine Hydrochloride solution* (without epinephrine).
Each gram of Ticarcillin should be reconstituted with 2 ml of Sterile Water for Injection, U.S.P., Sodium Chloride Injection, U.S.P. or 1% Lidocaine Hydrochloride solution* (without epinephrine) and **used promptly.** Each 2.6 ml of the resulting solution will then contain 1 Gm of Ticarcillin.
*[For full product information, refer to manufacturer's package insert for Lidocaine Hydrochloride.]
As with all intramuscular preparations, TICAR (Ticarcillin Disodium) should be injected well within the body of a relatively large muscle, using usual techniques and precautions.

**FIGURE 8-10**

Directions for use of ticarcillin disodium (Ticar). (Courtesy of SmithKline Beecham Laboratories.)

*(continued)*

Intramuscular Use: 125 mg vial: Add 1 ml Sterile Water for Injection, USP, or Bacteriostatic Water for Injection, USP (TUBEX® Sterile Cartridge-Needle Unit) to give a final concentration of 125 mg per ml. For fractional doses, withdraw the ampicillin sodium solution as follows:

| Dose | Withdraw |
|------|----------|
| 25 mg | 0.2 ml |
| 50 mg | 0.4 ml |
| 75 mg | 0.6 ml |
| 100 mg | 0.8 ml |
| 125 mg | 1 ml |

250 mg vial: Add 0.9 ml Sterile Water for Injection, USP, or Bacteriostatic Water for Injection, USP (TUBEX) to give a final concentration of 250 mg/ml. For fractional doses, withdraw the ampicillin sodium solution as follows:

| Dose | Withdraw |
|------|----------|
| 125 mg | 0.5 ml |
| 150 mg | 0.6 ml |
| 175 mg | 0.7 ml |
| 200 mg | 0.8 ml |
| 225 mg | 0.9 ml |
| 250 mg | 1 ml |

For dilution of 500-mg, 1-gram, and 2-gram vials, dissolve contents of a vial with the amount of Sterile water for Injection, USP, or Bacteriostatic Water for Injection, USP, listed in the table below:

| Label Claim | Recommended Amount of Diluent | Withdrawable Volume | Concentration in mg/ml |
|-------------|-------------------------------|---------------------|------------------------|
| 500 mg | 1.8 ml | 2.0 ml | 250 mg |
| 1.0 gram | 3.4 ml | 4.0 ml | 250 mg |
| 2.0 gram | 6.8 ml | 8.0 ml | 250 mg |

While the 1-gram and 2-gram vials are primarily for intravenous use, they may be administered intramuscularly when the 250-mg or 500-mg vials are unavailable. In such instances, dissolve in 3.4 or 6.8 ml Sterile Water for Injection, USP, or Bacteriostatic Water for Injection, USP, to give a final concentration of 250 mg/ml

The above solutions must be used within one hour after reconstitution.

## FIGURE 8-11

Reconstitution directions for ampicillin sodium (Omnipen®-N) for IM or IV injection. (Courtesy of Wyeth-Ayerst Laboratories, Philadelphia, PA.)

4. Order: Mefoxin 300 mg IM q4h
   Stock: vial of powder 1 gram (Fig. 8-12)

   **a.** Diluting fluid and number of milliliters:
   **b.** Solution and new stock:
   **c.** Rule and arithmetic:
   **d.** Amount to give:
   **e.** Write on label:
   **f.** Storage:

| — Preparation of Solution | | | |
|---------------------------|-----------------------------------|-------------------------------------|-----------------------------------------------|
| Strength | Amount of Diluent to be Added (mL) + + | Approximate Withdrawable Volume (mL) | Approximate Average Concentration (mg/mL) |
| 1 gram Vial | 2 (Intramuscular) | 2.5 | 400 |
| 2 gram Vial | 4 (Intramuscular) | 5 | 400 |
| 1 gram Vial | 10 (IV) | 10.5 | 95 |
| 2 gram Vial | 10 or 20 (IV) | 11.1 or 21.0 | 180 or 95 |
| 1 gram Infusion Bottle | 50 or 100 (IV) | 50 or 100 | 20 or 10 |
| 2 gram Infusion Bottle | 50 or 100 (IV) | 50 or 100 | 40 or 20 |
| 10 gram Bulk | 43 or 93 (IV) | 49 or 98.5 | 200 or 100 |

+ +Shake to dissolve and let stand until clear.

*Intramuscular*
MEFOXIN, as constituted with Sterile Water for Injection, Bacteriostatic Water for Injection, or 0.5 percent or 1 percent lidocaine hydrochloride solution (without epinephrine), maintains satisfactory potency for 24 hours at room temperature, for one week under refrigeration (below 5 C), and for at least 30 weeks in the frozen state.

## FIGURE 8-12

Directions to reconstitute Mefoxin (cefoxitin sodium). (Courtesy of Merck & Co.)

*(continued)*

**5.** Order:   cefazolin sodium 0.33 g IM q8h
   Stock:   vial of powder labeled 1 gram (see Fig. 8-3)

   **a.** Diluting fluid and number of milliliters:
   **b.** Solution and new stock:
   **c.** Rule and arithmetic:
   **d.** Amount to give:
   **e.** Write on label:
   **f.** Storage:

# Answers

## Self Test 1 Injections from Powders

1. You want 1 g. The stock is 1 g. When you dilute the powder, you will give the whole amount of fluid, *whatever the amount is*. The manufacturer states it will be 3.6 mL/1 g. If you solve the arithmetic you have:

*Formula Method*

$$\frac{D}{H} \times S = A$$

*Ratio Proportion Method*

$$\frac{1 \text{ mL}}{280 \text{ mg}} = \frac{x}{1000 \text{ mg}}$$

$$\frac{1000}{280} = x$$

$$\frac{1000 \text{ mg}}{280 \text{ mg}} \times 1 \text{ mL} = \frac{100}{28} \quad \begin{array}{r} 3.57 \\ 28\overline{)100.00} \\ \underline{84} \\ 160 \\ \underline{140} \\ 200 \\ \underline{196} \end{array} = 3.6 \text{ mL} = x$$

  a. 3 mL sterile water for injection
  b. 1 g in 3.6 mL. 280 mg/mL
  c. Not necessary
  d. Give 3.6 mL in two syringes.
  e. Discard the vial; it is empty.
  f. Discard the vial in appropriate receptacle.
2. a. 1.8 mL sterile water for injection
   b. 250 mg/mL

   *Formula Method*

   c. $\dfrac{D}{H} \times S = A \quad \dfrac{250 \text{ mg}}{250 \text{ mg}} \times 1 \text{ mL} = 1 \text{ mL}$

   *Ratio Proportion Method*

   $$\frac{1 \text{ mL}}{250 \text{ mg}} = \frac{x}{250 \text{ mg}}$$

   $$\frac{250}{250} = x$$

   $$1 \text{ mL} = x$$

   d. Give 1 mL IM
   e. Nothing! Read the last line: "The above solutions must be used within 1 hour after reconstitution." You must discard the remaining fluid!
   f. None

3. **a.** Choose 500 mg powder. (Can you see why?)
   **b.** Add 2 mL sterile water for injection.
   **c.** 225 mg/mL
   **d.** Not necessary: You want 225 mg; you made 225 mg/mL.

4. **a.** 3.0 mL sterile water for injection
   **b.** 280 mg/mL

   **e.** Give 1 mL IM.
   **f.** 225 mg/mL, date, initials
   **g.** Refrigerate. Stable for 96 hours

*Formula Method*

**c.** $\dfrac{D}{H} \times S = A \ \dfrac{500\ \text{mg}}{280\ \text{mg}} \times 1\text{mL} = \dfrac{50}{28}$

$$28\overline{)50.00} = 1.78$$
$$\underline{28}$$
$$220$$
$$\underline{196}$$
$$240$$
$$\underline{224}$$
$$16$$

$= 1.8\ \text{mL}$

*Ratio Proportion Method*

$$\dfrac{1\ \text{mL}}{280\ \text{mg}} = \dfrac{x}{500\ \text{mg}}$$

$$\dfrac{500}{280} = x$$

1.78 or 1.8 mL = x

   **d.** Give 1.8 mL IM.
   **e.** 280 mg/mL, date, initials
   **f.** Refrigerate. Stable for 7 days

5. **a.** Add 2 mL of sterile water for injection.
   **b.** 400 mg/mL

*Formula Method*

**c.** $\dfrac{D}{H} \times S = A \ \dfrac{\overset{1}{200\ \text{mg}}}{\underset{2}{400\ \text{mg}}} \times 1\ \text{mL} = \dfrac{1}{2}\ \text{mL}$ or 0.5 mL

*Ratio Proportion Method*

$$\dfrac{1\ \text{mL}}{400\ \text{mg}} = \dfrac{x}{200\ \text{mg}}$$

$$\dfrac{200}{400} = x$$

0.5 mL = x

   **d.** Give ½ mL (0.5 mL).
   **e.** 400 mg/mL, date, initials
   **f.** Refrigerate. Stable for 1 week

**6. a.** Add 2 mL sterile water for injection.
   **b.** 400 mg/mL

*Formula Method*

**c.** $\dfrac{D}{H} \times S = A$   0.6 g = 600 mg

$$\dfrac{\overset{3}{\cancel{600 \text{ mg}}}}{\underset{2}{\cancel{400 \text{ mg}}}} \times 1 \text{ mL} = \dfrac{3}{2} \, \overline{)3.0}^{\,1.5}$$

*Ratio Proportion Method*

$$\dfrac{1 \text{ mL}}{400 \text{ mg}} = \dfrac{x}{600 \text{ mg}}$$

$$\dfrac{600}{400} = x$$

$$1.5 \text{ mL} = x$$

   **d.** Give 1.5 mL IM.
   **e.** 400 mg/mL, date, initials
   **f.** Refrigerate. Stable for 1 week
**7. a.** Diluting fluid and number of milliliters: Add 2.5 mL sterile water for injection.
   **b.** Solution made and new stock: 20% solution means

20 g in 100 mL or reducing that $\dfrac{\overset{1}{\cancel{20 \text{ g}}}}{\underset{5}{\cancel{100 \text{ mL}}}} = \dfrac{1 \text{ g}}{5 \text{ mL}}$

New stock: 1 g = 5 mL; 1 g = 1000 mg; therefore, 1000 mg = 5 mL
   **c.** Rule and arithmetic:

*Formula Method*

$$\dfrac{D}{H} \times S = A \quad \dfrac{\overset{1}{\cancel{250 \text{ mg}}}}{\underset{4}{\cancel{1000 \text{ mg}}}} \times 5 \text{ mL} = \dfrac{5}{4} \, \overline{)5.0}^{\,1.25}$$

*Ratio Proportion Method*

$$\dfrac{5 \text{ mL}}{1000 \text{ mg}} = \dfrac{x}{250 \text{ mg}}$$

$$\dfrac{1250}{1000} = x$$

$$1.25 = x$$

   **d.** Amount to give 1.3 mL IM
   **e.** Write on label: Nothing. An ampule must be discarded.
   **f.** Storage: No. Discard in a suitable receptacle.

**8. a.** Diluting fluid and number of milliliters: Add 10 mL sterile water for injection.
  **b.** Solution and new stock: 100 mg/mL
  **c.** Rule and arithmetic:

*Formula Method*

$$\frac{D}{H} \times S = A$$

$$\frac{\overset{3}{\cancel{300 \text{ mg}}}}{\underset{1}{\cancel{100 \text{ mg}}}} \times 1 \text{ mL}$$

$$3 \text{ mL} = A$$

*Ratio Proportion Method*

$$\frac{1 \text{ mL}}{100 \text{ mg}} = \frac{x}{300 \text{ mg}}$$

$$\frac{300}{100} = x$$

$$3 \text{ mL} = x$$

  **d.** Amount to give: 3 mL IV
  **e.** 100 mg/mL, date, initials
  **f.** Refrigerate. Stable for 7 days

## Self Test 2 Mental Drill in Injection From Powder Problems

*Set A*

**1. a.** 4.6 mL sterile water for injection
   **b.** 200,000 units/mL
   **c.** Give 1.5 mL IM.
   **d.** 200,000 U/mL, date, initials
**2. a.** 2 mL diluent with the vial
   **b.** 100 mg = 2 mL
   **c.** Give entire amount (give 2 mL) IM.
   **d.** None. Discard empty vial.
**3. a.** 5 mL sterile water for injection
   **b.** 100 mg/mL
   **c.** 1 ½ mL or 1.5 mL IM
   **d.** 100 mg/mL, date, initials

**4. a.** 1.5 mL sterile water for injection
   **b.** 500 mg/cc
   **c.** Give ½ cc or 0.5 cc IM.
   **d.** 500 mg/cc, date, initials
**5. a.** 1.8 mL of sterile water for injection
   **b.** 250 mg/mL
   **c.** Give 1.6 mL IM.
   **d.** 250 mg/mL, date, initials

*Set B*

**1. a.** 3.0 mL sterile water for injection
   **b.** 280 mg/mL
   **c.** Give 0.3 mL IM (3-mL syringe) or 0.32 mL (1-mL precision syringe).
   **d.** 280 mg/mL, date, initials
**2. a.** 2 mL sterile water for injection
   **b.** 225 mg/mL
   **c.** 2 mL IM
   **d.** 225 mg/mL, date, initials
**3. a.** 1.8 mL sterile water for injection
   **b.** 250 mg/mL
   **c.** 1.6 mL
   **d.** 250 mg/mL, date, initials

**4. a.** 3 mL sterile water for injection
   **b.** 280 mg/mL
   **c.** 1.8 mL
   **d.** 280 mg/mL, date, initials
**5. a.** 2 mL sterile water for injection
   **b.** 400 mg/mL
   **c.** 1.3 mL IM
   **d.** 400 mg/mL, date, initials

# Calculation of Basic IV Drip Rates

## ▶ Overview

Administration of parenteral fluids and medications by the intravenous route is common medical practice and is a specialty within nursing and health care. Texts such as *Plumer's Principles and Practice of Intravenous Therapy* (Lippincott, 2001) present detailed and extensive information. This chapter presents basic knowledge—types of fluids, equipment, calculation of drip rates, and recording intake. Chapter 10 presents rules and calculations for special types of intravenous orders.

## ▶ Types of Intravenous Fluids

Intravenous fluids are packaged in sterile plastic bags or glass bottles. The nurse selects the IV fluid ordered and prepares the solution. Care is essential. An error in choosing the correct IV may result in serious fluid and electrolyte imbalance.

The written order for an IV may differ from the printed stock label. Always seek expert advice when in doubt about which solution to use.

Common abbreviations for IV fluids are D = dextrose; W = water; NS = normal (or isotonic) saline. Often a percent of these is indicated, for example D5W means 5% dextrose in water; .9%NS means .9% saline in water.

| | *Written Order* | *Stock Label* |
|---|---|---|
| **Example** | 1000 mL D5W | 1000 cc D5%W |
| | 500 mL D5S | 500 cc D5%.9NS |
| | 250 mL D5½NS | 250 cc D5W.45NS |
| | 500 mL D5⅓NS | 500 cc D5.33NS |
| | 500 mL NS | 500 cc .9%NS |
| | 1000 mL ½NS | 1000 cc .45%NS |

# ▶ Kinds of Intravenous Drip Factors

Intravenous fluids are administered through infusion sets that consist of plastic tubing attached at one end to the IV bag and at the other end to a needle or catheter inserted into a blood vessel. The top of the infusion set contains a chamber. Sets that contain a needle in the chamber are called *microdrip* because the drops are small. To deliver 1 mL of fluid to the patient, 60 drops must fall (60 gtt = 1 mL). All microdrip sets deliver 60 gtt/mL.

Infusion sets that do not have a needle in the chamber are called *macrodrip* (Fig. 9-1). Macrodrip amounts per mL differ according to the manufacturer.

For example, Baxter-Travenol macrodrip sets deliver 10 gtt/mL; Abbott sets deliver 15 gtts/mL. The package label will state the drops per milliliter (gtt/mL). You need to know this information to calculate IV drip rates.

The tubing for these sets includes a clamp that the nurse can open or close to regulate the drip rate; a second hand on a watch or clock is used to count the drops per minute (Fig. 9-2).

## *Infusion Pumps*

Electric infusion pumps also are used to deliver IV fluid. Some are easy to operate; others more elaborate. The nurse enters two pieces of information: the total number of milliliters to be infused and the number of milliliters per hour. Figure 9-3 shows a photo of the face of an infusion pump. IV tubing is connected to the pump. If an order read: "500 mL D5W IV. Run 50 mL/hr," the nurse would press Volume for Infusion, 500; Rate for Infusion, 50; and On. The pump would automatically deliver 50 mL/hr over a 10-hour period.

IV pumps can also run IVPB. If an order read: "Ampicillin 2 g IVPB in 100 mL NS over 1 hour," the nurse would press Secondary Volume, 100; Secondary Rate, 100; On. The pump would interrupt the main IV to administer the IVPB over 1 hour, then resume the primary flow.

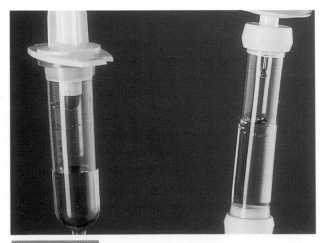

**FIGURE 9-1**
Drip chambers for macrodrip and microdrip IV tubing.

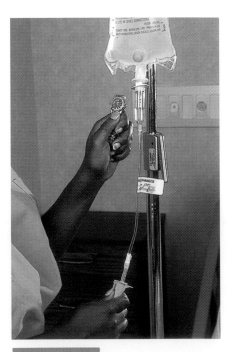

**FIGURE 9-2**
Timing the IV drip rate. (©B. Proud.)

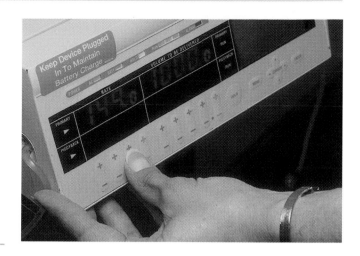

## FIGURE 9-3

IV rate is programmed into the infusion pump in mL/hr.

## Labeling IVs

Every IV must be identified so that any professional can check what fluid is infusing and the drip rate. The following information is a typical order:

Patient name, room, bed number and date

Order: 500 mL DW5½NS. Run 50 mL/hr

| Label | | | |
|---|---|---|---|
| Patient | James Latham | Room | 1411B |
| Date | 6/26 | Rate | 50 gtt/min |
| Order | 500 mL DW5½NS | Run | 50 mL/hr |
| Time | 10 A–8 P | Initials | CB |

Note that the physician orders 50 mL/hr. Since the IV fluid amount is 500 mL it will take 10 hours to complete; the time is 10 AM–8 PM (10 hours). Using microdrip tubing 50 mL/hr = 50 gtt/min, the rate set by the nurse. In the next section we will study how to calculate intravenous drip rates. Our goal is to deliver the amount of fluid ordered in the time ordered with a continuous and even drip rate.

## Calculating Basic IV Drip Rates

Routine IV orders contain the number of milliliters of fluid and the time of administration:

| **Example** | 250 mL D5W IV at 25 mL/hr | Fluid amount: 25 mL | Time: 1 hour |
|---|---|---|---|
| | 1000 mL Ringer's lactate IV 8 AM–8 PM | Fluid amount: 1000 mL | Time: 12 hours |
| | 500 mL D5½NS with 20 mEq KCl IV to run 75 mL/hr on a pump | Fluid amount: 500 mL | Time: 75 mL hour |

The equipment used by the nurse determines the drip factor and the calculations needed. With an infusion pump, calculations are in mL/hr because *the pump is set in mL/hr.* IV drips set in gtt/min depend on whether microdrip or macrodrip tubing is used.

**RULE**    Problems in IV calculations are solved in two steps. Step 1 is used to solve problems requiring an infusion pump and to simplify the arithmetic needed for microdrip and macrodrip. Step 2 will solve micro- and macrodrip problems. ■

Step 1. $\dfrac{\text{Total number of milliliters ordered}}{\text{number of hours to run}}$

= number of mL/hr

Step 2. $\dfrac{\text{Number of milliliters per hour} \times \text{tubing drip factor (TF)}}{\text{number of minutes}}$

= drops per minute

Note: Often the terms "drop factor," "drip factor" or "gtt factor" are used instead of "tubing drip factor." We use "TF" in this text to mean all these terms.

**Learning Aid**

Step 1. $\dfrac{\#\ mL}{\#\ hr} = mL/hr$

Step 2. $\dfrac{mL/hr \times TF}{\#\ min} = gtt/min$

Note that in Step 2 mL/hr is the answer to Step 1.

**Learning Aid**

Remember the abbreviation "gtt" is "drop."

## Explanation

**Step 1.** $\dfrac{\#\ mL}{\#\ hr} = mL/hr$

# mL: The physician will indicate the number of milliliters to be infused in the order.

# hr: The number of hours to run depends on the way the order is written. For example, if the order is written:

q8h = 8 hours at a time

10 AM–4 PM = 6 hours

25 mL/hr = the answer to Step 1. No calculation is required.

**Step 2.** $\dfrac{mL/hr \times TF}{\#\ min} = gtt/min$

mL/hr: the answer to Step 1.

TF: tubing drip factor is either microdrip (60 gtt = 1 mL) or macrodrip.

Depending on the manufacturer, macrodrip could be 10 gtt = 1 mL; 15 gtt = 1 mL; or 20 gtt = 1 mL.

# min: Number of minutes is always 60 for this problem. In Step 1 you found mL/hr, but you need gtt/min; because there are 60 minutes in an hour, divide by 60.

gtt/min: the drip factor calculated to deliver an even flow of fluid over a specified time. The nurse regulates the drip rate using a second hand on a watch or a clock. If the drip rate was calculated to be 80 gtt/min, the nurse would open the clamp and regulate the drip until there were 20 gtt in 15 seconds. This would provide 80 gtt/minute.

In the problems requiring calculation in this text, the drip factor will be given to you. In the clinical area, you must read the package label to identify the gtt/mL.

## Application of the Rule

**Example**

*EXAMPLE 1:*

Order: 1000 mL Ringer's lactate IV 8 AM–8 PM

Available: an infusion pump

Logic: 8 AM–8 PM is 12 hours for the IV to run. The infusion pump regulates the rate in milliliters per hour. Only Step 1 is necessary.

$$\frac{\# \text{ mL}}{\# \text{ hr}} = \text{mL/hr}$$

$$\frac{1000 \text{ mL}}{12 \text{ hr}} = \frac{1000}{12} \quad \begin{array}{r} 83.3 \\ \overline{)1000.0} \\ \underline{96} \\ 40 \\ \underline{36} \\ 40 \\ \underline{36} \end{array}$$

> **Learning Aid**
>
> Carry out arithmetic one decimal place and round off the answer to the nearest whole number.

Label the IV.

Set the pump as follows:

Total # mL: 1000

mL/hr: 83

*EXAMPLE 2:*

Order: 500 mL D5NS IV 12 N–4 PM

Available: microdrip at 60 gtt/mL; macrodrip at 20 gtt/mL

Logic: The IV will run 4 hours. Because no pump is available, the nurse must choose the drip factor; two steps are necessary. Solve for both drip factors and choose one.

**Step 1.** $\frac{\# \text{ mL}}{\# \text{ hr}} = \text{mL/hr}$

$$\frac{500}{4} \quad \begin{array}{r} 125. \\ \overline{)500.} \end{array} = 125 \text{ mL/hr}$$

**Step 2.** $\frac{\text{mL/hr} \times \text{TF}}{\# \text{ min}} = \text{gtt/min}$

> **Learning Aid**
>
> Note that the answer to Step 1 is 125 mL/hr.
> The answer to Step 2 is 125 gtt/min for microdrip. See next page.

Macrodrip

$$\frac{125 \times \overset{1}{\cancel{20}}}{\underset{3}{\cancel{60}}} = \frac{\cancel{125}}{3} \quad \begin{array}{r} 41.6 \\ 3\overline{)125.0} \\ \underline{12} \\ 5 \\ \underline{3} \\ 2\;0 \end{array}$$

Macrodrip at 42 gtt/min

Microdrip

$$\frac{125 \times \overset{1}{\cancel{60}}}{\underset{1}{\cancel{60}}} = 125 \text{ gtt/min}$$

Microdrip at 125 gtt/min

Logic: Answers are macrodrip at 42 gtt/min and microdrip at 125 gtt/min. Choose one. (See explanation for choosing the infusion set, following this discussion.)

Label the IV.

Set drip rate.

*EXAMPLE 3:*

Order: 500 mL D5⅓NS IVKVO for 24°

Available: microdrip at 60 gtt/mL; macrodrip 10 gtt/mL

Logic: Because no pump is available, choose the IV set. This is a two-step problem. The IV will run 24 hr.

**Step 1.** $\dfrac{\text{\# mL}}{\text{\# hr}} = \text{mL/hr}$

$$\frac{\cancel{500}}{24} \quad \begin{array}{r} 20.8 \\ 24\overline{)500.0} \\ \underline{48} \\ 20\;0 \\ \underline{19\;2} \end{array} = 21 \text{ mL/hr}$$

**Step 2.** $\dfrac{\text{mL/hr} \times \text{TF}}{\text{\# min}} = \text{gtt/min}$

Logic: The answer to Step 1 is 21 mL/hr. The number of minutes is 60. Work out the problem for micro- and macrodrip and make a nursing judgment about which tube to use.

Macrodrip

$$\frac{21 \times 10}{60} = \frac{21}{6} \quad \begin{array}{r} 3.5 \\ 6\overline{)21.0} \\ \underline{18} \\ 3\,0 \\ \underline{3\,0} \end{array}$$

Macrodrip at 4 gtt/min

Microdrip $\frac{21 \times 60}{60} = 21$ gtt/min

Logic: 4 gtt/min macrodrip is too slow. Choose microdrip. (See explanation for choosing the infusion set.)

Label the IV.

Select a microdrip infusion set.

Set the drip rate at 21 gtt/min.

---

## SELF TEST 1   Calculation of Drip Factors

*Calculate the drip factor for the following IV orders given in milliliters per hour or number of hours. Answers may be found at the end of the chapter.*

1. Order:    150 mL D5 .33NS IV q8h
   Available:  infusion pump

2. Order:    250 mL D5W; run at 25 L/hr
   Available:  infusion pump

3. Order:    1000 mL D5NS; run 100 mL/hr
   Available:  macrodrip (20 gtt/mL); microdrip (60 gtt/mL)

4. Order:    180 mL D5 ⅓ NS 12 N–6 PM
   Available:  macrodrip (10 gtt/mL); microdrip (60 gtt/mL)

5. Order:    1000 mL D5 .45S IV 4 PM–12 mid
   Available:  macrodrip (15 gtt/mL); microdrip (60 gtt/mL)

## Determining Hours an IV Will Run

It is helpful for the nurse to calculate approximately how long an IV will last so that the next IV can be prepared or new orders written. The rule is simple:

$$\frac{\text{Number of milliliters ordered}}{\text{Number of milliliters per hour}} = \text{number of hours to run}$$

---

**Learning Aid**

$$\frac{\#\ mL}{\#\ mL/hr} = \#\ hrs$$

---

**Example**     Order: 500 mL NS IV. Run 75 mL/hr.

Rule: $\dfrac{\#\ mL}{\#\ mL/hr} = \text{hrs}$

$$\frac{500\ mL}{75\ mL/hr} = 75 \overline{)500.00} \quad 6.67$$

$$\begin{array}{r} 450 \\ \hline 50\ 0 \\ 45\ 0 \\ \hline 5\ 00 \end{array}$$

The IV will last approximately 6.7 hours.

**Example**     Order: 1000 mL D5½ NS IV 8 AM–8 PM

No math necessary; 8 AM–8 PM = 12 hours

The IV will last 12 hours.

**Example**     Order: Aminophylline 500 mg in 250 mL D5W IV at 50 mL/hr

Rule: $\dfrac{\#\ mL}{\#\ mL/hr} = \#\ hr$

$$\frac{250\ mL}{50\ mL} = 5\ hrs$$

The IV will last 5 hours. Note that aminophylline must be added to the IV.

---

**SELF TEST 2**   **IV Infusions—Hours**

*Calculate the hours that the following IV orders will run. Answers are found at the end of this chapter.*

1. Order:   250 mL D5½ NS IV at 30 mL/hr      *8 hrs – 9hrs*

2. Order:   Ringer's lactate 500 mL IV. Run 60 mL/hr.   *8 - 9hrs*

3. Order:   1000 mL D5S IV 4 PM–2 AM *(10hrs)*   *100 ml/hr   10hrs*

4. Order:   1000 mL D5W IVKVO 24 hours   *24 hours*

5. Order:   500 mL D5½ S at 70 mL/hr   *7-8hrs*

## Choosing the Infusion Set

Experience will enable you to judge which IV tubing to use. Clinically you will be guided in making a choice. There is no problem when an electric infusion pump is used. The pump will deliver the amount programmed. There are specialized pumps in neonatal and intensive care units that can deliver 1 mL/hr and specialized syringe pumps that can deliver less than 1 mL/hr.

Some guidelines may be helpful when an IV pump is not available.

### Use Microdrip When

- The IV is to be administered over a long period.
- A small amount of fluid is to be infused.
- The macrodrops per minute are too few (Why? IV fluid flows by gravity. Blood flowing in the vein exerts a pressure. If the IV is too slow, blood pressure may force blood into the tube where it clots. The IV will stop.)

### Use Macrodrip When

- A large amount of fluid is ordered in a short time.
- The microdrips per minute are too many. Counting the drip rate becomes too difficult.

## Need for Continuous Observation

Many factors may interfere with the drip rate. Do not assume that once an IV is started it will continue to flow at the rate it was set. Check the IV frequently; IVs flow by gravity. As the amount of fluid decreases in the IV bag, pressure changes occur that may affect the rate. The patient's movements may kink the tube and shut off the flow, or the movements may change the position of the needle or catheter in the vein. The needle may be forced against the side of the blood vessel thereby changing the flow, or it may be forced out of the vessel, allowing fluid to enter the tissues (infiltration).

Infusion pumps have an alarm system that beeps to alert the nurse when the rate cannot be maintained or when the infusion is about to be completed.

## ▶ Adding Medications to IVs

When a continuous IV order includes a medication, add the medication to the IV and determine the rate of flow. In some institutions, the pharmacist adds the medications; in others, nurses add the medication.

## Medications Ordered Over Several Hours

**Example**

*EXAMPLE 1:*

Order: 1000 mL D5W with 20 mEq KCl IV 10 AM–10 PM

Available: vial of KCl 40 mEq/20 mL; microdrip (60 gtt/min); macrodrip (20 gtt/min)

*Formula Method*

Logic: $\dfrac{D}{H} \times S = A$  $\dfrac{\overset{1}{\cancel{20 \text{ mEq}}}}{\underset{\underset{1}{2}}{\cancel{40 \text{ mEq}}}} \times \overset{10}{\cancel{20}} \text{ mL} = 10 \text{ mL}$

Add 10 mL of KCl to the IV bag.

*Ratio-Proportion Method*

$$\frac{20 \text{ mL}}{40 \text{ mEq}} = \frac{x}{20 \text{ mEq}}$$

$$\frac{400}{40} = x$$

$$10 \text{ mL} = x$$

Use two steps to solve the drip factor.

Choose the tubing. The IV will run 12 hours.

**Step 1.** $\dfrac{\text{\# mL}}{\text{\# hr}} = \text{mL/hr}$ $\qquad \dfrac{1000}{12} = 83 \text{ mL/hr}$

**Step 2.** $\dfrac{\text{\# mL/hr} \times \text{TF}}{\text{\# min}} = \text{gtt/min}$

For macrodrip: $\dfrac{83 \times \overset{1}{\cancel{20}}}{\underset{3}{\cancel{60}}} = 28 \text{ gtt/min}$

For microdrip: mL/hr = gtt/min; hence, 83 gtt/min

Choose either drip rate.

Label the IV.

*EXAMPLE 2:*

Order: 5 MU penicillin G potassium in 1000 mL D5W IV q8h

Available: macrodrip (10 gtt/mL); microdrip (60 gtt/mL)

Logic: MU means million units. The order is for 5 million U of penicillin G potassium. Penicillin comes in 5 MU vials of powder. Directions say that the drug must be reconstituted with a minimum of 100 mL. The order states to add 5 MU to 1000 mL. The order is safe because you are adding 5 MU to 1000 mL. Use a 10-cc syringe to aseptically remove fluid from the 1000-mL bag of D5W and inject into the powder to make a solution. Withdraw the solution and inject into the bag. You now have 1000 mL D5W with the medication added. The IV will run 8 hours.

Two steps are needed:

**Step 1.** $\dfrac{\text{\# mL}}{\text{\# hr}} = \text{mL/hr}$ $\qquad \dfrac{\cancel{1000}\ 125}{8\ \overline{)1000.}} = 125 \text{ mL/hr}$

**Step 2.** $\dfrac{\text{\# mL/hr} \times \text{TF}}{\text{\# min}} = \text{gtt/min}$

Macrodrip: $\dfrac{125 \times \cancel{10}}{\cancel{60}} = \dfrac{\cancel{125}}{6\ \overline{)125.0}}\ \dfrac{20.8}{} = 21 \text{ gtt/min}$

Microdrip = 125 gtt/min; macrodrip = 21 gtt/min. Choose one.

Label the IV.

*EXAMPLE 3:*

Order: aminophylline 250 mg in 250 mL D5W IV; run at 50 cc/hr

Available: ampule of aminophylline labeled 1 g in 10 cc: Buretrol that delivers 60 gtt/mL (microdrip). See Figure 9-4.

Logic: The ampule of aminophylline has 1 g in 10 mL. This is equivalent to 1000 mg in 10 mL. You want 250 mg.

$$\frac{D}{H} \times S = A$$

*Formula Method*

$$\frac{\overset{1}{\cancel{250}}}{\underset{4}{\cancel{1000}}} \times 10 = \frac{\cancel{10}}{4} \quad \frac{2.5 \text{ mL}}{)10.0}$$

*Ratio-Proportion Method*

$$\frac{10 \text{ mL}}{1000 \text{ mg}} = \frac{x}{250 \text{ mg}}$$

$$\frac{2500}{1000} = x$$

$$2.5 \text{ mL} = x$$

Draw up 2.5 mL and inject into 250 mL D5W. You have 250 mg aminophylline in 250 mL D5W. Label the bag.

You want 50 cc/hr, and you have a Buretrol 60 gtt/mL.

$$\frac{\text{mL/hr} \times \text{TF}}{60} = \frac{50 \times \cancel{60}}{\cancel{60}} = 50 \text{ gtt/min}$$

Label the IV. Rate 50 cc/hr.

**Learning Aid**

The Buretrol is microdrip. No calculation is needed. mL/hr = gtt/min.

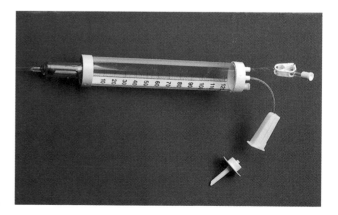

**FIGURE 9-4**

A Buretrol is an IV delivery system with tubing and a chamber that can hold 150 mL delivered as microdrip (1 mL = 60 drops). (This device is sometimes called a Volutrol.) The top of the Buretrol has a port so that a reservoir of fluid can be added. The Buretrol is a volume control because no more than 150 mL can be infused at one time. Because of the use of infusion pumps, it is rarely used.

**SELF TEST 3** | **IV Infustion Rates**

*Answers may be found at the end of the chapter.*

1. Order: 500 mL D5W IV with vitamin C 500 mg at 60 cc/hr
   Available: Ampule of vitamin C labeled 500 mg/2 mL; Microdrip tubing at 60 gtt/mL

2. Order: 250 mg hydrocortisone sodium succinate in 1000 mL D5W 8AM–12 mid
   Available: Vial of hydrocortisone sodium succinate labeled 250 mg with a 2-mL diluent; Microdrip tubing and macrodrip tubing at 20 gtt/mL

3. Order: aminophylline 250 mg in 250 mL D5W IV. Run 50 cc/hr.
   Available: Infusion pump Vial of aminophylline labeled 500 mg/10 mL

4. Order: 250 cc D5½ NS with KCl 10 mEq IV 12 N–6 PM
   Available: Microdrip tubing Vial of potassium chloride labeled 20 mEq/10 mL

## ▶ Medications for Intermittent Intravenous Administration

Some intravenous medications are not administered continuously but only intermittently such as q4h, q6h, or q8h. This route is termed intravenous piggyback or IVPB (Fig. 9-5).

Most of these drugs are prepared in powder form. The manufacturer specifies the type and amount of diluent needed to reconstitute the drug, which is connected by IV tubing to the main IV line.

The doctor may write a detailed order: vancomycin 0.5 g IVPB in 100 mL D5W over 1 hr. More often the doctor will write only the drug, route, and time interval, relying on the nurse to research the manufacturer's directions for the amount and type of diluent and the time for the infusion to run (e.g., Order: cefazolin 1 g IVPB q6h).

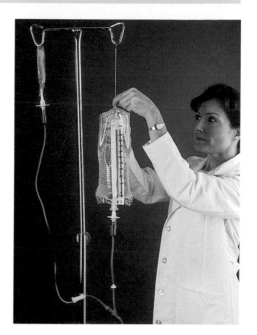

**FIGURE 9-5**

Photo of a primary IV line (right) and an IVPB (or secondary) line (left). Fluid flows continuously through the primary line into the patient's vein. At timed intervals medication placed in an intravenous piggyback bag (IVPB) is attached by tubing to the primary IV for delivery to the patient. The primary fluid is lowered and the IVPB fluid flows. After the IVPB has infused, the primary fluid begins infusing again.

## Explanation

The rule to solve IVPB problems is similar to the IV rule:

$$\frac{\# \, mL \times TF}{\# \, min} = gtt/min$$

# mL: The type and amount of diluent will be stated on the label or in the package insert. Nurses' drug references and the *Physicians Drug Reference (PDR)* also contain this information.

TF: The tubing for IVPB is called a secondary administration set and has a macrodrip factor. It is shorter than main line IV tubing. To solve IVPB problems we will use the tube factor 10 gtt = 1 mL. In the clinical setting, check the label for the tube factor.

# min: The manufacturer may or may not indicate the number of minutes needed for the IVPB medication to be infused. When the number is not given, a general rule to follow for adults is to allow 30 minutes for every 50 mL of solution.

**Example**

Order: cefazolin 1 g IVPB q6h

Stock: Package insert for IVPB dilution of cefazolin sodium: Reconstitute with 50 to 100 mL of Sodium Chloride injection or other solution listed under administration. Other solutions listed include: D5W, D10W, D5LR, D5NS.

Let's use 50 mL D5W. It is the most common IVPB diluent and we have 50 mL bags. No time for infusion is given in the directions for "piggyback" vials. Use 30 minutes for 50 mL.

$$\frac{\# \text{ mL} \times \text{TF}}{\# \text{ min}} = \text{gtt/min}$$

$\# \text{ mL} = 50 \text{ mL D5W}$

$\text{TF} = 10 \text{ gtt/mL}$ (For a secondary administration no set time for administration is given. Follow the general adult rule of 30 minutes for every 50 mL.)

$\# \text{ min} = 30$

$$\frac{50 \times 10}{30} = 16.6 = 17 \text{ gtt/min}$$

You are ready to prepare the IVPB. You have a vial of powder labeled 1 gram. You need the whole amount. You have a 50 mL bag of D5W. You need the whole amount. Use a reconstitution device to mix the powder and the diluent. A reconstitution device is a sterile implement containing two needles that connect the vial and the 50 mL bag. It enables the nurse to dilute the powder and place it in the IV bag without using a syringe (Fig. 9-6). Once the powder is reconstituted, label the IV bag.

| **Medication Added** | |
| --- | --- |
| **Patient**  *Tom Smith* | **Room**  *1503* |
| **Date**  *cefazolin 1g* | **Flow Rate**  *17 gtt/min* |
| **Base solution**  *50 mL D5W* | **Initials**  *RT* |
| **Time to Run**  *12 n–12:30 pm* | **Date**  *6/14* |

Note that the Time to Run is 12 N–12:30. Why? The order was q6h (6 AM–12 N–6 PM–12 M) and the time of infusion was 30 minutes.

It is time-consuming to look through package inserts for directions. Drug references such as *Lippincott's Nursing Drug Guide* provide concise information.

**Example**   Order: vancomycin 1 g IVPB 7 AM

Stock: 500 mg powder.

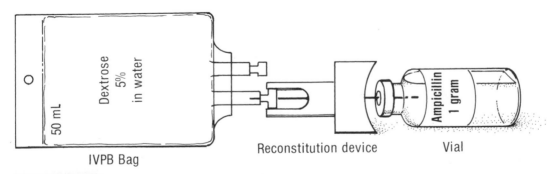

IVPB Bag        Reconstitution device        Vial

**FIGURE 9-6**

Reconstitution device. The IVPB bag is squeezed, forcing fluid into the vial of powder, which is then diluted. The three parts are turned to a vertical position—vial up, IVPB bag down. The IVPB bag is squeezed and released. This creates a negative pressure, allowing the diluted medication to flow into the IVPB bag.

Package insert directions: 250 mL (1 Gram)/05W.NS
2 hours (1 Gram)/7 days (REFRIGERATED)

Rule: $\dfrac{\#\,\text{mL} \times \text{TF}}{\#\,\text{min}} = \text{gtt/min}$

$$\frac{250 \times 10}{120} = \frac{250}{12} \quad 12\,\overline{)250.0}^{\;20.8} = 21$$

Use a reconstitution device to add 1 gram of vancomycin (2 vials of 500 mg) to 250 mL D5W. Label the IV. Set the rate at 21 gtt/min. The IVPB will run 2 hours.

**SELF TEST 4** | **IVPB Drip Factors**

*Solve these drip factors for IVPB problems. Answers may be found at the end of this chapter.*

1.     Order:   acyclovir 500 mg IVPB q8h
      Stock:   500 mg powder
Package directions:   100 mL/D5W.NS 1 hour/24 hours

2.     Order:   ceftazidime 1 g IVPB q12h
      Stock:   1 gram powder
Package directions:   50 mL (1 gram)/D5W.NS 15–30 minutes/7
            days (REFRIGERATED)

3.     Order:   cefotaxime 1 g IVPB q6h
      Stock:   1 gram powder
Package directions:   50 mL (1 gram)/D5W.NS 15–30 minutes/5
            days (REFRIGERATED)

## Admixture IVs

The institutional pharmacy may reconstitute and prepare IVPB solutions in a sterile environment using a laminar flow hood. This procedure saves nursing time: drugs are prepared, labeled, and screened for incompatibilities. However, the nurse is not relieved of responsibility. Check the diluent and volume with guidelines. Check the dose and the expiration date of the reconstituted solution. Note whether the admixture should be refrigerated before use or can remain at room temperature until hung. The nurse must calculate the drip rate and record this information on the IVPB label before hanging the bag.

## ▶ Changing the Intravenous Drip Rate

Setting the drip rate for an IV does not relieve the nurse of the responsibility to check the IV frequently. Many factors can interfere with the flow—kinking of the tube, movement of the client, the effect of gravity, or placement of the needle or catheter. If a discrepancy in flow exists, it may be necessary to recalculate the IV drip.

**Example**

As you make rounds, you check a client's IV. The label reads:

1000 mL D5W IV to run 8 AM–4 PM

The tubing is macrodrip (10 gtt/mL). Rate is set at 20 gtt/min.

It is now 1 PM. You note that there is 600 mL left in the IV. Should you change the drip?

Logic: **Step 1.** Calculate how many milliliters per hour.

$$\frac{1000}{8} = 125 \text{ mL/hr}$$

**Step 2.** It is now 1 PM. Therefore 5 hours have elapsed since the IV was started.

125 mL/hr
$\times$ 5 hr
$\overline{\quad}$
625 mL should have been delivered.

**Step 3.** Because there are 600 mL left in the IV, only 400 mL were delivered.

625 mL should have been delivered
400 mL were delivered
$\overline{\quad}$
225 mL behind

Conclusion: The nurse will have to make a judgment about whether to increase the IV drip on the basis of an assessment of the client's status. It may be necessary to consult with the physician.

## Recording Intake

An accurate account must be kept of parenteral intake as well as liquids taken orally, enterally (eg, tube feedings). Each institution will provide a flow sheet to record fluid input over a period of time specified.

---

**SELF TEST 5** | **Fluid Intake**

*Answer the following questions regarding fluid intake. Answers may be found at the end of this chapter.*

1. 900 mL of an IV solution is to infuse at 100 mL/hr. If it is 9 AM when the infusion starts, at what time will it be completed? 6 pm

2. A patient is receiving an antibiotic IVPB in 75 mL q6h plus a maintenance IV of 125 mL/hr. What is the 24-hour intake parenterally? 300 + 3000 = 3300

3. An IV of 1000 mL D5NS is infusing at 10 microdrips per minute. What is the parenteral intake for 8 hours? 4800

4. A doctor orders 500 mL aminophylline 0.5 g to infuse at 50 mL/hr. How many mg will the patient receive each hour? 10 mL

5. 20,000 units of heparin is added to 500 mL D5W, and the order is to infuse IV at 30 mL/hr. How many hours will the IV run?

*Solve these problems related to intravenous and IVPB drip rates. Aim for a high degree of accuracy. Answers may be found at the end of the chapter. Review material that you find difficult.*

1.  Order:  1500 mL D5W 8 AM–8 PM
    Available:  macrodrip tubing (10 gtt/mL)
    What is the drip rate?

    $$\frac{1500}{12} = \frac{125 \times 10}{60} \quad 20\text{–}21 \text{ gtt/min}$$

2.  Order:  250 mL D5 ½ NS IV KVO (give over 12 hours)  250  20–21 gtt/min
    Available:  microdrip tubing
    What is the drip rate?

3.  Order:  150 mL D5 ⅓ NS IV; run 20 mL/hr
    Available:  infusion pump

    $$\frac{150 \times}{20} = 7.5$$

    a.  What is the drip rate?
    b.  How long will the IV last?

4.  Order:  1000 mL D5S with 15 mEq KCl IV; run 100 mL/hr
    Available:  macrotubing (20 gtt/mL) and microdrip

    a.  How many hours will this run? 10
    b.  How many milliliters of KCl will you add to the IV if KCl comes in a vial labeled 40 mEq/20 mL?
    c.  What tubing will you use?
    d.  What are the gtt/min?

    $$\frac{100 \times 20}{60} = 33\text{–}34 \text{ gtt/min}$$

5.  Order:  aminophylline 1 g in 500 mL D5W IV at 75 mL/hr
    Available:  vial of aminophylline 1 g in 10 mL; infusion pump

    a.  How many mL of aminophylline should be added to the IV?
    b.  How will you set the drip rate?

6.  Order:  amikacin 0.4 g IVPB q8h
    Stock:  2 mL vial labeled 250 mg/mL
    See Table 9-2 for directions.

7.  Order:  500 mL D5 ½ S IV q8h
    Available:  microdrip tubing
    What are the gtt/min?

    $$\frac{62.5 \times 60}{60} = 62\text{–}63 \text{ gtt/min}$$

*Answers may be found at the end of this chapter.*

1. Order:   aqueous penicillin G 1 MU in 100 mL D5W IVPB q6h
   over 40 minutes (macrodrip tubing at 10 gtt/mL)
   Stock:   vial labeled 5 million units of powder. Directions say to
   inject 18 mL of sterile water for injection to yield 20 mL
   of solution. Reconstituted solution is stable for 1 week.

   a. How would you prepare the penicillin?
   b. What solution will you make?
   c. What amount of penicillin solution should be placed into the bag
   of 100 mL D5W?
   d. What is the drip factor for the IVPB?

2. 1000 mL of an IV solution is to infuse at 100 mL/hr. If the infusion
   starts at 8 AM, at what time will it be completed?

3. Order:   Gentamicin 60 mg IVPB in 50 mL D5W over 30 minutes
   using macrodrip (20 gtt/cc)
   Stock:   vial of gentamicin 40 mg/mL; 50-mL bag of D5W. Order
   is correct

   a. How many mL of gentamicin will you add to the 50-mL bag of
   D5W?
   b. What is the drip factor for the IVPB? Note microdrip factor.

4. Calculate the drip factor for 1500 mL D5 ½ NS to run 12 hours by
   macrodrip (10 gtt/mL).

5. Intralipid, 500 mL q6h, is ordered for a patient together with an IV
   that is infusing at 80 mL/hr. Calculate the 24-hour parenteral intake.

6. Order:   1000 mL D5W with 20 mEq KCl and 500 mg Vit C at 60
   mL/hr. No infusion pump is available.

   a. Approximately how many hours will the IV run?
   b. Which tubing will you choose—macrodrip at 10 gtt/mL or
   microdrip at 60 gtt/mL?
   c. What are the drops per minute (gtt/min) for the tubing that you
   choose?

**PROFICIENCY TEST 1**   Basic IV Problems

*Name:* _____

*There are 10 questions related to IV and IVPB calculations. If you have any difficulty doing these problems, review the information in Chapter 9 that explains this information. Answers will be found on page 350.*

1. Order:   1000 mL D5NS; run 150 mL/hr IV
   Stock:   IV bag of 1000 mL D5NS

   a. Approximately how many hours will the IV run?   6.6 hrs
   b. Which tubing will you choose—macrodrip (10 gtt/min) or
      microdrip (60 gtt/min)?
   c. What will be the drip rate?   25 gtt/min

2. Order:   100 mL Ringer's solution 12 noon–6 PM IV   16.6 per hr

   a. What size tubing will you use?   16.6 × 60
   b. What are the gtt/min?              ———————  ~ 17 gtt/min
                                            60

3. Order:   150 mL NS IV over 3 hours
   Stock:   bag of 250 mL normal saline for IV and macrotubing 15
            gtt/mL; microtubing (60 gtt/mL)

   a. What would you do to obtain 150 mL NS?
   b. What IV tubing would you use?
   c. What are the gtt/min?

4. Order:   500 mL D5W IVKVO. Solve for 24 hours. An infusion
            pump is available. What should be the setting on the
            infusion pump?

5. Order:   doxycycline 100 mg
            IVPB qd
   Stock:   100 mg powder. See Table 9-2 for directions.
   State the amount and type of IV fluid you will use and the time for
   infusion you will use.
   What are the gtt/min?

6.   Order:   aminophylline 500 mg in 250 mL D5W to run 8 hours   31.25 mL/hr
              IV
     Available:   vial of aminophylline labeled 1 gram in 10 mL;
                  microdrip tubing
     What is the drip rate?

7. A patient is receiving an IV at the rate of 125 mL/hr. The doctor
   orders cefoxitin 1 g in 75 mL D5W q6h.
   Calculate the 24-hour parenteral intake.

8. Order:   1000 mL D5 ½ NS to run at 90 mL/hr; infusion pump
            available

   a. What will be the pump setting?
   b. Approximately how long will the IV run?

*(continued)*

9. A doctor orders 500 mL of aminophylline 0.5 g to infuse at 50 mL/hr. How many milligrams will the patient receive each hour?

10. Order:    Bactrim 5 mL IVPB q6h
    Stock:    vial of 5 mL. Refer to Table 9-2 for directions.
              Main IV line is connected to an infusion pump. What will you do? Refer to Figure 9-4.

    a. State and type and amount of IV fluid you would use and the time for infusion.
    b. How would you program the infusion pump?

# Answers

### Self-Test 1 Calculation of Drip Factors

1. Logic: This is a continuous IV of 150 mL every 8 hours. There is a pump available. You only need Step 1.
   It will run 8 hr.

   $$\frac{\# \text{ mL}}{\# \text{ hr}} = \text{mL/hr} \qquad \frac{150 \text{ mL}}{8} \quad \frac{18.7 \text{ mL/hr}}{)150.0}$$

   $$\begin{array}{r} 8 \\ \hline 70 \\ 64 \\ \hline 6\,0 \\ 5\,6 \\ \hline \end{array}$$

   Label the IV. Set the pump:
   Total # mL: 150
   mL/hr: 19

2. Logic: This is a continuous IV. A pump is available. The order states mL/hr. There is no calculation needed. Label the IV. Set the pump as follows:
   Total # mL: 250
   mL/hr: 25

3. Logic: The order gives 100 mL/hr; mL/hr = gtt per minute microdrip, so you know the microdrip is 100 gtt/min. Work out the macrodrip factor and choose the tubing. You need Step 2.
   Macrodrip

   $$\text{Step 2.} \quad \frac{\text{mL/hr} \times \text{TF}}{\# \text{ min}} = \text{gtt/min}$$

   $$\frac{100 \times \overset{1}{\cancel{20}}}{\underset{3}{\cancel{60}}} = \frac{100}{3} = 33.3$$

   Macrodrip at 33 gtt/min
   Microdrip at 100 gtt/min
   Either drip rate could be used. Label the IV.

4. Logic: This is a small volume over several hours; use microdrip. Macrodrip would be too slow (5 gtt/min).

   $$\text{Step 1.} \quad \frac{\# \text{ mL}}{\# \text{ hr}} = \text{mL/hr} \qquad \frac{\overset{30}{\cancel{180}}}{\underset{1}{\cancel{8}}} = 30 \text{ mL/hr}$$

   $$\text{Step 2.} \quad \frac{\text{mL/hr} \times \text{TF}}{\# \text{ min}} = \text{gtt/min}$$

   Microdrip is 30 gtt/min because mL/hr = gtt/min.

5. Logic: This is a large volume over several hours; use macrodrip. Solve using two steps and decide.

   $$\text{Step 1.} \quad \frac{\# \text{ mL}}{\# \text{ hr}} = \text{mL/hr} \qquad \frac{\overset{125}{\cancel{1000}}}{\underset{1}{\cancel{8}}} = 125 \text{ mL}$$

   $$\text{Step 2.} \quad \frac{\text{mL/hr} \times \text{TF}}{\# \text{ min}} = \text{gtt/min}$$

   You know microdrip will be 125 gtt/min because mL/hr = gtt/min.
   Macrodrip

   $$\frac{125 \times \overset{1}{\cancel{15}}}{\underset{4}{\cancel{60}}} = \frac{\cancel{125}}{4} \quad \frac{31.2}{)125.0}$$

   $$\begin{array}{r} 12 \\ \hline 5 \\ 4 \\ \hline 1\,0 \\ 8 \\ \hline \end{array}$$

   Macrodrip at 31 gtt/min
   Microdrip at 125 gtt/min
   Use macrodrip.
   Label the IV.

### Self-Test 2 IV Infusions—hours

1. 8.3 hours approximately
2. 8.3 hours approximately
3. 10 hours (no math)
4. 24 hours (no math)
5. 7.1 hours approximately

## Self-Test 3 IV Infusion Rates

1. Logic: You want vitamin C 500 mg and the stock is 500 mg in 2 mL. Use a syringe to add the 2 mL to 500 mL D5W. You have microdrip available. The IV is to run at 60 cc/hr. Remember mL/hr = gtt/min for microdrip. No math necessary. Set the microdrip at 60 gtt/min. Label the IV.

2. Logic: You want 250 mg hydrocortisone sodium succinate, and it comes 250 mg with a 2 mL diluent. Use a syringe to reconstitute the hydrocortisone with 2 mL diluent and add it to the IV. 8 AM–12 MID is 16 hours. Microdrip tubing seems indicated. Solve using two steps.

   Step 1. $\dfrac{\#\,mL}{\#\,hr} = mL/hr$

$$\frac{1000}{16} \quad \frac{62.5}{)1000.0} = 63 \text{ mL/hr}$$
$$\frac{96}{40}$$
$$\frac{32}{8\ 0}$$
$$\frac{8\ 0}{}$$

   Step 2. mL/hr = gtt/min for microdrip. No math for microdrip. Microdrip = 63 gtt/min

   Macrodrip $\dfrac{mL/hr}{min} = gtt/min$

   $\dfrac{63 \times 20}{60} = 20.5 = 21 \text{ gtt/min}$

   Label the IV.
   Microdrip 63 gtt/min; macrodrip 21 gtt/min
   Choose one.

3. Logic: You want 250 mg aminophylline. Stock is 500 mg/10 mL.

   | *Formula Method* | *Ratio-Proportion Method* |
   |---|---|
   | $\dfrac{D}{H} \times S = A \quad \dfrac{250\ mg}{500\ mg} \times 10\ mL = 5\ mL$ | $\dfrac{10\ mL}{500\ mg} = \dfrac{x}{250\ mg}$ |
   | | $\dfrac{2500}{500} = x$ |
   | | $5 = x$ |

   Add 5 mL aminophylline to 250 mL D5W. Order is 50 cc/hr. You have an infusion pump. No math. Set the pump as follows:
   Total # mL: 250
   mL/hr: 50

**4.** Logic: You want KCl 10 mEq. Stock is 20 mEq/ 10 mL.

*Formula Method*

$$\frac{D}{H} \times S = A \qquad \frac{10\ mEq}{20\ mEq} \times 10\ mL = 5\ mL$$

*Ratio-Proportion Method*

$$\frac{10\ mL}{20\ mEq} = \frac{x}{10\ mEq}$$

$$\frac{100}{20} = x$$

$$5\ mL = x$$

Add 5 mL KCl to 250 mL D5W½NS. 12 N–6 PM is 6 hours. One step is needed because you have microdrip tubing.

$$\frac{\#\ mL}{\#\ hr} = mL/hr \qquad \frac{250}{6} \quad \frac{41.6}{)250.0} = 42\ mL/hr$$

$$\begin{array}{r} 24 \\ \hline 10 \\ 6 \\ \hline 40 \\ 36 \\ \hline \end{array}$$

mL/hr = gtt/min microdrip
Set the microdrip at 42 gtt/min.
Label the IV.

## Self-Test 4 IVPB Drip Factors

**1.** Logic: acyclovir comes in 500 mg powder. Use a reconstitution device to add the powder to 100 mL D5W; # min = 60; TF = 10 gtt/mL for IVPB

Rule: $\dfrac{\#\ mL \times TF}{\#\ min} = gtt/min$

$$\frac{100 \times 10}{60} = \frac{100}{6} \quad \frac{16.6}{)100.0} = 17\ gtt/min$$

Label the IVPB.
Set the rate at 17 gtt/min.

**2.** Logic: ceftazidime comes in a 1 gram powder. Use a reconstitution device to add the powder to 50 mL D5W; # min = 30; TF = 10 gtt/mL for IVPB

Rule: $\dfrac{\#\ mL \times TF}{\#\ min} = gtt/min$

$$\frac{50 \times 10}{60} = \frac{50}{3} = 16.6 = 17\ gtt/min$$

Label the IVPB.
Set the rate at 17 gtt/min.

**3.** Logic: cefotaxime comes as a 1 gram powder. Use a reconstitution device to add the powder to 50 mL D5W; # min = 30; TF = 10 gtt/mL for IVPB

Rule: $\dfrac{\#\ mL \times TF}{\#\ min} = gtt/min$

$$\frac{50 \times 10}{30} = 16.6 = 17\ gtt/min$$

Label the IVPB.
Set the rate at 17 gtt/min.

## Self-Test 5 Fluid Intake

1. Logic: 900 mL at 100 mL/hr = 9 hr to run. If the IV starts at 9 AM + 9 hr = 6 PM.
2. Logic: IVPB is 75 mL q6h or 4 times in 24 hr.

    $$\begin{array}{r} 75 \\ \times\ 4 \\ \hline 300\ \text{mL} \end{array}$$   The patient is receiving 125 mL for 24 hours.

    $$\begin{array}{r} 125\ \text{mL} \\ \times\ 24\ \text{hr} \\ \hline 500 \\ 250 \\ \hline 3000\ \text{mL} \end{array}$$   $$\begin{array}{r} 3000\ \text{mL} \\ +\ 300\ \text{mL} \\ \hline 3300\ \text{mL in 24 hr} \end{array}$$

3. Logic: IV is infusing at 10 microdrips/min. It takes 60 microdrips to make 1 mL, so 1 mL in 6 min, 10 mL in 60 min.

    $$\begin{array}{r} 10\ \text{mL in 60 min (1 hr)} \\ \times\ 8\ \text{hr} \\ \hline 80\ \text{mL in 8 hr} \end{array}$$

4. Logic: The IV is 0.5 g or 500 mg in 500 mL. This is equal to 1 mg/mL. The patient receives 50 mL/hr, so the patient receives 50 mg each hour.
5. Logic: The IV is infusing at 30 mL/hr and the solution is 500 mL.

    $$\frac{500\ \text{mL}}{30\ \text{mL/hr}} = \frac{50}{3} = 16.6\ \text{hr approximately}$$

## Self-Test 6 IV Drip Rates

1. $\frac{\#\ \text{mL}}{\#\ \text{hr}} = \text{mL/hr}$   $\frac{1500}{12} \quad \overset{125.}{)\overline{1500.}} = 125\ \text{mL/hr}$

    $$\begin{array}{r} 12 \\ \hline 30 \\ 24 \\ \hline 60 \\ 60 \end{array}$$

    *macro*

    $$\frac{\#\ \text{mL/hr} \times \text{TF}}{\#\ \text{min}} = \text{gtt/min} \quad \frac{125 \times 10}{60} = \frac{125}{6} \quad \overset{20.8}{)\overline{125.0}}$$

    $$\begin{array}{r} 12 \\ \hline 5\ 0 \\ 4\ 8 \end{array}$$

    = 21 gtt/min

2. $\frac{\#\ \text{mL}}{\#\ \text{hr}} = \text{mL/hr}$   $\frac{250}{12} \quad \overset{20.8}{)\overline{250.0}} = 21\ \text{mL/hr}$

    $$\begin{array}{r} 24 \\ \hline 10\ 0 \\ 9\ 6 \end{array}$$

    # mL/hr × TF = gtt/min  21 × 60 = 21 gtt/min

    You could also say mL/hr = gtt/min microdrip, so 21 mL/hr = 21 gtt/min.

3. $\frac{150\ \text{mL}}{20\ \text{mL/hr}} = \frac{15}{2} \quad \overset{7.5\ \text{hr}}{)\overline{15.0\ \text{hr}}}$

    a. The drip rate is 20 mL/hr. No math is necessary. Set the infusion pump.

    b. The IV will last approximately 7½ hours.

4. a. $\overset{10}{\dfrac{1000\ \text{mL}}{100\ \text{mL/hr}}} = 10\ \text{hr}$

    b. $\dfrac{D}{H} \times S = A$   $\dfrac{15\ \text{mEq}}{\underset{2}{40\ \text{mEq}}} \times \overset{1}{20}\ \text{mL} = \dfrac{15}{2} = 7.5\ \text{mL}$

    c. Microdrip. Order states to run at 100 mL/hr. mL/hr = gtt/min microdrip, so microdrip at 100 gtt/min

    Macrodrip. $\dfrac{100 \times \overset{1}{20}}{\underset{3}{60}} = \dfrac{100}{3} = 33\ \text{gtt/min}$

    Choose either tubing.

    d. 33 gtt/min macrodrip; 100 gtt/min microdrip

5. a. You desire 1 g. Aminophylline comes 1 g in 10 mL. Add 10 mL to the IV of 500 mL D5W and label.

    b. You have an infusion pump; there is no math.
    Set the pump:
    Total # mL: 500
    mL/hr: 75

**6.** $0.4 \text{ g} = 400 \text{ mg}$    $\dfrac{D}{H} \times S = A$

$$\dfrac{\overset{8}{\cancel{400} \text{ mg}}}{\underset{5}{\cancel{250} \text{ mg}}} \times 1 \text{ mL} = \dfrac{8}{5}\overset{1.6 \text{ mL}}{\overline{)8.0}}$$

Add 1.6 mL amikacin to 100 mL D5W;
TF = 10 gtt/mL for IVPB; # min = 30

$$\dfrac{\# \text{ mL} \times \text{TF}}{\# \text{ min}} = \text{gtt/min} \qquad \dfrac{100 \text{ mL} \times \cancel{10}}{\cancel{30}} = \dfrac{100}{3} = 33.3$$
$$= 33 \text{ gtt/min}$$

Label the IV.
Set the rate at 33 gtt/min.

**7.** $\dfrac{\# \text{ mL}}{\# \text{ hr}} = \text{mL/hr}$   $\dfrac{500}{8}\overset{62.5}{\overline{)500.0}} = 63 \text{ mL/hr}$

$\qquad \dfrac{48}{20}$
$\qquad \dfrac{16}{4\ 0}$
$\qquad \dfrac{}{4\ 0}$

You are using microdrip, so mL/hr = gtt/min.
Set the rate at 63 gtt/min.

## Self-Test 7 IV Problems

**1. a.** Add 18 mL of sterile water for injection to the vial of 5 million units (5 MU).
   **b.** Solution is 5 MU/20 mL.

   **c.** You want 1 MU so $\dfrac{D}{H} \times S = A$

   $$\dfrac{1 \text{ MU}}{\cancel{5} \text{ MU}} \times \overset{4}{\cancel{20}} \text{ mL} = 4 \text{ mL}$$

   **d.** $\dfrac{\# \text{ mL} \times \text{TF}}{\# \text{ min}} = \text{gtt/min}$   $\dfrac{\overset{25}{\cancel{100} \text{ mL}} \times \cancel{10}}{\underset{1}{\cancel{40}}} = 25 \text{ gtt/min}$

**2.** Logic: 1000 mL is infusing at 100 mL/hr, so the IV will take

$$\dfrac{\overset{10}{\cancel{1000}}}{\underset{1}{\cancel{100}}} = 10 \text{ hours to complete.}$$

If it starts at 8 AM, it should finish 10 hours later at 6 PM.

**3. a.** $\dfrac{D}{H} \times S = A$   $\dfrac{\overset{3}{\cancel{60} \text{ mg}}}{\underset{2}{\cancel{40} \text{ mg}}} \times 1 \text{ mL} = \dfrac{3}{2}\overset{1.5 \text{ mL}}{\overline{)3.0}}$

Add 1.5 mL gentamicin.

**b.** $\dfrac{\# \text{ mL} \times \text{TF}}{\# \text{ min}} = \text{gtt/min}$

$$\dfrac{50 \text{ mL} \times \cancel{20}}{30} = \dfrac{\cancel{100}}{3}\overset{33.3}{\overline{)100.00}} = 33 \text{ gtt/min}$$

**4.** Step 1. $\dfrac{\# \text{ mL}}{\# \text{ hr}} = \text{mL/hr}$

$$\dfrac{1500}{12}\overset{125.}{\overline{)1500.}} = 125 \text{ mL/hr}$$
$$\dfrac{12}{30}$$
$$\dfrac{24}{60}$$
$$\dfrac{60}{}$$

Step 2. $\dfrac{\# \text{ mL/hr} \times \text{TF}}{60} = \text{gtt/min}$

$$\dfrac{125 \times 10}{60} = \dfrac{\cancel{125}}{6}\overset{20.8}{\overline{)125.0}} = 21 \text{ gtt/min}$$
$$\dfrac{12}{5\ 0}$$
$$\dfrac{}{4\ 8}$$

**5.** Logic: Intralipid 500 mL q6h means the patient is receiving 500 mL four times every 24 hours.

$$\begin{array}{r} 500 \\ \times\ 4 \\ \hline 2000 \text{ mL} \end{array}$$

The IV is infusing 80 mL/hr. There are 24 hr in a day so

$$\begin{array}{r} 24 \\ \times\ 80 \\ \hline 1920 \end{array}$$

Adding these we have $\begin{array}{r} 2000 \text{ mL} \\ +\ 1920 \text{ mL} \\ \hline 3920 \text{ mL} \end{array}$

**6. a.** You have 1000 mL running at 60 mL/hr; therefore

$$60 \overline{)1000.0} = \text{approximately } 16\frac{1}{2} \text{ hours}$$

$$\begin{array}{r} 16.6 \\ 60 \overline{)1000.0} \\ \underline{60} \\ 400 \\ \underline{360} \\ 40\ 0 \end{array}$$

**b.** Logic: If you want 60 mL/hr and use microdrip tubing, the drip factor will be 60 gtt/min:

$$\frac{\# \text{ mL} \times \text{TF}}{60} = \frac{60 \times \cancel{60}}{\cancel{60}} = 60 \text{ gtt/min}$$

If you use macrodrip you have $\dfrac{\cancel{60} \times 10}{\cancel{60}}$

= 10 gtt/min

Because the IV will run over 16 hours, choose *microdrip tubing*.

**c.** The drip factor will be 60 gtt/min.

*Note:* It is not incorrect to choose the macrodrip at 10 gtt/min. However, because the IV will run so many hours, a good flow might help to keep the IV running.

# Special Types of Intravenous Calculations

CONTENT TO MASTER

▶ Rules and calculations for special IV orders
units/hr; mg/hr; g/hr; mL/hr; mg/min
milliunits/min; mcg/min; mg/kg/min

▶ Use of the body surface nomogram

▶ Calculating meters squared (m²) for IV medications

▶ Patient-controlled analgesia (PCA)

## ▶ Overview

In Chapter 9 we studied rules and calculations for microdrip and macrodrip factors, the use of the infusion pump, and IVPB orders.

In this chapter we consider rules and calculations for orders written in units, milliunits, and micrograms; how to calculate safety of doses based in kilograms of body weight and body surface area; and how orders for patient-controlled analgesia (PCA) are handled.

## ▶ Medications Ordered in Units/hr, mg/hr, or mL/hr

Patient medications may be administered as continuous IVs. Solutions for these medications are standardized to decrease possibility of error. Check guidelines to verify dose, dilution, and rate. If any doubts exist, consult with the prescribing physician.

### Units/hr—Rule and Calculation

The order will indicate the amount of drug to be added to IV fluid and the flow rate in units/hr.

**Example**

Order: heparin sodium 40,000 units in 1000 mL D5W IV. Infuse 800 units/hr on a pump.

Logic: We know the solution and the amount to administer. Because a pump will be used, the answer will be in mL/hr.

**Learning Aid**

An explanation of infusion pumps is given in Chapter 9.

$$\frac{\overset{20}{\cancel{800} \text{ units/hr}}}{\underset{\underset{1}{4}}{\cancel{40,000} \text{ units}}} \times \cancel{1000} \text{ mL} =$$

20 mL/hr on a pump

Note that units cancel out and the answer is mL/hr.

*Formula Method*

Rule: $\dfrac{D}{H} \times S = A$

*Ratio Proportion Method*

$$\frac{\text{x cc}}{800 \text{ units}} = \frac{1000 \text{ cc}}{40,000 \text{ units}}$$

$$\frac{\text{x}}{800} = .025$$

$$\text{x} = .025 \times 800$$

$$\text{x} = 20 \text{ mL/hr}$$

**Learning Aid**

Desire = 800 units/hr

Have = 40,000 units

Stock = 1000 mL D5W

**Example**

Order: heparin sodium 1100 units/hr IV

Available: infusion pump; standard solution of 25,000 units in 250 mL D5W

*Formula Method*

Rule: $\dfrac{D}{H} \times S = A$

$$\frac{1 \overset{11}{\cancel{100}} \text{ units/hr} \times 250 \text{ mL}}{\underset{\underset{1}{\cancel{100}}}{\cancel{25,000} \text{ units}}} =$$

11 mL/hr on a pump

*Ratio Proportion Method*

$$\frac{\text{x mL}}{1100 \text{ units}} = \frac{250 \text{ mL}}{25000}$$

$$\text{x mL} = \frac{27500}{25000}$$

$$\text{x} = 11 \text{ mL/hr}$$

**Learning Aid**

Standard solutions are prepared by pharmacy.

**Learning Aid**

Units cancel and the answer is mL/hr, the setting for the infusion pump.

**Example**

Order: Regular insulin 10 units/hr IV

Available: infusion pump; standard solution of 125 units Regular insulin in 250 mL NS

| *Formula Method* | *Ratio Proportion Method* |
|---|---|

*Formula Method*

$$\frac{D}{H} \times S = A$$

$$\frac{10 \text{ units} \times 250 \text{ mL}}{125 \text{ units}} = \frac{2500}{125} =$$

20 mL/hr on a pump

*Ratio Proportion Method*

$$\frac{x \text{ mL}}{10 \text{ units}} = \frac{250 \text{ mL}}{125}$$

$$x \text{ mL} = \frac{2500}{125}$$

$$x = 20 \text{ mL/hr}$$

## *mg/hr; g/hr—Rule and Calculation*

The order will indicate the amount of drug to be added to the IV fluid and the amount to administer.

**Example**

Order: calcium gluconate 2 g in 100 cc D5W. Run 0.25 g/hr IV

Logic: We know the solution and the amount of drug per hour; we can solve the problem and administer the drug in mL/hr.

*Formula Method*

Rule: $\dfrac{D}{H} \times S = A$

$$\frac{0.25 \text{ g/hr}}{\underset{1}{2 \text{ g}}} \times \overset{50}{\cancel{100}} \text{ mL (cc)} = 12.5$$

13 mL/hr on a pump

> **Learning Aid**
>
> $$\begin{array}{r} 0.25 \\ \times\ 50 \\ \hline 12.50 \end{array}$$
>
> Round off to the nearest whole number = 13.

*Ratio Proportion Method*

$$\frac{x \text{ mL}}{.25 \text{ g/hr}} = \frac{100 \text{ mL (cc)}}{2}$$

$$x = \frac{25}{2}$$

$$x = 12.5 \text{ or } 13 \text{ mL/hr}$$

**Example**

Order: aminophylline 250 mg in 250 mL D5W. Run 65 mg/hr IV.

*Formula Method*

Rule: $\dfrac{D}{H} \times S = A$

$$\frac{65 \text{ mg/hr}}{\underset{1}{250 \text{ mg}}} \times \cancel{250} \text{ mL} =$$

65 mL/hr on a pump

*Ratio Proportion Method*

$$\frac{x \text{ mL}}{65 \text{ mg}} = \frac{250 \text{ mL}}{250 \text{ mg}}$$

$$x = 65 \text{ mL/hr}$$

## mL/hr—Rule and Calculation

The order indicates the amount of the drug to be added to an IV and the time to run.

**Example**

Order: KCl 10 mEq in 200 mL D5W over 24 hours via pump

Logic: First add KCl to the IV.

KCl comes in a vial labeled 20 mEq per 40 mL; add 20 mL KCl. The order states to administer 200 mL over 24 hours.

Infusion pumps are set in mL/hr.

Rule: $\dfrac{\text{\# mL}}{\text{\# hr}} = \text{mL/hr}$

**Learning Aid**

The rule $\dfrac{D}{H} \times S = A$ is used to determine the amount of KCl needed.

$$\dfrac{\overset{1}{\cancel{10}}\text{ mEq}}{\underset{2}{\cancel{20}}\text{ mEq}} \times \overset{20}{\cancel{40}} \text{ mL} = 20 \text{ mL}$$

$$\dfrac{200 \text{ mL}}{24 \text{ hr}} \quad 24 \text{ hr} \overline{)\begin{array}{r} 8.3 \\ 200.0 \\ \underline{192\phantom{.0}} \\ 8\,0 \\ \underline{7\,2} \\ 8 \end{array}}$$

Set pump at 8 mL/hr.

**Learning Aid**

Chapter 9 presents rules to determine IV drip rates.

**Example**

Order: nitroglycerin 50 mg in 250 mL D5W over 24 hours via pump

Logic: Nitroglycerin is prepared by the pharmacy as standard solution of 50 mg in 250 mL D5W. We only need to calculate mL/hr.

Rule: $\dfrac{\text{\# mL}}{\text{\# hr}} = \text{mL/hr}$

$$\dfrac{250 \text{ mL}}{24 \text{ hr}} \quad 24 \text{ hr} \overline{)\begin{array}{r} 10.4 \\ 250.0 \\ \underline{24\phantom{.0}} \\ 10\,0 \\ \underline{9\,6} \end{array}}$$

Set pump at 10 mL/hr.

## mg/min—Rule and Calculation

The order will indicate the amount of drug to add to IV fluid. These medications are administered through an IV pump set in mL/hr.

**Learning Aid**

The word "minute" can be abbreviated min or mt. We will use min.

**Example**

Order: bretylium 1 mg/min IV

Available: infusion pump; standard solution of 1 g in 500 mL D5W

Logic: The order calls for 1 mg/min. We need mL/hr for the pump.

*Formula Method*

1 mg/min = 60 mg/hr

Rule: $\dfrac{D}{H} \times S = A$

$$\dfrac{\overset{30}{\cancel{60 \text{ mg/hr}}}}{\underset{\underset{1}{2}}{\cancel{1000 \text{ mg}}}} \times \cancel{500} \text{ mL} = 30 \text{ mL/hr}$$

Set pump at 30 mL/hr.

*Ratio Proportion Method*

$$\dfrac{x \text{ mL}}{60 \text{ mg}} = \dfrac{500 \text{ mL}}{1000 \text{ mg}}$$

$$x = \dfrac{30000}{1000}$$

$$x = 30 \text{ mL/hr}$$

---

## SELF TEST 1   Infusion Rates

*Solve the following problems. Answers may be found at the end of this chapter.*

1. Order:     heparin sodium 800 units/hr IV
   Available: infusion pump; standard solution of 25,000 units in 250 mL D5W

2. Order:     acyclovir 500 mg in 100 mL D5W IV over 1 hr
   Available: pump; acyclovir vials of 500 mg

3. Order:     Amicar 24 g in 1000 mL D5W over 24 hr IV
   Available: infusion pump; vials of Amicar labeled 5 g per 20 cc

4. Order:     diltiazem 125 mg in 100 mL D5W at 10 mg/hr IV
   Available: infusion pump; vial of diltiazem labeled 5 mg/mL

5. Order:     furosemide 100 mg in 100 mL D5W. Infuse 4 mg/hr
   Available: infusion pump; vial of furosemide labeled 10 mg/cc

6. Order:     Regular Insulin 15 units/hr IV
   Available: Standard solution of 125 units in 250 mL NS; Infusion Pump

   a. What is the drip rate?

   b. How many hours will this IV run?

# ▶ Medications Ordered in mcg/min, mcg/kg/min, or milliunits/min

In intensive care units, powerful drugs are administered in extremely small amounts called micrograms (1 mg = 1000 mcg). The orders for these drugs differ from any we have studied.

| Example | Order: Renal dose dopamine 2 mcg/kg/min |
|---|---|

Order: Titrate levophed to maintain arterial mean pressure above 65 and below 95

In this section we will learn how to calculate doses in micrograms and in milliunits and how kilograms are used in determining doses.

## mcg/min—Rule and Calculations

Drugs ordered in mcg/min are standardized solutions prepared by a pharmacist. They are administered using infusion pumps that deliver medication in mL/hr.

Drugs ordered in mcg/min are calculated using the microdrip tubing factor (60 gtt = 1 mL). We learned in Chapter 9 that *mL/hr = microdrips per min*. We solve mcg/min problems with an answer in mcg/min and report the answer in mL/hr to set the pump flow.

There are five steps in solving mcg/min:

1. Reduce the # in the standard solution.

2. Change mg to mcg.

3. Reduce the # in the solution to mcg/1 mL.

4. Substitute 60 gtt for the mL.

5. $\dfrac{D}{H} \times S = A$

| Example | Order: dopamine 400 mcg/min IV |
|---|---|

Available: infusion pump; standard solution 400 mg in 250 mL D5W

**Step 1.** Reduce the numbers in the standard solution.

$$\frac{\overset{8}{\cancel{400}} \text{ mg}}{\underset{5}{\cancel{250}} \text{ mL}} = 8 \text{ mg/5 mL}$$

**Step 2.** Change mg to mcg.
8 mg = 8000 mcg. Solution is 8000 mcg/5 mL.

**Step 3.** Reduce # in solution to mcg/1 mL.

$$\frac{\overset{1600}{\cancel{8000}} \text{ mcg}}{\underset{1}{\cancel{5}} \text{ mL}} = 1600 \text{ mcg/mL}$$

**Step 4.** Substitute 60 gtt for the mL.
1600 mcg/60 gtt

**Learning Aid**

D = order: 400 mcg/min

H = 1600 mcg

S = 60 gtt

**Step 5.** $\dfrac{D}{H} \times S = A$

$$\dfrac{\overset{1}{\cancel{400 \text{ mcg/min}}}}{\underset{4}{\cancel{1600 \text{ mcg}}}} \times \overset{15}{\cancel{60}} \text{ gtt} = 15 \text{ gtt microdrop}$$

To set the infusion pump, you must input

a. Total # mL ordered

b. mL/hr to run

Set the pump:

Total # mL: 250 (standard solutions)

mL/hr: 15

**Learning Aid**

When using an infusion pump, gtt/min = mL/hr. The pump can be set only in mL/hr.

**Example**

Order: Aramine 60 mcg/min IV

Available: infusion pump; standard solution 50 mg in 250 mL D5W

**Step 1.** Reduce # in standard solution.

$$\dfrac{\overset{1}{\cancel{50 \text{ mg}}}}{\underset{5}{\cancel{250 \text{ mL}}}} = 1 \text{ mg/5 mL}$$

**Step 2.** Change mg to mcg.
1 mg = 1000 mcg. Solution is 1000 mcg/5 mL.

**Step 3.** Reduce # in solution.

$$\dfrac{\overset{200}{\cancel{1000 \text{ mcg}}}}{\underset{1}{\cancel{5 \text{ mL}}}} = 200 \text{ mcg/mL}$$

**Step 4.** Substitute 60 gtt for the mL.
200 mcg/60 gtt

**Learning Aid**

1 mL = 60 gtt microdrip

Step 5. $\dfrac{D}{H} \times S = A$

$$\dfrac{\overset{3}{\cancel{60}} \text{ mcg/min}}{\underset{1}{\underset{\cancel{3}}{\cancel{200} \text{ mcg}}}} \times \cancel{60} \text{ gtt} =$$

18 gtt/min = 18 mL/hr

Set the pump:

Total # mL: 250 (standard solution)

mL/hr: 18

## mcg/kg/min—Rule and Calculation

**Example**    Order: dopamine 2 mcg/kg/min

Available: infusion pump; standard solution 200 mg in 250 mL D5W. Client weighs 176 lbs.

Note that this order is somewhat different. We are to give 2 mcg per kilogram of body weight. First we must weigh the patient, convert pounds to kilograms if the scale is not in kilograms, then multiply the kg by 2 mcg. Once we have determined this answer, we follow the steps given above.

The patient weighs 176 lb.

$$\dfrac{176 \text{ lb}}{2.2} \quad \overset{8\,0.}{\overline{)176.0}} = 80 \text{ kg}$$

$$\begin{array}{r} 80 \text{ kg} \\ \times\, 2 \text{ mcg} \\ \hline 160 \text{ mcg} \end{array}$$   The order now is 160 mcg/min.

1. Reduce # in standard solution.

$$\dfrac{\overset{4}{\cancel{200}} \text{ mg}}{\underset{5}{\cancel{250}} \text{ mL}} = 4 \text{ mg/5 mL}$$

2. Change mg to mcg.
   4 mg = 4000 mcg. Solution is 4000 mcg/5 mL.

3. Reduce # in the solution.

$$\dfrac{\overset{800}{\cancel{4000}} \text{ mcg}}{\underset{1}{\cancel{5} \text{ mL}}} = 800 \text{ mcg/mL}$$

4. Substitute 60 gtt for the mL.
   800 mcg/60 gtt

5. $\dfrac{D}{H} \times S = A$

$$\dfrac{\overset{2}{\cancel{160} \text{ mcg/min}}}{\underset{1}{\cancel{800} \text{ mcg}}} \times \cancel{60} \text{ gtt} = 12$$

12 gtt/min = 12 mL/hr

Set the pump:

Total # mL: 250 (standard solution)

mL/hr: 12

## milliunits/min—Rule and Calculation

In obstetrics, labor can be initiated using a Pitocin drip. The standard solution is 10 units in 1 liter. Because 1 unit = 1000 milliunits, these problems are solved in the same way as mcg/min.

**Example**    Order: Pitocin drip 2 milliunits/min IV

Available: infusion pump; standard solution 10 units in Ringer's solution 1 liter

1. Reduce # in standard solution.

$$\dfrac{\cancel{10} \text{ units}}{\cancel{1000} \text{ mL}} = 1 \text{ unit/100 mL}$$

2. Change units to milliunits.
1 unit = 1000 milliunits. Solution is 1000 milliunits in 100 mL.

3. Reduce the # in the solution.

$$\dfrac{\cancel{1000} \text{ milliunits}}{\cancel{100} \text{ mL}} = 10 \text{ milliunits/mL}$$

4. Substitute 60 gtt for the mL.
10 milliunits/60 gtt

5. $\dfrac{D}{H} \times S = A$

$$\dfrac{\overset{1}{\cancel{2 \text{ milliunits/min}}}}{\underset{\underset{1}{\cancel{5}}}{\cancel{10 \text{ milliunits}}}} \times \overset{12}{\cancel{60}} \text{ gtt} =$$

12 gtt/min = 12 mL/hr

Set the pump:

Total # mL = 1000 mL
(standard solution)

mL/hr = 12

> **Learning Aid**
>
> D = order: 2 milliunits/min
>
> H = 10 milliunits
>
> S = 60 gtt

| SELF TEST 2 | Infusion Rates for Drugs Ordered in mcg/min, mcg/kg/min, milliunits/min |
|---|---|

*Answers may be found at the end of the chapter.*

**1.**    Order:     dopamine double strength
                    800 mcg/min IV
        Available:  Standard solution 800 mg in 250 mL D5W
                    Infusion pump

**2.**    Order:     norepinephrine bitartrate
                    12 mcg/min IV
        Available:  Standard solution of 4 mg in 250 mL D5W
                    Infusion pump

**3.**    Order:     dobutamine 5 mcg/kg/min IV
        Available:  Patient weight—220 lb
                    Standard solution of 1 gram in 250 mL D5W
                    Infusion pump

**4.**    Order:     dobutamine 7 mcg/kg/min IV
        Available:  Patient weight—70 kg
                    Standard solution of 500 mg in 250 mL D5W
                    Infusion pump

**5.**    Order:     nitroglycerin 10 mcg/min IV
        Available:  Standard solution of 50 mg in 250 mL D5W
                    Infusion pump

**6.**    Order:     Pitocin drip 1 milliunit/min IV
        Available:  infusion pump; standard solution 20 units/1000 mL
                    Ringer's solution

**7.**    Order:     isoproterenol titrated at 4 mcg/min IV
        Available:  infusion pump; solution 2 mg/in 250 mL D5W

**8.**    Order:     esmolol 50 mcg/kg/min IV
        Available:  infusion pump; 2.5 g in 250 mL D5W; weight 58 kg

**9.**    Order:     bretylium 1 mg/min IV
        Available:  infusion pump; solution of 1 g in 500 mL D5W

## ▶ Body Surface Nomogram

Antineoplastic drugs used in cancer chemotherapy have a narrow therapeutic range. Dosage errors can lead to devastating effects. Calculation of these drugs is based on body surface area (BSA) in square meters ($m^2$). This method is considered more precise than mg/kg/body weight.

BSA can be estimated by using a three-columned chart called a nomogram (Fig. 10-1). Height is marked in the first column, weight in the third column. A line is drawn between these two marks. The point at which the line intersects the middle column indicates estimated body surface in meters squared. A different BSA chart is used for children because of differences in growth.

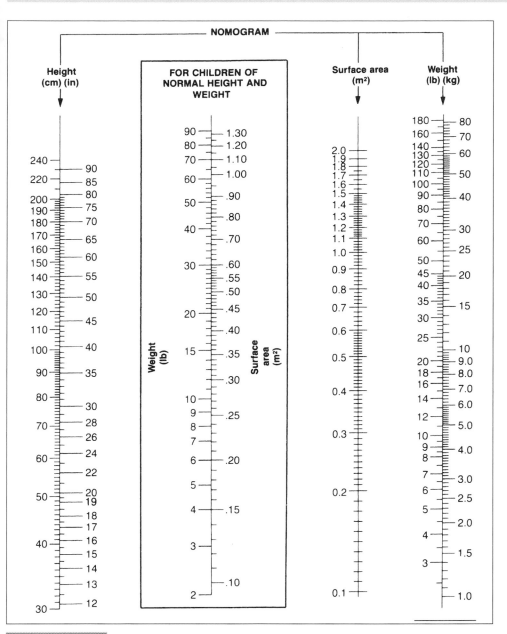

**FIGURE 10-1**

Body surface area (BSA) is critical when calculating dosages for pediatric patients or for drugs that are extremely potent and need to be given in precise amounts. The nomogram shown here lets you plot the patient's height and weight to determine the BSA. Here's how it works:

- Locate the patient's height in the left column of the nomogram and the weight in the right column.
- Use a ruler to draw a straight line connecting the two points. The point where the line intersects the surface area column indicates the patient's BSA in square meters.
- For an average-sized child, use the simplified nomogram in the box. Just find the child's weight in pounds on the left side of the scale, and then read the corresponding BSA on the right side.

| DIAGNOSIS: _ANAL CANCER_ | PROTOCOL NAME/NUMBER: _____ |
|---|---|
| PATIENT'S HEIGHT: _6'2_ cm | WEIGHT: _186_ Kg or BSA: _2.1_ m² |
| VENOUS ACCESS: | DEEP ☐    PERIPHERAL ☒ |

| | DRUG | PROTOCOL DOSAGE | PATIENTS DOSAGE | ROUTE AND DILUENT | FREQUENCY AND / OR DOSAGE | # OF DAYS |
|---|---|---|---|---|---|---|
| 1. | MITOMYCIN | 12 mg/m² | 24 mg | IVP × 1 m  9/08 | | |
| 2. | 5FU | 1000 mg/m² | 2000 mg | in 1000 cc of NS as a continuous infusion QD × 4 days on 9/08, 9/09, 9/10, 9/11 | | |
| 3. | | | | | | |

**FIGURE 10-2**

Portion of doctor's order form for chemotherapy. The doctor writes the patient's height and weight and calculates the BSA as 2.1 m². The protocol dosage is the guide used to determine the patient's dose. For mitomycin the protocol is 12 mg/m² × 2 m² = 24 mg. For 5FU the protocol dose is 1000 mg/m² × 2 m² = 2000 mg.

The oncologist, a physician who specializes in treating cancer, lists the patient's height, weight, body surface area; gives the protocol (drug requirement based on BSA in m²); and then the order. Figure 10-2 shows a partial order sheet for chemotherapy. The pharmacist and the nurse validate the order before preparation.

Determination of BSA in m² is easier, faster, and more accurate using either a manual sliding calculator or a battery-operated calculator. These can be purchased commercially or obtained from companies manufacturing antineoplastics.

## m²–Rule and Calculation

Oncology drugs are prepared by a pharmacist or specially trained technician who is gowned, gloved, and masked, and who works under a laminar flow hood. When the medication reaches the unit, it is the nurse's responsibility to check the dose for accuracy before administration and to use an infusion pump for IV orders.

**Example**

Hgt 6'0″   Wgt 175 lbs.   BSA 2.0 m²

Order: Cisplatin 160 mg (80 mg/m²) IV in 1 L NS with 2 mg magnesium sulfate over 2 hours

**Logic: 1.** Check the BSA using the nomogram in Figure 10-1. It is correct. Protocol calls for 80 mg/m²; 160 mg is correct.

**2.** IV is prepared by the pharmacy. Determine the rate of infusion.

$$\frac{\# \text{ mL}}{\# \text{ hr}} = \text{mL/hr} \qquad \frac{\overset{500}{\cancel{1000}}}{\underset{1}{\cancel{2}}} = 500 \text{ mL/hr}$$

Set the pump:

Total # mL: 1000

    mL/hr: 500

*Solve the following problems. Answers are found at the end of this chapter. Use the nomogram in Figure 10-1.*

1. Hgt 6'0"    Wgt 165 lbs   BSA 1.96 m²
   Order:        Doxil 39 mg (20 mg/m²) in D5W 250 mL to infuse
                 over ½ hour

   a. Is BSA correct?
   b. Is dose correct?
   c. How should the pump be set?

2. Hgt 165 cm Wgt 70 kg   BSA 1.77 m²
   Order:        CCNU 230 mg po (130 mg/m²) once q 6 weeks

   a. Is BSA correct?
   b. Is dose correct?
   c. CCNU comes in tabs of 100 mg and 10 mg. What is the dose?

3. Hgt 6'2"    Wgt 170 lbs   BSA 2.0 m²
   Order:        daunorubicin 80 mg (40 mg/m²) in D5W cc/cc over 1
                 hour IV
   Available:    IV bag labeled 80 mg in 80 mL D5W. Infuse in rapidly
                 flowing IV.

   a. Is BSA correct?
   b. Is dose correct?
   c. How should the pump be set? (See IVPB administration in
      Chapter 9)

4. Hgt 72"    Wgt 200 lbs   BSA 2.1 m²
   Order:        etoposide 400 mg po qd × 3 (200 mg/m²)
   Available:   Capsules of 50 mg

   a. Is BSA correct?
   b. Is dose correct?
   c. How many capsules should be poured?

5. Hgt 5'3"    Wgt 130 lbs   BSA 1.6 m²
   Order:        Taxol 216 mg (135 mg/m²) in D5W ½ L glass bottle
                 over 3 hours

   a. Is BSA correct?
   b. Is dose correct?
   c. How should the pump be set?

## ▶ Patient-Controlled Analgesia (PCA)

PCA is an intravenous method of pain control that allows a patient to self-administer a pre-set dose of pain medication. The physician prescribes the narcotic dose and concentration, the basal rate, lockout time, and total maximum hourly dose.

Basal rate is the amount of medication that is infused continuously each hour. PCA dose is the amount of medication infused when the patient activates the button control. Lockout time or delay is the interval during which the patient cannot initiate another dose after giving a self-dose. Lockout prevents overdosage. Total hourly dose is the maximum amount of medication the patient can receive in an hour. All this information is written by the physician on an order form.

Figure 10-3 shows a narcotic PCA medication record. Morphine concentration is 1 mg/cc. The pharmacy dispenses a 100 mL NS bag with 100 mL morphine. The patient continuously receives 0.5 mg by infusion pump and can give self 1.5 mg by pressing the PCA button. Eight minutes must elapse before another PCA dose can be delivered. Note that at 12 N the nurse charted that the patient made three attempts but received only two injections. This indicates that 8 minutes had not elapsed before one of the attempts.

The nurse's responsibility is to assess the patient every hour, noting how the patient scores his pain, the number of PCA attempts, and the total hourly dose received, as well as the cumulative dose, the patient's level of consciousness, and side effects and respirations.

### Saint Vincent's Hospital and Medical Center
NARCOTIC / PCA
MEDICATION ADMINISTRATION RECORD

#### PCA Charting Legend

| Pain | Sedation Scale | Side Effects |
|------|----------------|--------------|
| 0      10<br>0 - no pain<br>10 - excruciating | 0 - alert<br>1 - sleepy but arousable<br>2 - somnolent, difficult to arouse<br>3 - minimal or no response | N - nausea<br>V - vomiting<br>I - itching<br>R - respiratory depression<br>U - urinary retention |

Date: From 8 a.m.....   To 8 a.m.....   **PHYSICIAN'S ORDER**

| INIT. | TIME | Drug | Concentration | Basal Rate | PCA Dose | Delay | I Hour Limit |
|-------|------|------|---------------|-----------|----------|-------|--------------|
| m | 114 | Morphine | 1 mg/cc | 0.5 mg | 1.5 mg | 8 min | 11.5 mg |
| | | | | | | | |

4 — Patient Identified Pain Score Goal

**NURSING ASSESSMENT**

| Time | Pain Score | PCA Injections/Attempts | Total Dose This Hour | Cumulative Dose | Level of Consciousness | Side Effects | Respirations | Comments | Initials |
|------|-----------|------------------------|----------------------|-----------------|------------------------|--------------|--------------|----------|----------|
| 12 N | 7 | 2 - 3 | 3.5 mg | 3.5 mg | O | Ø | 18 | | m |
| 1 P | 7 | 1 - 3 | 2 mg | 5.5 mg | O | Ø | 18 | | m |
| 2 P | 7 | 3 - 4 | 5 mg | 10.5 mg | O | Ø | 18 | | m |
| 3 P | 8 | 2 - 2 | 3.5 mg | 14 mg | O | Ø | 18 | | m |
| 4 P | 8 | 3 - 6 | 5 mg | 19 mg | O | N | 18 | | m |
| 5 P | 6 | 4 - 7 | 6.5 mg | 25.5 mg | O | N | 18 | | m |
| 6 P | 6 | 3 - 5 | 5 mg | 30.5 mg | O | N | 18 | | m |
| 7 P | 8 | 3 - 3 | 5 mg | 35.5 mg | O | V | 18 | | m |
| 8 P | 8 | 4 - 5 | 6.5 mg | 42 mg | I | Ø | 18 | | m |
| 9 P | 8 | 2 - 3 | 3.5 mg | 45.5 mg | I | Ø | 18 | | m |
| 10 P | 7 | 3 - 5 | 5 mg | 50.5 mg | I | Ø | 18 | | m |
| 11 P | 7 | 5 - 6 | 8 mg | 58.5 mg | i | Ø | 18 | | m |
| 12 m | 7 | 4 - 4 | 6.5 mg | 65 mg | i | Ø | 18 | | m |
| 1 A | 6 | 3 - 3 | 5 mg | 70 mg | i | Ø | 18 | | m |
| 2 A | 6 | 2 - 3 | 3.5 mg | 73.5 mg | i | Ø | 16 | | m |
| 3 A | 5 | 1 - 1 | 2 mg | 75.5 mg | i | U | 16 | | m |
| 4 A | 4 | 0 - 0 | 0 | 75.5 mg | I | U | 16 | | m |
| 5 A | 4 | 0 - 0 | 0 | 75.5 mg | I | Ø | 16 | | m |
| 6 A | 4 | 0 - 0 | 0 | 75.5 mg | O | Ø | 16 | | m |
| 7 A | 4 | 3 - 4 | 5 mg | 80.5 mg | O | Ø | 18 | | m |
| 8 A | 5 | 3 - 3 | 5 mg | 85.5 mg | O | Ø | 20 | | m |
| 9 A | 4 | 2 - 3 | 3.5 mg | 89 mg | O | Ø | 20 | | m |
| 10 A | 4 | 2 - 2 | 3.5 mg | 92.5 mg | O | Ø | 20 | | m |
| 11 A | 4 | 2 - 2 | 3.5 mg | 96 mg | O | Ø | 20 | | m |

| Initials | Signature | | Initials | Signature |
|----------|-----------|---|----------|-----------|
| m | Josephine Musto | | | |

**FIGURE 10-3**

Sample PCA medication record. (Courtesy of Saint Vincent's Hospital and Medical Center.)

*Solve these problems. Answers may be found at the end of the chapter.*

1.    Order:    Start labetalol 0.5 mg/min on pump.
      Available:    infusion pump; standard solution of 200 mg in 200
                    mL D5W
      What is the pump setting?

2.    Order:    aminophylline 250 mg in 250 mL D5W at 75 mg/hr IV
      Available:    infusion pump; vial of aminophylline labeled 250
                    mg/10 mL
      How much drug is needed? What is the pump setting?

3.    Order:    Bretylol 2 g in 500 mL D5W at 4 mg/min IV
      Available:    infusion pump; standard solution of 2 g in 500 mL
                    D5W
      What is the pump setting?

4.    Order:    acyclovir 400 mg in 100 cc D5W over 2 hours
      Available:    infusion pump; 500 mg vials of acyclovir with 10 cc
                    diluent; makes 50 mg/cc
      How much drug is needed? What is the pump setting?

5.    Order:    urokinase 5000 units/hr for 5 hrs IV
      Available:    infusion pump; vials of 5000 units
      Directions:    Dissolve urokinase in 1 cc sterile water. Add to 250
                    mL D5W.
      How much drug is needed? What is the pump setting?

6.    Order:    $MgSO_4$ 3 g in 500 cc D5W at 166 cc/hr IV
      Available:    infusion pump; 50% solution of $MgSO_4$
      How much drug is needed? What is the pump setting?

7.    Order:    nitroglycerin 80 mcg/min IV
      Available:    infusion pump; standard solution of 50 mg in 250 mL
                    D5W
      What is the pump setting?

8.    Order:    dobutamine 6 mcg/kg/min IV
      Available:    infusion pump; solution 500 mg/250 mL D5W;
                    weight 180 lbs
      Change lbs to kg. What is the pump setting?

9.    Order:    Pitocin 2 milliunits/min IV
      Available:    infusion pump; solution of 20 units in 1000 mL
                    Ringer's solution
      What is the pump setting?

10.   Hgt 60″    Wgt 128.5 lbs    BSA 1.55 $m^2$
      Order:    cisplatin 124 mg (80 mg/$m^2$) in 1 L NS to infuse
                over 4 hours

      a. Is BSA correct? Check Figure 10-1.
      b. Is dose correct?
      c. How should the pump be set?

## TEST YOUR CLINICAL SAVVY

A very sick patient in the intensive care unit is receiving Heparin, insulin, calcium gluconate, and potassium chloride IV (intravenously).

A. Why would an infusion pump be needed with these medications?

B. Why would medications that are based on body weight require the use of a pump? Why would medications based on BSA (body surface area) require an infusion pump?

C. Can any of these medications be regulated with standard roller clamp tubing? What would be the advantage? What would be the contraindication?

**PROFICIENCY TEST 1**   Special IV Calculations

*Name:* _____

*Solve these problems. Aim at a high degree of accuracy. Answers will be found on page 352.*

**1.**   Order:   Regular insulin 15 units/hr IV
   Available:   infusion pump; standard solution 125 units in 250 cc NS
   What is the pump setting?

**2.**   Order:   heparin sodium 1500 units/hr IV
   Available:   infusion pump; standard solution 25000 units in 500 mL D5W IV
   What is the pump setting?

**3.**   Order:   bretylium tosylate 2 g in 500 mL D5W at 2 mg/min IV
   Available:   infusion pump; standard solution of 2 g in 500 mL D5W
   What is the pump setting?

**4.**   Order:   diltiazem 125 mg in 100 mL D5W at 5 mg/hr IV
   Available:   infusion pump; vial of diltiazem labeled 5 mg/mL
   What is the pump setting? How much drug is needed?

**5.**   Order:   lidocaine 4 mg/min IV
   Available:   infusion pump; standard solution of 2 g in 500 mL D5W
   What is the pump setting?

**6.**   Order:   KCl 40 mEq/L at 10 mEq/hr IV
   Available:   infusion pump; vial of KCl labeled 20 mEq/10 mL
   How much KCl should be added? What is the pump setting?

**7.**   Order:   procainamide 1 mg/min IV
   Available:   infusion pump; standard solution of 2 g in 500 mL D5W
   What is the pump setting?

**8.**   Order:   amphotericin B 50 mg in 500 mL D5W over 6 hrs IV
   Available:   infusion pump; vial of 50 mg
   How should the drug be added to the IV? What is the pump setting?

**9.**   Order:   vasopressin 18 units/hr IV. Solution 200 units in 500 cc D5W
   Available:   infusion pump; vial of vasopressin labeled 20 units/mL
   How much drug is needed? What is the pump setting?

**10.**   Order:   dobutamine 250 mg/min IV
   Available:   infusion pump; solution of 500 mg in 500 mL D5W
   What is the pump setting?

*(continued)*

**11.**    Order:    Renal dose dopamine 2.5 mcg/kg/min
   Available:   infusion pump; solution 400 mg in 250 mL D5W
                   Weight 60 kg
   What is the pump setting?

**12.**    Order:    Pitocin 2 milliunits/min IV
   Available:   infusion pump; solution of 10 units in 1000 mL
                   Ringer's solution
   What is the pump setting?

**13.**   Hgt 5'3"   Wgt 143 lbs   BSA 1.7 m$^2$
   Order:   ARAc 170 mg (100 mg/m$^2$) in 1 L D5W over 24
               hours

   **a.** Is BSA correct (use Figure 10-1 to check)?
   **b.** Is dose correct?
   **c.** How should the pump be set?

# Answers

## Self Test 1 Infusion Rates

### Formula Method

**1.** $\dfrac{D}{H} \times S = A$

$$\dfrac{\overset{8}{\cancel{800 \text{ units/hr}}}}{\underset{\underset{1}{100}}{\cancel{25{,}000 \text{ units}}}} \times \overset{1}{\cancel{250}} \text{ mL} = 8 \text{ mL/hr on a pump}$$

### Ratio Proportion Method

$$\dfrac{x \text{ mL}}{800 \text{ units}} = \dfrac{250 \text{ mL}}{25000 \text{ units}}$$

$$\dfrac{x \text{ mL}}{800 \text{ units}} = 0.01$$

$$x \text{ mL} = 0.01 \times 800$$

$$x = 8 \text{ mL/hr on a pump}$$

**2.** Add 500 mg acyclovir to 100 mL D5W using a reconstitution device (see Chapter 9).

$$\dfrac{\# \text{ mL}}{\# \text{ hr}} = \text{mL/hr}$$

$$\dfrac{100 \text{ mL}}{1 \text{ hr}} \quad \text{no math necessary. Set pump at 100 mL/hr.}$$

**3. a.** Add Amicar to IV.

### Formula Method

$$\dfrac{D}{H} \times S = A$$

$$\dfrac{24 \cancel{\text{ g}}}{\cancel{5 \text{ g}}} \times \overset{4}{\cancel{20}} \text{ mL} = 96 \text{ mL}$$

(Note: Adding 96 mL to 1000 mL D5W = 1096 mL.)

Use 5 vials. Empty 4 completely.
Take 16 mL from the last vial.
20 cc × 4 vials = 80 cc + 16 cc = 96 mL

### Ratio Proportion Method

$$\dfrac{x \text{ mL}}{24 \text{ g}} = \dfrac{20 \text{ mL (cc)}}{5 \text{ g}}$$

$$x = \dfrac{480}{5}$$

$$x = 96 \text{ mL}$$

**b.** $\dfrac{\# \text{ mL}}{\# \text{ hr}} = \text{mL/hr}$

$$\dfrac{1000 \text{ mL}}{24 \text{ hr}} \quad 24\overline{)1000.0}^{\,41.6}$$

$$\begin{array}{r} 96 \\ \hline 40 \\ 24 \\ \hline 16\,0 \\ 14\,4 \end{array}$$

Set pump at 42 mL/hr.
Remove 96 mL D5W from the IV bag before adding the amicar.
This results in 1000 mL.

**4. a.** Add diltiazem to IV.

*Formula Method*

$$\frac{D}{H} \times S = A$$

$$\frac{\overset{25}{\cancel{125}\ \text{mg}}}{\cancel{5}\ \text{mg}} \times 1\ \text{mL} = 25\ \text{mL}$$

(Note: Adding 25 mL to 100 mL D5W = 125 mL. Remove 25 mL D5W from the IV bag before adding the diltiazem. This results in 100 mL.)

Add 25 mL to IV bag.

*Ratio Proportion Method*

$$\frac{x\ \text{mL}}{125\ \text{mg}} = \frac{1\ \text{mL}}{5\ \text{mg}}$$

$$x = \frac{125}{5}$$

$$x = 25\ \text{mL}$$

*Formula Method*

**b.**
$$\frac{D}{H} \times S = A$$

$$\frac{\overset{2}{\cancel{10}\ \text{mg/hr}}}{\underset{1}{\underset{\cancel{5}}{\cancel{125}\ \text{mg}}}} \times \overset{4}{\cancel{100}}\ \text{mL} = 8\ \text{mL/hr}$$

*Ratio Proportion Method*

$$\frac{x\ \text{mL}}{10\ \text{mg}} = \frac{100\ \text{mL}}{125\ \text{mg}}$$

$$x = \frac{1000}{125}$$

$$x = 8\ \text{mL/hr}$$

**5. a.** Add furosemide to IV.

*Formula Method*

$$\frac{D}{H} \times S = A$$

$$\frac{\overset{10}{\cancel{100}\ \text{mg}}}{\underset{1}{\cancel{10}\ \text{mg}}} \times 1\ \text{cc} = 10\ \text{cc}$$

(Note: Adding 10 mL to 100 mL D5W = 100 mL. Remove 10 mL D5W from the IV bag before adding the furosemide. This results in 100 mL.)

Add 10 cc to the IV bag.

*Ratio Proportion Method*

$$\frac{x\ \text{mL}}{100\ \text{mg}} = \frac{1\ \text{mL}}{10\ \text{mg}}$$

$$x = 10\ \text{cc}$$

**b.** Logic. Because the solution is 100 mg/100 mL (1:1) and the order reads 4 mg/hr, the pump should be set at 4 mL/hr. Let's prove this!

*Formula Method*

$$\frac{D}{H} \times S = A$$

$$\frac{4\ \text{mg/hr}}{\underset{1}{\cancel{100}\ \text{mg}}} \times \overset{1}{\cancel{100}}\ \text{mL} = 4\ \text{mL/hr}$$

*Ratio Proportion Method*

$$\frac{x\ \text{mL}}{4\ \text{mg}} = \frac{100\ \text{mL}}{100\ \text{mg}}$$

$$x = 4\ \text{mL/hr}$$

**6. a.** *Formula Method*

$$\frac{D}{H} \times S = A$$

$$\frac{15 \text{ units/hr}}{125 \text{ units}} \times 250 \text{ mL}$$

$$0.12 \times 250 \text{ mL} = 30 \text{ mL/hr}$$

*Ratio Proportion Method*

$$\frac{x \text{ mL}}{15 \text{ units}} = \frac{250 \text{ mL}}{125}$$

$$x \text{ mL} = 30 \text{ mL/hr}$$

**b.** Logic: The total volume of medication is 125 units and the client receives 15 units/hr.

$$\frac{125}{15} \overset{8.33}{)125.} = \text{approximately 8 hours}$$
$$\underline{120}$$
$$5.0$$
$$\underline{4\,5}$$
$$50$$

## Self Test 2 Infusion Rates for Drugs Ordered in mcg/min, mcg/kg/min, milliunits/min

**1.** Order: 800 mcg/min
Standard solution = 800 in 250 mL D5W

Step 1. $\dfrac{\overset{16}{\cancel{800} \text{ mg}}}{\underset{5}{\cancel{250} \text{ mL}}} = 16 \text{ mg/5 mL}$

Step 2. 16 mg = 16,000 mcg
16,000 mcg/5 mL

Step 3. $\dfrac{\overset{3200}{\cancel{16,000} \text{ mcg}}}{\underset{1}{\cancel{5} \text{ mL}}} = 3200 \text{ mcg/mL}$

Step 4. 3200 mcg/60 gtt

Step 5. $\dfrac{\overset{1}{\cancel{800} \text{ mcg/min}}}{\underset{1}{\underset{4}{\cancel{3200} \text{ mcg}}}} \times \overset{15}{\cancel{60}} \text{ gtt} = 15 \text{ gtt/min}$

$$= 15 \text{ mL/hr}$$

Set the pump:
Total # mL: 250 (standard solution) mL: 15

**2.** Order: 12 mcg/min
Standard solution = 4 mg in 250 mL D5W
Step 1. Skip this step for easier calculation.
Step 2. 4 mg = 4000 mcg. Solution is 4000 mcg/250 mL.

Step 3. $\dfrac{\overset{16}{\overset{80}{\cancel{4000} \text{ mcg}}}}{\underset{1}{\underset{5}{\cancel{250} \text{ mL}}}} = 16 \text{ mcg/mL}$

Step 4. 16 mcg/60 gtt

Step 5. $\dfrac{\overset{3}{\cancel{12} \text{ mcg/min}}}{\underset{1}{\underset{4}{\cancel{16} \text{ mcg}}}} \times \overset{15}{\cancel{60}} \text{ gtt} = 45$

$$45 \text{ gtt/min} = 45 \text{ mL/hr}$$

Set the pump:
Total # mL: 250
mL/hr: 45

**3.** Order: 5 mcg/kg/min
Weight 220 lb
Standard solution = 1 g in 250 mL
Convert lb to kg.

$$\frac{220 \text{ lb}}{2.2 \text{ kg}} \overset{100.0}{)220.0} = 100 \text{ kg}$$

To obtain the order in mcg:

Multiply 100 kg
$$\underline{\times 5} \text{ mcg/kg/min}$$
$$500 \text{ mcg/min—Order}$$

Step 1. 1 g = 1000 mg. Solution is 1000 mg/250 mL.

Step 2. $\dfrac{\overset{4}{\cancel{1000} \text{ mg}}}{\underset{1}{\cancel{250} \text{ mL}}} = 4 \text{ mg/mL}$

Step 2. 4 mg = 4000 mcg. Solution is 4000 mcg/mL.
Step 3. not needed.
Step 4. 4000 mcg/60 gtt

Step 5. $\dfrac{\overset{5}{\cancel{500}\text{ mcg/min}}}{\underset{2}{\cancel{4000}\text{ mcg}}} \times \overset{3}{\cancel{60}}\text{ gtt}$

$= \dfrac{15}{2} = 7.5 = 8$ gtt/min

8 gtt/min = 8 mL/hr

Set the pump:
Total # mL: 250 (standard solution)
mL/hr: 8

4. Order: 7 mcg/kg/min
Standard solution = 500 mg in 250 mL D5W
Patient's weight 70 kg

$$70 \text{ kg}$$
The patient weighs $\underline{\times\ 7}$ mcg/kg/min
$$490 \text{ mcg/min—order}$$

Step 1. $\dfrac{\overset{2}{\cancel{500}\text{ mg}}}{\underset{1}{\cancel{250}\text{ mL}}} = 2$ mg/mL

Step 2. 2 mg = 2000 mcg. Solution is 2000 mcg/mL.

Step 3. not needed

Step 4. 2000 mcg/60 gtt

Step 5. $\dfrac{\overset{}{\cancel{490}\text{ mcg/min}}}{\underset{10}{\underset{\cancel{100}}{\cancel{2000}\text{ mcg}}}} \times \overset{3}{\cancel{60}}\text{ gtt} = 49 \times 3$

$= \dfrac{147}{10} = 14.7 = 15$

15 gtt/min = 15 mL/hr

Set the pump:
Total # mL: 250 (standard solution)
mL/hr: 15

5. Order: 10 mcg/min
Standard solution: 50 mg in 250 mL

Step 1. $\dfrac{\overset{1}{\cancel{50}\text{ mg}}}{\underset{5}{\cancel{250}\text{ mL}}} = 1$ mg/5 mL

Step 2. 1 mg = 1000 mcg. Solution 1000 mcg/5 mL

Step 3. $\dfrac{\overset{200}{\cancel{1000}\text{ mcg}}}{\underset{1}{\cancel{5}\text{ mL}}} = 200$ mcg/mL

Step 4. 200 mcg/60 gtt

Step 5. $\dfrac{\overset{}{\cancel{10}\text{ mcg/min}}}{\underset{1}{\cancel{200}\text{ mcg}}} \times \overset{3}{\cancel{60}}\text{ gtt} = 3$

3 gtt/min = 3 mL/hr

Set the pump:
Total # mL: 250
mL/hr: 3

6. Order: 1 milliunit/min
Standard solution: 20 units in 1000 mL Ringer's solution

Step 1. $\dfrac{\overset{1}{\cancel{20}\text{ units}}}{\underset{50}{\cancel{1000}\text{ mL}}} = 1$ unit/50 mL

Step 2. 1 unit = 1000 milliunits
Solution is 1000 milliunits/50 mL

Step 3. $\dfrac{\overset{20}{\cancel{1000}\text{ milliunits}}}{\underset{1}{\cancel{50}\text{ mL}}} = 20$ milliunits/mL

Step 4. 20 milliunits/60 gtt

Step 5. $\dfrac{\cancel{1}\text{ milliunit/min}}{\underset{1}{\cancel{20}\text{ milliunits}}} \times \overset{3}{\cancel{60}}\text{ gtt} = 3$ gtt/min

3 gtt/min = 3 mL/hr Set the pump:
Total # mL: 1000
mL/hr: 3

7. Order: 4 mcg/min
Solution: 2 mg in 250 mL
Step 1. not necessary. Math easier.
Step 2. 2 mg = 2000 mcg. Solution is 2000 mcg/250 mL.

Step 3. $\dfrac{\overset{8}{\cancel{2000}\text{ mcg}}}{\underset{1}{\cancel{250}\text{ mL}}} = 8$ mcg/mL

Step 4. 8 mcg/60 gtt

Step 5. $\dfrac{\cancel{4}\text{ mcg/min}}{\underset{1}{\underset{2}{\cancel{8}\text{ mcg}}}} \times \overset{30}{\cancel{60}}\text{ gtt} = 30$

30 gtt/min = 30 mL/hr
Set the pump:
Total # mL: 250
mL/hr: 30

8. Order: 50 mcg/kg/min
Solution: 2.5 g in 250 mL
Weight: 58 kg
$$58 \text{ kg} \times 50 \text{ mcg} = 2900 \text{ mcg (order)}$$

Step 1. 2.5 g $= \dfrac{\overset{10}{\cancel{2500}\text{ mg}}}{\underset{1}{\cancel{250}\text{ mL}}} = 10$ mg/mL

Step 2. 10 mg = 10,000 mcg. Solution is 10,000 mcg/mL.

Step 3. not needed

Step 4. 10,000 mcg/60 gtt

Step 5. $\dfrac{2900 \text{ mcg/min}}{10,000 \text{ mcg}} \times 60 \text{ gtt} = \dfrac{174}{10} = 17.4$

$\qquad$ 17 gtt/min = 17 mL/hr

Set the pump:

Total # mL: 250

mL/hr: 17

9. Order: 1 mg/min = 1000 mcg/min

Solution: 1 g in 500 mL

Step 1.  1 g = 1000 mg; $\dfrac{\overset{2}{1000} \text{ mg}}{\underset{1}{500} \text{ mL}} = 2 \text{ mg/mL}$

## Self Test 3 Use of Nomogram

1. **a.** Check BSA on nomogram. It is correct.
   **b.** Dose is correct; 20 mg/m² × 1.96 = 39 mg
   **c.** Order calls for 250 mL over ½ hr, but pump is set in mL/hr. Double 250 mL.
      Setting: Total # mL = 250; mL/hr = 500.
      The pump will deliver 250 mL in ½ hour.
2. **a.** correct
   **b.** correct; 130 mg/m² × 1.77 = 230 mg
   **c.** Pour two 100 mg tabs and three 10 mg tabs.
3. **a.** yes, correct
   **b.** correct; 40 mg/m² × 2 = 80 mg
   **c.** Rapidly flowing IV is the primary line. Set the secondary pump: total # mL = 80; mL/hr = 80 (see Chapter 9 for IVPB).

## Self Test 4 Infusion Problems

1. Logic: A pump is needed. This is set in mL/hr. The order calls for 0.5 mg/min. Because there are 60 minutes in an hour, multiply 0.5 mg × 60 = 30 mg/hr. The standard solution is 200 mg in 200 mL. This is a 1:1 solution, so 30 mg/hr = 30 mL/hr.

   Proof: $\dfrac{D}{H} \times S = A$

   $\dfrac{30 \text{ mg/hr}}{200 \text{ mg}} \times \overset{1}{200} \text{ mL} = 30 \text{ mL/hr}$

   Total # mL: 200
   mL/hr: 30

2. Logic: Aminophylline comes 250 mg/10 mL. Remove 10 mL from the IV bag and add 10 mL drug. Order is 75 mg/hr. You have 250 mg in 250 mL (a 1:1 solution), therefore set the pump at 75 mL/hr.

Step 2.  2 mg = 2000 mcg. Solution is 2000 mcg/mL.

Step 3. not needed

Step 4. 2000 mcg/60 gtt

Step 5. $\dfrac{1000 \text{ mcg/min}}{\underset{1}{2000} \text{ mcg}} \times 60 \text{ gtt} = 30$

$\qquad$ 30 gtt/min = 30 mL/hr

Set the pump:

Total # mL: 500

mL/hr: 30

4. **a.** 72″ = 6 ft; BSA is correct
   **b.** correct; 200 mg/m² × 2 = 400 mg
   **c.** $\dfrac{D}{H} \times S = A$  $\dfrac{\overset{8}{400} \text{ mg}}{50 \text{ mg}} \times 1 \text{ cap} = 8 \text{ capsules}$
5. **a.** correct
   **b.** correct; 135 mg/m² × 1.6 = 216 mg
   **c.** ½ L = 500 mL over 3 hrs; $\dfrac{500}{3} \; \overset{166.6}{3)500} = 167$

   Set the pump: Total # mL = 500; mL/hr = 167.

Proof: $\dfrac{D}{H} \times S = A$

$\dfrac{75 \text{ mg/hr}}{250 \text{ mg}} \times \overset{1}{250} \text{ mL} = 75 \text{ mL/hr}$

Total # mL: 250
mL/hr: 75

3. 2 g = 2000 mg
   Logic: A pump is needed and is set in mL/hr. Order calls for 4 mg/min; there are 60 minutes in an hour; 60 × 4 = 240 mg/hr.

$\dfrac{D}{H} \times S = A$

$\dfrac{\overset{60}{240} \text{ mg/hr}}{\underset{1}{2000} \text{ mg}} \times \overset{1}{500} \text{ mL} = 60 \text{ mL/hr}$

Total # mL: 500
mL/hr: 60

4. Add acyclovir.

$$\frac{D}{H} \times S = A$$

$$\frac{\overset{8}{\cancel{400}\text{ mg}}}{\cancel{50}\text{ mg}} \times 1 \text{ cc} = 8 \text{ cc}$$

Remove 8 mL of fluid from the IV bag and add 8 mL of drug. This is now 400 mg/100 cc.

$$\frac{\#\text{ mL}}{\#\text{ hr}} = \text{mL/hr}$$

$$\frac{\overset{50}{\cancel{100}\text{ mL}}}{\underset{1}{\cancel{2}\text{ hr}}} = 50 \text{ mL/hr on a pump}$$

Total # mL: 100
mL/hr: 50

5. Logic: 5000 units/hr × 5 hrs = 25,000 units in 250 mL D5W. Need 5 vials. Dissolve each with 1 cc sterile water. Remove 5 cc from the IV bag and add the 5 cc of urokinase.

$$\frac{D}{H} \times S = A$$

$$\frac{\cancel{5000}\text{ units/hr}}{\underset{\underset{1}{100}}{\cancel{25,000}\text{ units}}} \times \cancel{250} \text{ mL} = 50 \text{ mL/hr on a pump}$$

Total # mL: 250
mL/hr: 50

6. Logic: $MgSO_4$ comes in a 50% solution = 50 g in 100 mL.

$$\frac{D}{H} \times S = A$$

$$\frac{3\text{ g}}{\cancel{50}\text{ g}} \times \overset{2}{\cancel{100}} \text{ mL} = 6 \text{ mL}$$

Add 6 mL of $MgSO_4$ to IV bag.
No math necessary. Order is 166 cc/hr. Set pump at 166 mL/hr.
Total # mL: 500
mL/hr: 166

7. Order: 80 mcg/min
Solution: 50 mg in 250 mL

Step 1. $\dfrac{\cancel{50}\text{ mg}}{\underset{5}{\cancel{250}\text{ mL}}} = 1 \text{ mg/5 mL}$

Step 2. 1 mg = 1000 mcg. Solution is 1000 mcg/5 mL.

Step 3. $\dfrac{\overset{200}{\cancel{1000}\text{ mcg}}}{\underset{1}{\cancel{5}\text{ mL}}} = 200 \text{ mcg/mL}$

Step 4. 200 mcg/60 gtt

Step 5. $\dfrac{\overset{4}{\cancel{80}\text{ mcg/min}}}{\underset{1}{\cancel{200}\text{ mcg}}} \times \cancel{60} \text{ gtt} = 24$

24 gtt/min = 24 mL/hr
Set pump:
Total # mL: 250
mL/hr: 24

8. Order: 6 mcg/kg/min
Solution: 500 mg/250 mL
Weight: 180 lbs

a. Change lbs to kg $\dfrac{180 \text{ lbs}}{2.2} \underset{\underset{\text{---}}{\underset{176}{\underset{40}{\underset{22}{18\ 0}}}}}{\overset{8\ 1.8}{\overline{)180.0\ 0}}} = 82 \text{ kg}$

b. 6 mcg/kg × 82 kg = 492 mcg (order now)

Step 1. $\dfrac{\overset{2}{\cancel{500}\text{ mg}}}{\underset{1}{\cancel{250}\text{ mL}}} = 2 \text{ mg/mL}$

Step 2. 2 mg = 2000 mcg. Solution is 2000 mcg/mL.

Step 3. not necessary

Step 4. 2000 mcg/60 gtt

Step 5. $\dfrac{492\text{ mcg/min}}{\underset{100}{\cancel{2000}\text{ mcg}}} \times \overset{3}{\cancel{60}} \text{ gtt} = \dfrac{1476}{100} \quad \overset{14.76}{100 \overline{)1476.00}}$

= 15
15 gtt/min = 15 mL/hr
Set pump:
Total # mL: 250
mL/hr: 15

9. Order: 2 milliunits/min
Stock: 20 units in 1000 mL

Step 1. $\dfrac{\overset{1}{\cancel{20}\text{ units}}}{\underset{50}{\cancel{1000}\text{ mL}}} = 1 \text{ unit/50 mL}$

Step 2. 1 unit = 1000 milliunits. Solution is 1000 milliunits/50 mL.

Step 3. $\dfrac{\overset{20}{\cancel{1000}\text{ milliunits}}}{\underset{1}{\cancel{50}\text{ mL}}} = 20 \text{ milliunits/mL}$

Step 4.  20 milliunits/60 gtt

Step 5.  $\dfrac{\overset{2}{\cancel{\text{milliunits/min}}}}{\underset{\underset{1}{\cancel{10}}}{\cancel{20\ \text{milliunits}}}} \times \overset{6}{\cancel{60}}\ \text{gtt} = 6$

6 gtt/min = 6 mL/hr
Set pump
Total # mL: 1000
mL/hr: 6

10. **a.** 60″ is 5 ft; correct
 **b.** correct; 1.55 BSA × 80 mg
 **c.** 1 L = 1000 mL;

$\dfrac{\#\ \text{mL}}{\#\ \text{hr}} = \dfrac{\overset{250}{\cancel{1000}}\ \text{mL}}{\underset{1}{\cancel{4}}\ \text{hrs}} = 250\ \text{mL/hr}$

Set the pump:
Total # mL: 1000
mL/hr: 250

# Dosage Problems for Infants and Children

## ▶ Overview

In previous chapters we discussed calculations for adult medications administered orally and parenterally. This chapter considers dosage for infants and children. Wide variations in age, weight, growth, and development within this group require special care in computation. Pediatric doses are often minute, and a slight error can result in serious harm.

Before preparing and administering a pediatric medication, the nurse determines that the dose is safe for the child. Safe means that the amount ordered is not an overdose or an underdose. An overdose can produce toxic effects; underdose may lead to therapeutic failure. When a discrepancy is noted, the nurse consults the physician who ordered the drug.

Children's medications are usually given by mouth in a liquid form or intravenously. Injections are not common except for immunizations. Pediatric injections are calculated to the nearest hundredth and administered using a 1 mL precision (tuberculin) syringe. For IV therapy microdrip, Buretrols or other volume control sets and infusion pumps are used. Most institutions will have guidelines for pediatric infusions; when guidelines are not available the nurse must consult a reliable *pediatric* reference. Adult guidelines are not safe for children.

Recall these equivalents as you begin this chapter:

| | |
|---|---|
| 1 g = 1000 mg | 16 oz = 1 lb |
| 1 kg = 2.2 lb | microdrip = 60 gtt/mL |
| 1 mg = 1000 mcg | > = greater than |
| 1 tsp = 5 mL | < = less than |
| 1 oz = 30 mL | q4° = every four hours |

# ▶ Dosage Based on mg/kg and Body Surface Area

The dose of most pediatric drugs is based on mg/kg body weight or body surface area (BSA) in meters squared ($m^2$). We will learn how to convert pounds to kilograms, to use a nomogram to calculate body surface area, to estimate the safety of a dose, and, finally, to determine the dose. *The use of a calculator is advisable.*

## Steps and Rule—mg/kg Body Weight

*EXAMPLE 1* A child weighing 33 lbs is ordered Augmentin 150 mg po q8h. Figure 11-1 shows the label for Augmentin, which comes as a dry powder. The accompanying prescribing information states that children ≤ 40 kg receive 6.7–13.3 mg/kg q8h. We need to convert 33 lbs to kg, calculate the low and high safe dose, determine if the dose ordered is within the safe range, and prepare the dose. These are the steps:

| | |
|---|---|
| **STEP 1.** | Convert lb to kg by dividing by 2.2. |
| **STEP 2.** | Determine the safe dose range in mg/kg using a reference. |
| **STEP 3.** | Decide if the ordered dose is safe by comparing the order with the safe dose range listed in the reference. |
| **STEP 4.** | Calculate the dose needed. |

**Step 1.** Convert lb to kg. Divide lb by 2.2

```
       1 5.
2.2 )33.0
     22
     11 0
     11 0
```

The child weighs 15 kg.

### Learning Aid

2.2 lb = 1 kg

$$\frac{2.2\ lb}{1\ kg} = \frac{33\ lb}{x\ kg}$$

$2.2x = 33$

$$x = \frac{33}{2.2}$$

Therefore, to obtain kg divide lb by 2.2.

**AUGMENTIN®**
125mg/5mL

NSN 6505-01-340-0847
**Directions for mixing:**
Tap bottle until all powder flows freely. Add approximately 2/3 of total water for reconstitution (total = 67 mL); shake vigorously to wet powder. Add remaining water; again shake vigorously.
**Dosage:** See accompanying prescribing information.

*Keep tightly closed.*
*Shake well before using.*
*Must be refrigerated.*
*Discard after 10 days.*

**125mg/5mL**
NDC 0029-6085-39

**AUGMENTIN®**
AMOXICILLIN/
CLAVULANATE POTASSIUM
FOR ORAL SUSPENSION
When reconstituted, each 5 mL contains:
**AMOXICILLIN, 125 MG,**
as the trihydrate
**CLAVULANIC ACID, 31.25 MG,**
as clavulanate potassium

**75mL** *(when reconstituted)*

SB SmithKline Beecham

Use only if inner seal is intact.
**Net contents:** Equivalent to 1.875 g amoxicillin and 0.469 g clavulanic acid. Store dry powder at room temperature.
**SmithKline Beecham Pharmaceuticals**
Philadelphia, PA 19101

Rx only

LOT

EXP.

9405804-H

3 0029-6085-39 3

**Step 2.** Determine the safe dose range.
Literature states dose should be between 6.7–12.3 mg/kg q8h.

| *Low Dose* | *High Dose* |
|---|---|
| 6.7 mg | 13.3 mg |
| × 15 kg | × 15 kg |
| 100.5 (calculator) | 199.5 = 200 mg (calculator) |

**Step 3.** Is the dose safe? The safe range is 100–200 mg q8h. The dose ordered (150 mg q8h) is safe because it falls within the 100–200 mg range.

**Step 4.** Calculate the dose.
The label states that 134 mL of water should be added gradually (see Fig. 11-1) to make a concentration of 125 mg/5 mL.

*Formula Method*               *Ratio Proportion Method*

Rule: $\dfrac{D}{H} \times S = A$     $\dfrac{\overset{6}{\cancel{150}}\text{ mg}}{\underset{\underset{1}{\cancel{5}}}{\cancel{125}\text{ mg}}} \times \overset{1}{\cancel{5}}\text{ mL} = 6\text{ mL}$     $\dfrac{5\text{ mL}}{125\text{ mg}} = \dfrac{\text{x mL}}{150}$

$\dfrac{150 \times \overset{1}{\cancel{5}}}{\underset{25}{\cancel{125}}} = \text{x}$

Give 6 mL.                    6 mL = x

This dose can be measured with a calibrated safety dropper or oral syringe. See Figure 11-2 for examples of this equipment. Techniques and procedures to administer pediatric medications are beyond the scope of this workbook. Please consult a pediatric nursing textbook.

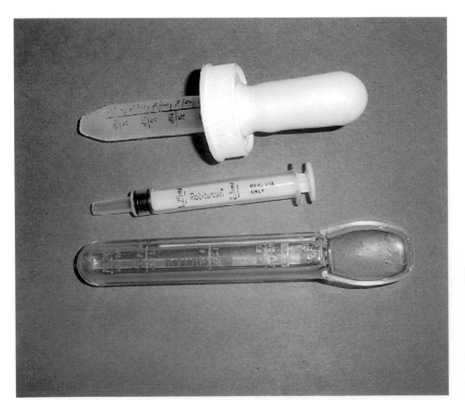

**FIGURE 11-2**

Examples of equipment used to obtain pediatric doses: *(top)* a safety dropper calculated in mL and teaspoons; *(center)* an oral syringe calculated in mL; and *(bottom)* a medication spoon calculated in mL and teaspoons.

*EXAMPLE 2* A child weighing 16 lb 10 oz is ordered Lasix 15 mg po bid (Fig. 11-3). Is the dose safe? What amount should be poured?

**Step 1.** Convert lb to kg.

**a.** Change the oz to part of a lb.

$$\frac{10\ \text{oz.}}{16} \quad \begin{array}{r} .62\ \text{lb} \\ \overline{\smash{\big)}10.00} \\ \underline{9\ 6} \\ 40 \\ \underline{32} \end{array}$$

> ### Learning Aid
>
> Equivalent is 16 oz = 1 lb. Change oz to a part of a lb by dividing by 16. Carry arithmetic out to two places and round off.

Child's weight is 0.6 lb + 16 lb = 16.6 lb

**b.** Change lb to kg.

$$\frac{16.6\ \text{lb}}{2.2} \quad \begin{array}{r} 7.54 = 7.54\ \text{kg} \\ \overline{\smash{\big)}16.6\ 00} \\ \underline{15\ 4} \\ 1\ 2\ 0 \\ \underline{1\ 1\ 0} \\ 1\ 00 \\ \underline{88} \\ 12 \end{array}$$

**Step 2.** Determine the safe dose range in mg/kg.

The package insert states: The initial dose of oral Lasix (furosemide) in infants and children is 2 mg/kg body weight, given as a single dose. If the diuretic response is not satisfactory after the initial dose, dosage may be increased by 1 or 2 mg/kg no sooner than 6 to 8 hours after the previous dose. Doses greater than 6 mg/kg body weight are not recommended.

| *Single Dose* | *High Range* |
|---|---|
| 7.54 kg | 7.54 kg |
| $\times$ 2 mg | $\times$ 6 |
| 15.08 mg/day | 45.24 mg/day |

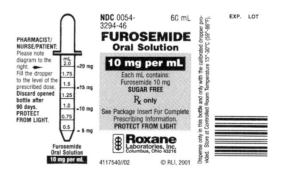

**FIGURE 11-3**

Label for furosemide. (Used with permission of Roxane Laboratories, Inc.)

**Step 3.** Decide if the ordered dose is safe. The order is 15 mg po bid. The 15 mg meets the requirement for a single dose. The order is bid which means twice in a day, so 15 mg × 2 = 30 mg. The child will receive 30 mg in a day. The high range is 45 mg, so the dose is safe.

**Step 4.** Calculate the dose needed. The stock is 10 mg/mL.

<table>
<tr><td>*Formula Method*</td><td>*Ratio Proportion Method*</td></tr>
</table>

$$\frac{D}{H} \times S = A \quad \frac{\overset{3}{\cancel{15\ mg}}}{\underset{2}{\cancel{10\ mg}}} \times 1\ mL = \frac{3}{2} = 1.5\ mL$$

$$\frac{1\ mL}{10\ mg} = \frac{x}{15\ mg}$$

$$\frac{15}{10} = x$$

$$1.5\ mL = x$$

The label states that Lasix comes with a calibrated safety dropper. The dropper can be used to obtain the dose of 1.5 mL.

*EXAMPLE 3* A child weighing 48 lbs is ordered Tegopen (cloxacillin) 250 mg po q6h. Literature states for children > 20 kg dose should be 250–500 mg q6h.

**Step 1.** Convert lb to kg.

$$\frac{48}{2.2} = 21.8\ kg\ (calculator)$$

**Step 2.** Determine the safe dose range.
No math needed. Literature states if the child's weight is above 20 kg, dose should be 250–500 mg q6h.

**Step 3.** The child is above 20 kg. Dose is safe.

**Step 4.** Calculate the amount needed.

<table>
<tr><td>*Formula Method*</td><td>*Ratio Proportion Method*</td></tr>
</table>

$$\frac{D}{H} \times S = A \quad \frac{\overset{2}{\cancel{250\ mg}}}{\underset{1}{\cancel{125\ mg}}} \times 5\ mL = 10\ mL$$

Give 10 mL.

$$\frac{5\ mL}{125\ mg} = \frac{x}{250\ mg}$$

$$\frac{1250}{125} = x$$

$$10\ mL = x$$

---

**SELF TEST 1**    **Converting pounds to kilograms**

*Convert pounds to kilograms. Answers will be found at the end of the chapter.*

**1.** 30 lb = _____ kg        **4.** 22 lb = _____ kg

**2.** 15 lb 5 oz = _____ kg     **5.** 54 lb 8 oz = _____ kg

**3.** 7¼ lb = _____ kg

*In these practice problems, determine if the doses are safe and calculate the amount needed. Answers may be found at the end of the chapter. You may find it helpful to use a calculator.*

1. Child weighs 20 lb.

   Order:    Amoxil 60 mg po q 8 h
   Stock:    See Figure 11-4

2. Order:    Augmentin 175 mg po q8h
   Patient:  child weighing 29 lb

   Stock:    Literature states: 40 mg/kg/day in divided doses; bottle of
             125 mg/5 mL

3. Order:    Ferrous sulfate 200 mg po tid

   Stock:    bottle of 125 mg/5 mL
   Child is 9 years old and weighs 30 kg.
   Literature states: children 6–12 years old, 600 mg divided doses tid

   a. Is the dose safe?
   b. How many milliliters would you pour?

4. Order:    Tylenol 80 mg po q4° prn for temp 100.9°F and above

   Stock:    chewable tablets 80 mg
   Child is 6 years old; weighs 20.5 kg.
   Literature states for child 6–8 years give four chewable tablets. May
   repeat four or five times daily. Not to exceed five doses in 24 hours.
   Is dose safe?

5. Order:    diazepam 1 mg IM q3–4h prn

   Stock:    vial 5 mg/1 mL
             Infant 30 days old
             Literature states: child < 6 mo
             IM 1–2.5 mg tid or qid

   a. Is dose safe?
   b. How much will you prepare?

AMOXIL®
125mg/5mL

**125mg/5mL**
NDC 0029-6008-22

**Directions for mixing:** Tap bottle
until all powder flows freely. Add
approximately 1/3 total amount of
water for reconstitution (total=116 mL);
shake vigorously to wet powder.
Add remaining water; again shake
vigorously. Each 5 mL (1 teaspoonful)
will contain amoxicillin trihydrate
equivalent to 125 mg amoxicillin.
**Usual Adult Dosage:** 250 to
500 mg every 8 hours.
**Usual Child Dosage:** 20 to
40 mg/kg/day in divided doses every
8 hours, depending on age, weight and
infection severity. See accompanying
prescribing information.

**AMOXIL®**
AMOXICILLIN
FOR ORAL
SUSPENSION

**150mL**
*(when reconstituted)*

**Keep tightly closed.**
**Shake well before using.**
**Refrigeration preferable but not required.**
**Discard suspension after 14 days.**

SB SmithKline Beecham

NSN 6505-01-011-1464
**Net contents:** Equivalent to 3.75 grams amoxicillin.
Store dry powder at room temperature.
**SmithKline Beecham Pharmaceuticals**
Philadelphia, PA 19101

Rx only

3 0029-6008-22 4

LOT
EXP.                9405813-F

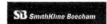

FIGURE 11-4

Label for amoxicillin (Amoxil). (Courtesy of GlaxoSmithKline.)

## Determining BSA in m²

A second method to determine pediatric dosage is to calculate body surface area (BSA) in meters squared ($m^2$) using a chart called a nomogram (Fig. 11-5). Height is marked in the left column, weight in the right column. A line is drawn between these two marks. The point at which the line intersects the middle column indicates BSA in $m^2$.

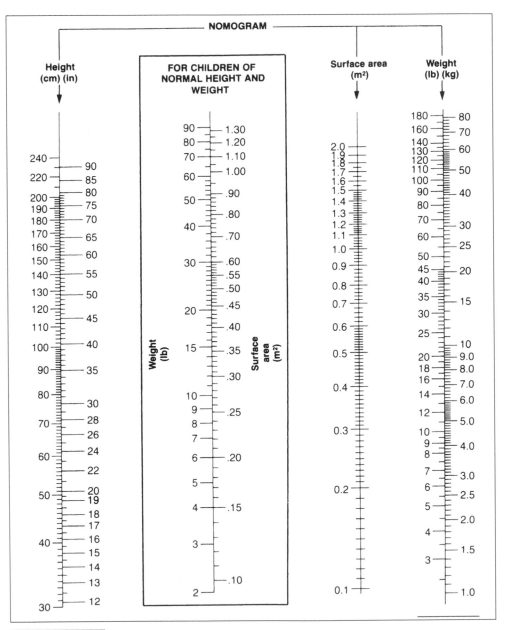

**FIGURE 11-5**

To determine the surface area, draw a straight line between the point representing the patient's height on the left vertical scale to the point representing the patient's weight on the right vertical scale. The point at which this line intersects the middle vertical scale represents the surface area in square meters. (A) Nomogram for adults and children. (continued)

| Height | | Surface Area | Weight | |
|---|---|---|---|---|
| Feet | Centimeters | Square meters | Pounds | Kilograms |

**FIGURE 11-5 (Continued)**

(B) Nomogram for infants and toddlers.

Because of differences in growth, different charts are used for infants and young children than for older children and adults. If a child weighs more than 65 lbs or is more than 3 ft tall, the adult nomogram should be used. Trace these BSAs using Figure 11-5:

**Example**

1. An infant with a height of 12 inches weighing 15 lbs has a BSA of 0.19 $m^2$.

2. A child 4'2" weighing 130 lbs has a BSA of 1.36 $m^2$.

Determining BSA is easier and faster with a battery-operated calculator or with a manual slide calculator. Figure 11-6 shows how a slide calculator is used.

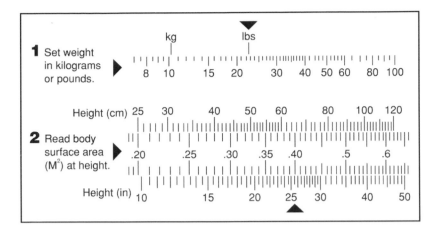

**FIGURE 11-6**
A manual slide calculator. The weight is set first. Note the arrow pointing to 23 lbs. Then find the height of 25½ inches, indicated by an arrow. The line above the height is the BSA = 0.4 m². 

**SELF TEST 3** | **Determining BSA**

*Convert height and weight to BSA in m² using Figure 11-5. Answers may be found at the end of this chapter*

| Height | Weight | BSA in m² |
|--------|--------|-----------|
| **1.** 36 in | 26 lbs | _____ |
| **2.** 80 cm | 13 kg | _____ |
| **3.** 50 in | 75 lbs | _____ |
| **4.** 17 in | 9 lbs | _____ |

## Steps and Rule—m² Medication Orders

*EXAMPLE 1* A 6-year-old child weighing 21 kg with a height of 116 cm has an order for propylthiouracil 50 mg po q6h.

Literature: initial dose 150–200 mg/m²/24 hr

Stock: 50-mg tab

| | |
|---|---|
| **STEP 1.** | Find the BSA in m². |
| **STEP 2.** | Determine the safe dose using a reference. |
| **STEP 3.** | Decide if the ordered dose is safe. |
| **STEP 4.** | Calculate the dose needed. |

**Step 1.** See Figure 11-5.
Height 116 cm; weight 21 kg; BSA = 0.82 m$^2$

**Step 2.** Safe dose is 150–200 mg/m$^2$/24 hr.

| *Low Dose* | *High Dose* |
|---|---|
| 150 mg | 200 mg |
| × 0.82 m$^2$ | × 0.82 m$^2$ |
| 123 mg (calculator) | 164 mg (calculator) |

Safe dose is 123 mg–164 mg/24 hr.

**Step 3.** Order is 50 mg q8h = 50 × 3 doses = 150 mg.
Dose is within guidelines; safe.

**Step 4.** *Formula Method*  　　　　　　　　　　*Ratio Proportion Method*

$$\frac{D}{H} \times S = A \qquad \frac{\cancel{50\ mg}}{\underset{1}{\cancel{50\ mg}}} \times 1\ tab = 1\ tab \qquad\qquad \frac{1\ tab}{50\ mg} = \frac{x}{50\ mg}$$

Give 1 tab.  　　　　　　　　　　　　　　　　　　　1 tab = x

*EXAMPLE 2* A 2-year-old child weighing 27 lbs 12 oz, height 35 in., is prescribed leucovorin calcium 5.5 mg po q6h × 72 hr.
　　Literature: Dose for rescue after methotrexate therapy is 10 mg/m$^2$/dose q6h × 72 hr.
　　Stock: 1 mg/mL reconstituted by the pharmacy

**Step 1.** Use Figure 11-5.
Height 35 in; weight 27 lbs 12 oz
Make weight 27¾ lbs.

### Learning Aid

To use the nomogram convert oz to lb.
16 oz = 1 lb

$$\therefore \frac{\overset{3}{\cancel{12}}}{\underset{4}{\cancel{16}}} = 3/4\ lb$$

**Step 2.** Safe dose is 10 mg/m$^2$/dose q6h.

$$\begin{array}{r} 10\ mg \\ \times\ 0.55\ m^2 \\ \hline 5.5\ mg = \text{safe dose q 6 h} \end{array}$$

**Step 3.** Order is 5.5 mg q6h. Dose is safe.

**Step 4.** *Formula Method*  　　　　　　　　　　*Ratio Proportion Method*

$$\frac{D}{H} \times S = A \qquad \frac{5.5\ mg}{\cancel{1\ mg}} \times 1\ mL = 5.5\ mL \qquad\qquad \frac{1\ mL}{1\ mg} = \frac{x}{5.5\ mg}$$

Give 5.5 mL.  　　　　　　　　　　　　　　　　　　5.5 mL = x

*In these problems, determine if the dose is safe using the nomogram in Figure 11-5 and calculate the amount needed. Answers may be found at the end of the chapter. You will find it helpful to use a calculator.*

1. Child:       8 yrs; height 50 in; weight 55 lbs
   Literature:  Dose 100–200 mg/m$^2$/24 h divided q 8–12 h
   Order:       flecainide 50 mg po q8h

   Stock:       50-mg tabs

2. Child:       12 yrs; height 59 in; weight 88 lbs

   Order:       methotrexate 12.5 mg po q week
   Literature:  10 mg/m$^2$/dose as needed weekly to control fever and
                joint inflammation in rheumatoid arthritis
   Stock:       2.5-mg tab

3. Infant:      12 mo; height 30 in; weight 22 lb 8 oz.
   Order:       prednisone 5 mg po q12h
   Literature:  immunosuppressive dose 6–30 mg/m$^2$/24 hr

   Stock:       5 mg/5 mL syrup

# Dosage for Parenteral Medications

Intravenous medications are administered when a child cannot maintain an oral fluid intake, has a fluid electrolyte imbalance, or requires IV medication. Buretrols or other volume control units are used to administer IV fluids; they are calibrated and hold no more than 100 to 150 mL at a time. This reduces the possibility of fluid overload. Infusion pumps are also used to provide a second safeguard. In neonatal areas, syringe pumps can deliver IV fluid ranging from 1 to 60 mL.

Dosages for IV medications are calculated in mg/kg. In pediatrics, drugs are administered in small amounts of diluent; a pediatric reference must be consulted to determine the minimum safe amount (Table 11-1). Institutions may provide guidelines to aid the nurse in preparing IVs.

*Drugs for IVPB must be initially diluted following the manufacturer's directions.* Once the initial dilution is made, the amount of drug required to obtain the dose is withdrawn from the vial then diluted further. IV solutions in pediatrics usually range from 10 to 20 mL for smaller children and infants requiring IVPB medications. This amount of fluid will fill the tubing from the Buretrol to the patient. When the Buretrol is empty of the IV medication, most of the drug will be in the tubing. For this reason an IV flush of 20 mL must be added to the Buretrol *after* the medication is infused to ensure that the patient receives the drug.

In this section we will consider the calculation of pediatric doses for IV and IVPB administration. These problems may seem complex. However, their solution requires a step-by-step analysis that is easily learned and applied.

### TABLE 11-1 Sample of a Table Listing the Safe Dosage Range for Pediatric Medications

| Drug | Dose and Route |
|---|---|
| Ampicillin | Neonate<br><7 days: 50–150 mg/kg/24h<br>q8–12h IM or IV<br>>7 days: 75–200 mg/kg/24h<br>q8–9h IM or IV<br>Child—moderate, mild infections<br>50–100 mg/kg/24h given q6h po |
| Cefotaxime | Neonate<br><1 wk: 100 mg/kg/24h given q12h IM or IV<br>1–4 wk: 150 mg/kg/24h given q8h IM or IV<br>Infant and child (<50 kg)<br>50–200 mg/kg/24h given q4–6h IV or IM |
| Chloral hydrate | Children<br>Sedative: 5–15 mg/kg/dose q8h po or pr<br>Hypnotic: 50–75 mg/kg/dose po or pr |
| Meperidine HCl | po, IM, IV, SC<br>Children: 1–1.5 mg/kg/dose q3–4h prn<br>Max. dose 100 mg |
| Penicillin G | Newborn: 50,000 units/kg × 1 IM |
| Benzathine | Infants/children: 50,000 units/kg × 1 IM<br>Max. 2.4 MU<br>Rheumatic fever prophylaxis<br>600,000 units q2 weeks or 1.2 MU q month IM |

## STEPS TO SOLVE PARENTERAL PEDIATRIC MEDICATIONS

1. Decide if the dose is safe; check a pediatric reference.
2. Decide if the dilution ordered meets the minimum pediatric safety standard (Table 11-2).
3. Prepare the medication according to directions.
4. Draw up the dose and dilute further as needed.
5. Set the pump in mL/hr. If the infusion time is 30 minutes, set the pump for double the amount because the pump delivers mL/hr.

   **Example**    The order is 10 mL over 30 minutes. Set the pump for 20 mL/hr. It will deliver 10 mL in 30 minutes.

6. When the IV is completed, add a flush of 20 mL to the Buretrol to clear the tubing of the medication. Be sure to chart the flush as fluid intake.

| TABLE 11-2 | Sample of a Dilution Table for Pediatric Antibiotics | | |
|---|---|---|---|
| **Antibiotic** | **Recommended Final Concentration IV** | | **Recommendation Duration of IV** |
| Ampicillin | 50 mg/mL | | 10–30 min |
| Cefotaxime | 50 mg/mL | | 10–30 min |
| Clindamycin | 6–12 mg/mL | | 15–30 min |
| Gentamicin | 2 mg/mL | | 15–30 min |
| Penicillin G | Infants: 50,000 units/mL Large child: 100,000 units/mL | | 10–30 min |
| Pentamidine | 2.5 mg/mL | | 1 hr |

**Example**

*EXAMPLE 1:*

Child 4 years old; 17 kg

Order: Tazicef 280 mg IV q8h in 10 mL D5⅓NS

Reference: Safe dose 30–50 mg/kg/day
          Concentration for IV use: 50 mg/mL over 30 minutes

Stock: 1 gram powder. Directions: Dilute with 10 mL sterile water for injection to make 95 mg/mL; stable for 7 days if refrigerated.

1. Safe dose is 30 to 50 mg/kg/day.

   | *Low Range* | *High Range* |
   |---|---|
   | 30 mg | 50 mg |
   | $\times$17 mg | $\times$17 mg |
   | 510 mg/day | 850 mg/day |

   Order is 280 mg q8h (3 doses).
   280 mg $\times$ 3 = 840 mg. Dose falls within the range and is safe.

2. Minimum safe dilution is 50 mg/mL. Dose is 280 mg.

   $$50 \overline{)280.}$$
   $$\underline{250}$$
   $$300$$
   $$\underline{300}$$

   5.6 = 6 mL is the minimum dilution. The order of 10 mL is safe because it is more than the minimum.

3. Dilute 1 g with 10 mL sterile water to make 95 mg/mL.

**Formula Method**

$$\frac{D}{H} \times S = A$$

$$\frac{280 \text{ mg}}{95 \text{ mg}} \times 1 \text{ mL}$$

**Ratio Proportion Method**

$$\frac{1 \text{ mL}}{95 \text{ mg}} = \frac{x}{280 \text{ mg}}$$

$$\frac{280}{95} = x$$

2.9 mL = x

= 2.9 mL. Withdraw 2.9 mL; label the vial and store in the refrigerator.

4. Run about 5 mL D5⅓NS into the Buretrol. Add the 2.9 mL drug. Add more D5⅓NS to make 10 mL.

5. Set the pump at 20. This is 20 mL/hr; the pump will deliver 10 mL in 30 minutes.

6. When the IV is completed, add a 20-mL flush of D5⅓NS to clear the IV tubing of medication.

*EXAMPLE 2:*

Infant 4.3 kg

Order: ampicillin 100 mg IV q6h in 10 cc D5⅓NS

Reference: Safe dose 75–200 mg/kg/24h given q6–8h IV
    Concentration for IV use: 50 mg/mL over 10–30 min
Stock: vial of powder labeled 500 mg. Directions: Add 1.8 mL of sterile water for injection to make 250 mg/mL; use within 1 hr.

1. Safe dose is 75 to 200 mg/kg/24h given q6–8h.

| **Low Range** | **High Range** |
|---|---|
| 75 mg | 200 mg |
| × 4.3 kg | × 4.3 kg |
| 322.5 mg/24h | 860 mg/24h |

Order is 100 mg q6h (4 doses).
100 mg × 4 doses = 400 mg. This is within the range. The dose is safe.

2. Minimum safe dilution is 50 mg/mL (see Table 11-2). Dose is 100 mg.

$$50 \overline{)100}$$   2 mL is the minimum dilution; 10 mL is safe.

3. Add 1.8 mL sterile water for injection to 500 mg powder to make 250 mg/mL.

**Formula Method**

$$\frac{D}{H} \times S = A$$

$$\frac{\cancel{100} \text{ mg}}{\cancel{250} \text{ mg}} \times 1 \text{ mL} = \frac{2}{5} = 0.4 \text{ mL}$$

**Ratio Proportion Method**

$$\frac{1 \text{ mL}}{250 \text{ mg}} = \frac{x}{100 \text{ mg}}$$

$$\frac{100}{250} = x$$

0.4 mL = x

Withdraw 0.4 mL from the vial. Discard the remainder (directions say to use within 1 hr).

4. Add about 5 mL D5⅓NS to the Buretrol. Add 0.4 mL drug. Add more D5⅓NS to make 10 cc.

5. Set the pump at 20. This means 20 mL/hr; the pump will deliver 10 mL in 30 min.

6. When the IV is finished, add 20 mL flush of D5⅓NS to the Buretrol to clear the tubing of medication.

*EXAMPLE 3:*

Infant 3 mo; 6 kg

Order: nafcillin 150 mg IV q8h in 10 mL D5⅓NS

Reference: Safe dose 100–200 mg/kg/24h given q6h
        Concentration for IV use: 6 mg/mL over 30–60 min

Stock: 500 mg vial of powder. Directions: Add 1.7 mL sterile water for injection to make 500 mg/2 mL. Stable for 48 hrs if refrigerated.

1. Safe dose is 100 to 200 mg/kg/24h given q6h.

| *Low Range* | *High Range* |
|---|---|
| 100 mg | 200 mg |
| ×6 kg | ×6 kg |
| 600 mg/24h | 1200 mg/24h |

Order is 150 mg q8h (3 doses) = 450 mg/24h.
The dose is below range and is q8h. Reference states q6h.

2. Minimum safe dilution is 6 mg/mL. Order is 150 mg. Divide 150 by 6.

25 = 25 mL. The dilution of 10 mL does not meet concentration requirements.
6 )150 mg

Should be 25 mL.

Consult with the physician regarding the dose, the times of administration, and the dilution. Do not prepare the dose.

## SELF TEST 5    Parenteral Medication Calculations

*In these practice problems determine if the dose is safe, calculate the amount needed and state how the order will be administered. Answers may be found at the end of this chapter. Follow the steps used in the examples.*

1. Infant 6 mo; 8 kg
    Order:    cefuroxime 200 mg IV q6h in 10 mL D5¼NS
    Reference: Safe dose 50–100 mg/kg/24h given q6–8h
             Concentration for IV use: 50 mg/mL over 30 min
    Stock:    750 mg vial of powder. Directions: Dilute with 8 mL sterile water for injection to make 90 mg/mL; stable for 3 days if refrigerated.

*(continued)*

## SELF TEST 5 | Parenteral Medication Calculations (Continued)

2. Child 3 years; 15 kg
   Order:      Bactrim (as TMP/SMX) 75 mg IV q12h in 75 mL
               D5W over 1 hr
   Reference:  Safe dose for a child 8–10 mg/kg/24h given q12h
               Concentration for IV use: 1 mL in 15–25 mL (stock is
               a liquid).
   Stock:      vial labeled 80 mg/5 mL

3. Child 12 yr; 40 kg
   Order:      tobramycin 100 mg IV q8h in 50 mL D5⅓NS
   Reference:  Safe dose 6–7.5 mg/kg/24h given q8h
               Concentration for IV use: 2 mg/mL over 15–30 min
   Stock:      Vial 80 mg/2 mL

4. Child 5 yr; 18 kg
   Order:      cefotaxime 900 mg IV q6h in 25 mL D5⅓NS
   Reference:  Safe dose 50–200 mg/kg/24h given q6h
               Concentration for IV use: 50 mg/mL; give over 30
               min.
   Stock:      1 g powder. Directions: Dilute with 10 mL sterile
               water for injection to make 95 mg/mL. Stable in the
               refrigerator 10 days.

## T EST YOUR CLINICAL SAVVY

You are working in a pediatric unit and taking care of 5-year-old Georgia Smith. Although she is a sweet girl during most of the time you are taking care of her, she has her moments when she will not do anything she doesn't want to do. She is receiving IV fluids and an oral medication that has an aftertaste.

A. What could you do to help her take the medication? Are there other alternatives you could use regarding the medication? What would you suggest to the family to promote easier compliance?

B. Besides reducing the possibility of fluid overload, what are some other reasons IV infusion pumps are used with children?

Another patient, 11-year-old Sean McBrady, is unable to swallow pills. What are some alternatives to the medication? What would you suggest to the family and patient to promote easier administration?

Name: _____

*Here is a mix of oral and parenteral pediatric orders. For each problem, determine the safe dose and calculate the amount to be given. If you experience any difficulty, review the content. Answers will be found on page 356.*

**1.** Newborn: weighs 4 kg
    Order: vitamin K 1 mg IM $\times$ 1 dose
  Reference: Prophylaxis and treatment: 0.5–1 mg/dose IM, SC,
           IV $\times$ 1
    Stock: Vial 10 mg/mL

**2.** Infant 1 yr: 10 kg
    Order: Augmentin 125 mg po q8h
  Reference: Safe dose amoxicillin-clavulanic acid: 20–40 mg/kg/24h
          given q8h po
    Stock: 125 mg/5 mL

**3.** Infant 10 mo: 10 kg
    Order: benzathine penicillin 500,000 units IM $\times$ 1 dose
  Reference: Safe dose 50,000 units/kg $\times$ 1 IM. Max. 2.4 MU
    Stock: Vial labeled 600,000 units/mL

**4.** Infant 3.6 kg
    Order: gentamicin 9 mg IV q8h in 10 mL D5¼NS
  Reference: Safe dose 2.5 mg/kg/dose q8h
         Concentration for IV 2 mg/mL given over 15–30 min
    Stock: Vial 40 mg/mL

**5.** Infant 6.7 kg
    Order: Colace Syrup 10 mg po bid
  Reference: Infants and children under 3: 10–40 mg
    Stock: 20 mg/5 mL

**6.** Infant 5.5 kg
    Order: vancomycin 54 mg IV q8h in 12 mL D5¼NS
  Reference: Safe dose 10 mg/kg q8h IV
         Concentration for IV 5 mg/mL; infuse over 1 hr.
    Stock: 500 mg powder
         Directions: Add 10 mL sterile water for injection to give
         50 mg/mL. Stable in the refrigerator 14 days

**7.** Infant 6.7 kg
    Order: chloral hydrate 350 mg po prior to electroencephalogram
        (EEG)
  Reference: Hypnotic for children: 50–75 mg/kg/dose po
    Stock: 500 mg/5 mL

*(continued)*

**PROFICIENCY TEST 1**    **Infants and Children Dosage Problems (Continued)**

**8.** Child 3 yr; 9.9 kg
    Order:   theophylline 65 mg qid via ngt
 Reference:   22 mg/kg/24h given q6h
    Stock:   bottle labeled 80 mg/15 mL

**9.** Child 8 yr; 24 kg
    Order:   Fortaz 2 g IVPB q8h in 50 mL D5⅓NS
 Reference:   Safe dose 2–6 g/24h given q8–12h IV
              Concentration for IV 50 mg/mL over 15–30 min
    Stock:   2 g vial of powder
              Dilute initially with 10 mL sterile water for injection.

**10.** Child 35 lb
    Order:   meperidine HCl 20 mg IM stat
 Reference:   Children: usual dose 0.5 mg/lb to 1 mg/lb
    Stock:   50 mg/mL

# Answers

## Self-Test 1 Converting Pounds to Kilograms

**1.** 13.64 kg (calculator)

**2.** $\dfrac{5\ oz}{16\ oz}$ = 0.31 lbs (calculator)

Weight 15.31 lbs
Change to kilograms.

$\dfrac{15.31}{2.2}$ = 6.96 kg (calculator)

**3.** 1/4 lb = 0.25 lb

Weight to 7.25 lb
Change to kilograms.

$\dfrac{7.25}{2.2}$ = 3.3 kg (calculator)

**4.** 10 kg (calculator)

**5.** $\dfrac{8\ oz}{16}$ = 0.5 lb

Weight is 54.5 lb.
Change to kilograms.

$\dfrac{54.5\ lb}{2.2}$ = 24.77 kg

## Self-Test 2 Dosage Calculations

**1.** Step 1.
$$\begin{array}{r} 20 \qquad 9.0\ kg \\ 2.2\ \overline{)20.0.0} \\ \underline{19\ 8} \\ 2\ 0 \end{array}$$

Label states: 20–40 mg/kg/day in divided doses q 8 h.

Step 2. *Low range:*
$$\begin{array}{r} 9.0\ kg \\ \times\ 20\ mg \\ \hline 180\ mg/day \end{array}$$

*High range:*
$$\begin{array}{r} 9.0\ kg \\ \times\ 40\ mg \\ \hline 360.0\ mg/day \end{array}$$

Step 3. 60 mg × 3 doses = 180 mg/day
The order is safe.

Step 4. **Formula Method**

$$\dfrac{\overset{12}{\cancel{60\ mg}}}{\underset{\overset{25}{5}}{\cancel{125\ mg}}} \times \cancel{5}\ mL = \dfrac{12}{5}\quad \begin{array}{r} 2.4 \\ 5\ \overline{)12.0} \\ \underline{10} \\ 20 \\ \underline{20} \end{array}$$

Give 2.4 mL.

**Ratio Proportion Method**

$$\dfrac{5\ mL}{125\ mg} = \dfrac{x\ mL}{60\ mg}$$

$$\dfrac{300}{125} = x$$

2.4 mL = x

**2.** Step 1.  29 lb = 13.18 kg (calculator)

Step 2.        40 mg

    $\times$ 13.18 kg

            527 mg (calculator) = safe dose

Step 3.  175 mg

    $\times$ 3

    525 mg = child's dose. Order is safe.

Step 4. *Formula Method*

$$\frac{D}{H} \times S = A \qquad \frac{\overset{7}{\cancel{175}\ \text{mg}}}{\underset{\underset{1}{\cancel{25}}}{\cancel{125}\ \text{mg}}} \times \cancel{5}\overset{1}{}\ \text{mL} = 7$$

Give 7 mL po q8h.

*Ratio Proportion Method*

$$\frac{5\ \text{mL}}{125\ \text{mg}} = \frac{x\ \text{mL}}{175\ \text{mg}}$$

$$\frac{875}{125} = x$$

7 mL = x

**3.** **a.** It was not necessary to use a rule. The literature was clear. Children 6–12 years should receive 600 mg divided into three doses, which equals 200 mg/dose: the ordered dose is safe.

**b.** *Formula Method*

$$\frac{D}{H} \times S = A \qquad \frac{200}{125} \times 5 = \frac{1000}{125} \quad \overset{8.0\ \text{mL}}{125\overline{)1000.}}$$

Give 8 mL.

*Ratio Proportion Method*

$$\frac{5\ \text{mL}}{125\ \text{mg}} = \frac{x}{200}$$

$$\frac{1000}{125} = x$$

8.0 mL = x

**4.** Tylenol 80 mg seems low. Literature says a child of 6 should receive four chewable tablets. This would be 320 mg. Check with the physician.

**5.** **a.** The literature states that children under 6 months can receive 1–2.5 mg IM three to four times a day. The individual dose for the infant is 1 mg. This is safe, but the physician wrote q3–4h prn for the time. This would allow six to eight doses per 24 hours. The nurse can give the first dose but should clarify the times with the doctor.

**b.** *Formula Method*

$$\frac{D}{H} \times S = A \qquad \frac{1\ \text{mg}}{5\ \text{mg}} \times 1\ \text{mL} = 0.2\ \text{mL IM}$$

*Ratio Proportion Method*

$$\frac{1\ \text{mL}}{5\ \text{mg}} = \frac{x\ \text{mL}}{1\ \text{mg}}$$

0.2 mL = x

## Self-Test 3 Determining BSA

**1.** $0.54 \text{ m}^2$
**2.** $0.51 \text{ m}^2$

**3.** $1.08 \text{ m}^2$ (adult nomogram)
**4.** $0.19 \text{ m}^2$

## Self-Test 4 Use of the Nomogram

**1.** Step 1. Find the BSA in $\text{m}^2 = 0.94$.
Step 2. Determine safe dose.

| Low Dose | High Dose |
|---|---|
| 100 mg | 200 mg |
| $\times 0.94$ | $\times 0.94$ |
| 94 mg | 188 mg |

Safe dose is 94–188 mg over 24 hr.
Step 3. Is order safe?

$50 \text{ mg q8h} = 50 \text{ mg} \times 3 = 150 \text{ mg/24 hrs}$

Dose is safe.
Step 4. Order is 50 mg. Stock is 50 mg. Give 1 tab.

**2.** Step 1. Find the BSA in $\text{m}^2 = 1.29$.

Step 2. Safe dose is

| 10 mg |
|---|
| $\times 1.29$ |
| 12.9 mg |

Step 3. Is order safe? Yes; 12.5 mg is below the maximum.

Step 4. *Formula Method*

$\dfrac{D}{H} \times S = A \qquad \dfrac{\overset{5}{\cancel{12.5 \text{ mg}}}}{\underset{1}{\cancel{2.5 \text{ mg}}}} \times 1 \text{ tab} = 5 \text{ tabs}$

*Ratio Proportion Method*

$\dfrac{1 \text{ tab}}{2.5 \text{ mg}} = \dfrac{x \text{ tab}}{12.5 \text{ mg}}$

$\dfrac{12.5}{2.5} = x$

$5 \text{ tabs} = x$

**3.** Step 1. Find the BSA in m2 $= 0.46$.
Step 2. Safe dose is 6.30 mg/m2/24 hr.

| Low Dose | High Dose |
|---|---|
| 6 mg | 30 mg |
| $\times 0.46$ | $\times 0.46$ |
| 2.76 mg | 13.8 mg |

Safe dose is 2.8 mg to 13.8 mg over 24 hr.
Step 3. Order is 5 mg $\times$ 12 hr = 10 mg. Dose is safe.
Step 4. Order is 5 mg; stock is 5 mg/5 mL. Give 5 mL.

## Self-Test 5 Parenteral Medication Calculations

**1.** Step 1. Safe dose is 50–100 mg/kg/24h.

| Low Range | High Range |
|---|---|
| 50 mg | 100 mg |
| × 8 kg | × 8 kg |
| 400 mg/24 hr | 800 mg/24 hr |

Order is 200 mg q6h (4 doses).

200 mg × 4 = 800 mg/24 h.
Dose is safe.

Step 2. Minimum safe dilution is 50 mg/mL.

4 mL is the minimum dilution;

$50\overline{)200\text{ mg}}$

10 mL is safe.

Step 3. Dilute 750 mg with 8 mL sterile water to make 90 mg/mL.

*Formula Method*

$\dfrac{D}{H} \times S = A \quad \dfrac{200\text{ mg}}{90\text{ mg}} \times 1\text{ mL} = 2.2\text{ mL (calculator)}$

*Ratio Proportion Method*

$\dfrac{1\text{ mL}}{90\text{ mg}} = \dfrac{x\text{ mL}}{200\text{ mg}}$

$\dfrac{200}{90} = x$

$2.2\text{ mL} = x$

Withdraw 2.2 mL of the drug into a syringe. Label the remainder and store in the refrigerator.

Step 4. Add about 5 mL D5¼NS to the Buretrol. Add the 2.2 mL of drug. Add more D5$\frac{1}{4}$NS to make 10 mL.

Step 5. Set the pump at 20. This means 20 mL/hr. The pump will deliver 10 mL in 30 min.

Step 6. When the IV is finished, add a 20 mL flush of D5¼NS to clear the tubing of medication.

**2.** Step 1. Safe dose is 8–10 mg/kg/24h given q12h.

| Low Range | High Range |
|---|---|
| 8 mg | 10 mg |
| × 15 kg | × 15 kg |
| 120 mg/24 hr | 150 mg/24 hr |

Order is 75 mg q12h (2 doses) = 150 mg/24h. Dose is safe.

Step 2. Minimum safe dilution is 1 mL in 15–25 mL. The drug comes as a liquid 80 mg/5 mL.

**Formula Method**

$$\frac{D}{H} \times S = A \qquad \frac{75 \text{ mg}}{80 \text{ mg}} \times 5 \text{ mL} = 4.7 \text{ mL (calculator)}$$

**Ratio Proportion Method**

$$\frac{5 \text{ mL}}{80 \text{ mg}} = \frac{x \text{ mL}}{75 \text{ mg}}$$

$$\frac{375}{80} = x$$

4.7 mL
$\underline{\times \ 15}$ mL (minimum dilution factor)
70.5 mL is the safe dilution.

4.7 mL = x

Step 3. 75 mL D5W is a safe concentration (more than 70.5 mL).

Step 4. Draw up 4.7 mL drug into a syringe. Discard the remainder.

Step 5. Add about 50 mL D5W to the Buretrol. Add the 4.7 mL medication. Now add D5W until 75 mL is reached. Order is to administer over 1 hr. Set the pump at 75.

Step 6. When the IV is completed, add a 20 mL flush of D5W to clear the tubing of medication.

**3.** Step 1. Safe dose range is 6–7.5 mg/kg/24h given q8h.

| Low Range | High Range |
|---|---|
| 6 mg | 7.5 mg |
| $\underline{\times \ 40}$ kg | $\underline{\times \ 40}$ kg |
| 240 mg/24 hr | 300 mg/24 hr |

Order is 100 mg q8h (3 doses).
        100 mg $\times$ 3 = 300 mg. Dose is
        safe.

Step 2. Minimum safe dilution is 2 mg/mL.

$$2 \text{ mg} \overline{)100 \text{ mg}}^{\ 50 \text{ mL}}$$

is the safe minimum dilution. Order is 50 mL.

Step 3. We need 100 mg of tobramycin. Stock is
80 mg per 2 mL. We will need two
ampules. Use the first ampule (2 mL) and
20 mg from the second ampule.

*Formula Method*                  *Ratio Proportion Method*

$\dfrac{D}{H} \times S = A$                  $\dfrac{2 \text{ ml}}{80 \text{ mg}} = \dfrac{x \text{ ml}}{20 \text{ mg}}$

$\dfrac{20 \text{ mg}}{80 \text{ mg}} \times 2 \text{ mL} = \dfrac{1}{2} = 0.5 \text{ mL}$          $\dfrac{40}{80} = x$

$+ \ 2 \text{ mL} = 2.5 \text{ mL}$          $.5 \text{ mL} + 2 \text{ mL} = 2.5 \text{ mL}$

Step 4. Draw up 2.5 mL tobramycin into a
syringe. Add about 30 mL D5⅓NS into
the Buretrol.
Add the 2.5 mL medication. Now add
more D5⅓NS to make a total of 50 mL.

Step 5. Set the pump at 100. The pump will
deliver 50 mL over 30 min.

Step 6. When the IV is finished, add a 20-mL
flush of D5⅓NS to clear the tubing of
medication.

**4.** Step 1. Safe dose is 50–200 mg/kg/24h given
q6h.

*Low Range*          *High Range*

   50 mg                  200 mg

$\times$ 18 kg              $\times$  18 kg

  900 mg/24 hr        3600 mg/24 hr

Order is 900 mg q6h (4 doses).
900 mg $\times$ 4 = 3600 mg/24h.
Dose is safe.

Step 2. Minimum safe dilution is 50 mg/mL.

$$50 \text{ mg} \overline{)900 \text{ mg}}^{\,18}$$

18 mL is the minimum safe dilution.
25 mL is safe.

Step 3.  1 g powder. Dilute with 10 mL to make
95 mg/mL.

*Formula Method*

$$\frac{D}{H} \times S = A \quad \frac{900\ mg}{95\ mg} \times 1\ mL = 9.5\ mL\ drug\ (calculator)$$

*Ratio Proportion Method*

$$\frac{1\ mL}{95\ mg} = \frac{x\ mL}{900\ mg}$$

$$\frac{900}{95} = x$$

$$9.5\ mL = x$$

Draw up the 9.5 mL in a syringe.
Discard the remainder. Amount too small
to keep.

Step 4.  Add about 10 mL of D5⅓NS to the
Buretrol. Add the 9.5 mL medication.
Add D5⅓NS to make a total of 25 mL.

Step 5.  Set the pump at 50. The pump will
deliver 25 mL in 30 min.

Step 6.  When the IV is finished, add a flush of
20 mL D5⅓NS to clear the tubing of
medication.

# Information Basic to Administering Drugs

In previous chapters we learned drug forms and preparations, how to read prescriptions, and how to calculate dosages. This chapter provides the opportunity to focus on some of the nurse's responsibilities for drug therapy—drug knowledge, legal and ethical considerations, and finally, specific points that may prove helpful in giving medications.

## ▶ Drug Knowledge

Nursing drug handbooks are the best references for the nurse practitioner who needs a variety of information specifically designed to help assess, manage, evaluate, and teach the patient. The following headings represent the kind of information found in a nursing handbook.

| | |
|---|---|
| Generic and trade names | Side and adverse effects |
| Classification | Contraindications and precautions |
| Pregnancy category | Interactions and incompatibilities |
| Dosage and route | Nursing implications |
| Action | Signs of effectiveness |
| Indications | Patient teaching |

## Generic and Trade Names

The generic name is the official name given a drug. A drug has only one generic name in the United States. The letters USP (United States Pharmacopeia) following a generic name indicate that the drug meets government standards for purity and assay.

A trade name is the brand name under which a company manufactures a generic drug. A drug may have several trade names but only one generic name. The trade name is capitalized and is followed by the symbol ®. The generic name is not capitalized.

Consumer groups have advocated that drugs be prescribed by generic name only so that the pharmacist may dispense the least expensive drug available on the market. The nurse should understand that generic drugs, manufactured by different companies, are not exactly the same. The active ingredient in the drug meets standards of uniformity and purity, but manufacturers use different fillers and dyes. These substances can cause adverse effects (eg, severe nausea caused by the dye used in coloring). Additionally when a pharmacist dispenses a different trade name, the patient may become confused and distressed about receiving medication that appears unlike previous doses. The active ingredient is the same, but size, shape, or color may vary.

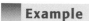 **Example**   The generic name of Nubain® is nalbuphine.

## Classification

The drug class is a quick reference to the therapeutic action, use, and adverse effect of a drug. As the nurse develops a knowledge base, the drug class will identify general nursing implications and precautions in administering a drug.

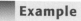 **Example**   Classification of nalbuphine is opioid analgesic. This drug will relieve pain. It is also an agonist/antagonist and will decrease the effect of other opioids.

## Pregnancy Category

The U.S. Federal Drug Administration (FDA) has established the following categories:

A. No risk to the fetus in any trimester

B. No adverse effect demonstrated in animals; no human studies available

C. Animals studies have shown adverse reactions. No human studies are available. Given only after risks to the fetus have been considered

D. Definite fetal risk exists; may be given in spite of risk to the fetus if needed for a life-threatening condition

X. Absolute fetal abnormality; not to be used anytime in pregnancy

A nurse administering a drug to a woman of childbearing age should be aware of the pregnancy category of a drug so that he/she can teach the patient and protect the fetus. In addition, this knowledge will aid in discussing the use of over-the-counter (OTC) drugs in pregnancy.

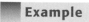 **Example**   Nubain is pregnancy category C. Consider fetal risk before administering to a pregnant woman.

## Dosage and Route

Information about the dosage and route of administration is crucial to protect against medication error. Most handbooks give a dosage range for adults, the elderly, and children.

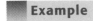 **Example**  Nalbuphine—IM, SC, IV (adults)

Usual dose—10 mg q 3–6 h. Single dose not to exceed 20 mg. Total daily dose not to exceed 160 mg. Dose in children not determined.

## Action

Information explains how the drug is known or believed to act to produce a therapeutic effect. This knowledge aids in understanding whether a drug should be taken with food or between meals; with other drugs or alone; orally or parenterally.

Patients with liver or kidney disease may not be able to metabolize or excrete certain drugs. The drug accumulates in the body, leading to adverse effects. The nurse who knows drug action can better assess, manage, and evaluate drug therapy.

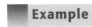 **Example**  Nalbuphine binds to opiate receptors in the central nervous system (CNS) and alters perception of and response to painful stimuli.

## Indications

Information gives the reasons for using the drug. This information aids in observing for expected effects and therapeutic response, as well as indicating what side and adverse effects might occur. One of the most common questions asked of nurses is "Why am I getting this drug?" The nurse relates the use of the drug to the expected effect.

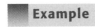 **Example**  Nalbuphine is used for moderate to severe pain.

## Side and Adverse Effects

Side effects are nontherapeutic reactions to a drug that are transient and may not require any nursing intervention. Adverse effects are nontherapeutic effects that may be harmful to the patient and that require lowering the dosage or discontinuing the drug. An example of a side effect is drowsiness, which occurs with some antihistamines. An example of an adverse effect is a serious decrease in white blood cells that results in lowered resistance to infection. The nurse must observe for these effects, know how to manage them, and teach the patient necessary information.

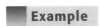 **Example**  Nalbuphine side effects: sedation, headache, dizziness, nausea, vomiting, dry mouth, sweating

Nalbuphine adverse effects: in high doses hypotension, miosis, dependency, dysphoria

## Contraindications and Precautions

These refer to conditions in which a drug should be given with caution or not given at all. For example, patients who have exhibited a previous reaction to penicillin should be cautioned against taking it again. Certain antibiotics must be administered with caution to patients who have poor kidney function. The nurse has a responsibility to know this information to safeguard the patient and carry out effective nursing care.

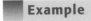 **Example**  Nalbuphine is contraindicated if hypersensitivity to the drug exists or if the patient has dependency on other opioids. Use cautiously in head trauma; increased intracranial pressure (ICP), severe respiratory disease; undiagnosed abdominal pain; pregnancy (depressed respirations in newborn). Safety is not established in children.

## Interactions and Incompatibilities

When more than one drug is administered at a time, unexpected or nontherapeutic responses may occur. Some interactions are desirable. For example, naloxone (Narcan) is a narcotic antagonist that reverses the effects of a morphine overdose. Other interactions, however, are undesirable. For example, aspirin should not be taken with an oral anticoagulant because the possibility of an adverse effect increases.

Some drugs may be incompatible and should not be mixed. This information is especially important when medications are combined for injection in IV administration. Chemical incompatibility is usually indicated by a visible sign such as precipitation or color change. Physical incompatibility can occur without any visible sign; therefore, the nurse should check a suitable reference before combining drugs. A good rule of thumb is: When in doubt, do not mix.

Interactions also may occur between drugs and certain foods. Calcium present in dairy products interferes with the absorption of tetracycline. Foods high in vitamin $B_6$ can decrease the effect of an anti-Parkinson drug. Foods high in tyramine, such as wine and cheese, can precipitate a hypertensive crisis in patients taking monoamine oxidase (MAO) inhibitors.

Cigarette smoke can increase liver metabolism of drugs and decrease drug effectiveness. Even individuals who are passively exposed to cigarette smoke may require higher doses of medication.

**Example**     Nalbuphine produces additive CNS depression with alcohol, antihistamines, and sedative/hypnotics; can produce withdrawal in patients dependent on opioids and diminish analgesic effect; exercise care if given to patients receiving MAO inhibitors. Severe reactions are possible.

## Nursing Implications

The nurse needs this information to administer the drug safely and to assess, manage, and teach the patient.

**Example**     Some nursing implications related to nalbuphine include: assess pain before and 1 hour following the dose; assess BP, pulse, respirations before and periodically after the dose; assess for dependency and tolerance.

## Signs of Effectiveness

Few drug references actually list this heading, yet the nurse is expected to evaluate the drug regimen and to record and report observations. Knowledge of the drug's class, its action, and its use leads to an understanding of expected therapeutic outcomes.

For example, ampicillin sodium is a broad-spectrum antibiotic that is used for urinary, respiratory, and other infections. Signs of effectiveness might include normal temperature; the laboratory report of the white blood cell (WBC) count indicating a normal result; clear urine; no pain on urination; no WBC in urine, decreased pus in an infected wound; wound healing; a patient who is more alert and interested in surroundings; improved appetite.

**Example**     Nalbuphine—relief of pain; sedation

## Patient Teaching

The patient has a right to know the name and dose of the drug, why the drug is ordered, and what effects to expect or watch for. In addition, the patient who is to take a drug at home needs specific information. This is a professional responsibility shared by the physician, the nurse, and the pharmacist.

# ▶ Pharmacokinetics

When a drug is taken orally, it is absorbed through the villi of the small intestine, distributed to the cells by the bloodstream, metabolized to a greater or lesser extent, and then excreted from the body. Pharmacokinetics includes absorption, distribution, biotransformation, and excretion.

## *Absorption*

Absorption of an oral drug depends on the degree of stomach acidity, the time it takes for the stomach to empty, whether or not food is present, the amount of contact with villi in the small intestine, and blood flow to the villi.

Absorption of a drug may be affected in many ways. Enteric-coated (EC) tablets are not meant to dissolve in the acidic stomach. They ordinarily pass through the stomach to the duodenum. When an antacid is administered with an EC tablet, the pH of the stomach is raised, and the tablet may dissolve prematurely. The drug may become less potent or it may irritate the gastric lining. Timed-release EC capsules that dissolve prematurely can deliver a huge dose of drug, causing adverse effects.

Laxatives increase gastrointestinal movement and decrease the time a drug is in contact with the villi of the small intestine where most absorption occurs. The presence of food in the stomach can impair absorption. Penicillin is a good example of a drug that should be taken on an empty stomach. Foods that contain calcium, such as milk and cheese, form a complex with some drugs and inhibit absorption.

## *Distribution*

Distribution is the movement of a drug through body fluids, chiefly the bloodstream, to cells. Drugs do not travel freely in the blood. Most travel attached to plasma proteins, especially albumin. Drugs that are free can attach to cells on which they produce an effect.

When more than one drug is present in the bloodstream, they may compete for protein-binding sites. One drug may displace another. The displaced drug is now free to act with the cells, and its effect will be more pronounced. Aspirin is a common drug for displacement; it should not be given with oral anticoagulants, which are 99% bound to albumin. Aspirin displaces the anticoagulant; more is free to act at the cellular level, and the toxic effect of bleeding may occur.

## *Biotransformation*

This refers to the chemical change of a drug to a form that can be excreted. Most biotransformation occurs in the liver. Because oral drugs are carried first to the liver, this process begins when the drug is absorbed. Here, too, one drug can interfere with the effects of another. Barbiturates increase the liver enzyme activity. Because drugs are metabolized more quickly, their effect is reduced. Conversely, acetaminophen (Tylenol) will block the breakdown of penicillin in the liver, thereby increasing its activity.

## *Excretion*

Excretion refers to the removal of a drug from the body. The major organ of excretion is the kidney. Drug interactions may also occur at this level; for example, probenecid inhibits the excretion of penicillin and increases its length of action; furosemide (Lasix), a diuretic, blocks the excretion of aspirin and can lead to adverse effects by aspirin.

Drug interactions are not necessarily harmful. For example, narcotic antagonists are used to reverse the adverse effects of general anesthetics. This action is termed *antagonism. Synergism* is a term used when a second drug increases the intensity or prolongs the effect of a first drug. For example, a narcotic and a minor tranquilizer produce more pain relief than the narcotic alone. The nurse administering medications needs to be aware of possible interactions and evaluate the patient's response.

To minimize adverse interactions, the nurse should know the patient's drug profile, give as low a dose as possible, know the actions and adverse effects of the drugs administered, and monitor the patient. Some drug interactions may take several weeks to develop.

## Tolerance

When a pain or sleeping medication is given frequently, the liver enzymes become skilled in biotransforming more quickly. Less drug is available, thus the drug is less effective in relieving pain or aiding sleep. Some nurses call this reaction "addiction" because the patient complains that the drug is not working and asks for more. In fact, it is a physiologic response. The patient requires more of the drug or a drug with a different molecular structure.

## Cumulation

When biotransformation or excretion is inhibited, as can occur in liver or kidney disease, the drug accumulates in the body and an adverse effect can occur. Cumulation can also result from taking too much drug or from taking a drug too frequently.

Other factors that affect drug action include:

- Weight: Larger individuals need a higher dose.

- Age: Extremes of life respond more strongly. The livers and kidneys of infants are not well developed; in the elderly, systems are less efficient.

- Pathologic conditions: especially of liver and kidney.

- Hypersensitivity to a drug: allergic reaction.

- Psychological and emotional state: Depression or anxiety can decrease or increase body metabolism and affect drug action.

Adverse reactions may occur in any system or organ. Drug knowledge will enhance the nurse's observational skills and lead to responsible and appropriate intervention.

## Half-Life

Half-life of a drug correlates roughly with its duration of action and gives an indication of how often the drug may be given to continue therapeutic effect. For example, piroxicam has a duration of 48–72 hours and is given po as a single dose once a day; carisoprodol has a half-life of 4–6 hours and is administered 3–4 times daily.

# ▶ Legal Considerations

There are two types of law that affect nursing practice—criminal and civil.

## Criminal Law

Criminal law relates to offenses against the general public that are detrimental to society as a whole. Criminal actions are prosecuted by governmental authorities. If the defendant is judged guilty, the penalty may be a fine, imprisonment, or both.

Nurses must know the scope of nursing practice in the state in which they function. They should be familiar with government regulations—federal, state, and local—that affect nursing. The policies and procedures of the agency in which they practice also have legal status. Failure to follow guidelines or lack of knowledge can lead to liability.

Criminal charges include unlawful use, possession, or administration of a controlled substance. The Comprehensive Drug Abuse, Prevention and Control Act of 1970 classified drugs that are subject to abuse into one of five schedules according to their medical usefulness and abuse potential.

*Schedule I* drugs have no valid use and are not available for prescription use (eg, LSD).

*Schedule II* drugs have a valid medical use and are available for prescriptions but exhibit a high abuse potential. Misuse can lead to physical and psychological dependence. Labels for these drugs are marked with the symbol ⓘ. An order for a narcotic in a hospital setting might be valid for 3 days. When the 3 days have elapsed, the order must be rewritten. A nurse who administers a controlled drug after the order has expired commits a medication error.

*Schedule III, IV, and V* drugs are classed as having less abuse potential than Schedule II drugs, but they can cause some physical and psychological dependence. Note that ⓘⓘⓘ, ⓘⓥ and ⓥ symbols identify these drugs. A few examples of these drugs are Percodan, Fiorinal, diazepam (Valium), Tylenol #3 (Tylenol with Codeine).

Schedule II, III, IV and V drugs are kept locked on nursing units. A locked narcotic cabinet or cart is used, and a record is kept for each narcotic administered. The Pyxis® system is being used in many hospitals, which is a computerized locked cabinet that dispenses controlled substances. Controlled drugs are counted each shift, and discrepancies are reported. Government and institutional policies specify how these drugs are stored and protected.

Nurses who become impaired (unable to function) owing to alcohol or drug abuse leave themselves open to criminal action, as well as to disciplinary action by the state board of nursing. Many states have laws requiring mandatory reporting of impaired nurses.

## Civil Law

Civil law is concerned with the legal rights and duties of private persons. When an individual believes that a wrong was committed against him or her personally, that individual can sue for damages in the form of money.

The legal wrong is called a *tort*. *Malpractice* refers to negligence on the part of the nurse. There are four elements of negligence:

1. A claim that the nurse owed the patient a special duty of care, that is, a nurse-patient relationship existed.

2. A claim that the nurse was required to meet a specific standard of care in carrying out the action or function. To prove or disprove this element, both sides bring in expert witnesses to testify.

3. A claim that the nurse failed to meet the required standard.

4. A claim that harm or injury resulted for which compensation is sought.

The nurse–patient relationship is a legal status that is created the moment a nurse actually provides nursing care to another person.

For administration of medications, *a nurse is required by law to exercise the degree of skill and care that a reasonably prudent nurse with similar training and experience, practicing in the same community, would exercise under the same or similar circumstances.* When a nursing student performs duties that are customarily performed by a registered nurse, the courts have held the nursing student to the higher standard of care of the registered nurse.

Mistakes in administering medications are among the most common causes of malpractice. Liability may result from administering the wrong dose, giving a medication to a wrong patient, giving a drug at the wrong time, or failing to administer a drug at the right time or in the proper manner.

A frequent cause of medication errors is misreading the physician's order or failing to check with the physician when the order is questionable. Faulty technique in administering medications, especially injections that result in injury to the patient, is another common medication error.

Not all malpractice is a result of negligence. Malpractice claims are also founded on the daily interaction between the nurse and the patient; consequently, the nurse's personality plays a major role in fostering or preventing malpractice claims. All nurses should be familiar with the principles of psychology. The surest way to prevent claims is to recognize the patient as a human being who has emotional, as well as physical, needs and to respond to these needs in a humane and competent manner.

Should an error occur, primary consideration must be given to the patient. The nurse notifies the physician and the immediate nursing supervisor; students notify the instructor. Error-in-medication forms are filled out and appropriate action is taken under the direction of the physician.

To prevent malpractice claims, the nurse must render, as consistently as possible, the best possible care to patients. Every nurse involved in direct care should regard prevention of malpractice claims as an integral part of daily nursing responsibilities for two fundamental reasons:

1. Such measures result in higher quality care.

2. All affirmative measures taken to minimize malpractice will minimize the nurse's exposure to personal liability.

How can liability claims be avoided?

- Know and follow institutional policies and procedures.

- Look up what you do not know.

- Do not leave medicines at the bedside.

- Chart carefully.

- Listen to the patient: "I never took that before," and the like.

- Check.

- *Double check* when a dose seems high. Most oral tablet doses range from $\frac{1}{2}$ to 2 tablets.

- Most injections are less than 3 mL.

- Label any powder you dilute. Label any IV bag you use.

- When necessary, seek advice from competent professionals.

- Do not administer drugs poured by another nurse.

- Keep drug knowledge up to date: Attend continuing education programs; update nursing skills.

It is possible to render high-quality nursing care and never commit a medication error. Safe, effective drug therapy is a combination of knowledge, skill, carefulness, and caring.

## ▶ Ethical Principles in Drug Administration

A moral as well as legal dimension is involved in the administration of medications. Nurses are responsible for their actions.

The American Nurses Association Code of Ethics contains several statements that apply to drug therapy. Briefly stated, they are:

1. The nurse provides services with respect for the human dignity and the uniqueness of the patient.

2. The nurse safeguards the patient's right to privacy.

3. The nurse acts to safeguard the patient from incompetent, unethical, or illegal practice.

4. The nurse assumes responsibility and accountability for nursing judgments and actions.

5. The nurse maintains competence in nursing.

Several principles can be used as guides when an ethical decision must be made. These principles are autonomy, truthfulness, beneficence, nonmaleficence, confidentiality, justice, and fidelity.

## Autonomy

Autonomy is self-determination. It is a form of personal liberty in which an individual has the freedom to decide, knows the facts and understands them, and acts without outside force, deceit, or constraints. For the patient, this implies a right to be informed about drug therapy and a right to refuse medication. For the nurse, autonomy brings a responsibility to discuss drug information with the patient and to accept the patient's right to refuse. Autonomy also gives the nurse the right to refuse to participate in any drug therapy deemed to be unethical or unsafe for the patient.

## Truthfulness

The nurse has the obligation not to lie. Telling the truth, however, is not the same as telling the *whole* truth. Ethically it is sometimes difficult to decide what may be concealed and what must be revealed.

In drug research the patient has a right to informed consent—to be told the truth before signing as a participant. Double-blind studies are employed in determining effectiveness. Patients are randomly assigned to an experimental group that receives the drug or to a control group that receives a placebo (a preparation devoid of pharmacologic effect). Neither the patient nor the nurse knows to which group he or she is assigned. The patient must receive full disclosure of risks and benefits and understand the research design to participate freely.

## Beneficence

This principle holds that the nurse should act in the best interests of the patient. Actions are limited by the respect due to the freedom of the patient and the right of the patient to self-determination. Conflict can arise when the nurse decides what is best for the patient and violates the patient's rights.

## Nonmaleficience

This principle holds that the nurse must not inflict harm on the patient and must prevent harm whenever possible. In drug therapy every medication has the risk of inducing some undesirable side and/or adverse effect. Chemotherapy may reduce the size of a tumor but cause nausea, vomiting, decreased white cell count, etc. The nurse anticipates what untoward effects of drugs may occur and acts to minimize them.

## Confidentiality

Confidentiality is respect for information learned from professional involvement with patients. A patient's drug therapy and responses should be discussed only with those individuals who have a right to know, that is, other professionals caring for the patient. The extent to which the family or significant others have a right to know depends on the specific situation and wishes of the patient. These varying interests may cause conflict.

## Justice

Justice refers to the patient's right to receive the right drug, the right dose, by the right route, at the right time. In addition, the patient has a right to the nurse's careful assessment, management, and evaluation of drug therapy and to those nursing actions that promote the patient's safety and well-being. The nurse's obligation is to maintain a high standard of care.

## Fidelity

A nurse should keep promises made to the patient. Statements such as "I'll be right back" and "I'll check the chart and let you know" create a covenant that should be respected.

# ▶ Specific Points That May Be Helpful in Giving Medications

### Three Checks and Five Rights

The nurse always observes the three checks and five rights of medication administration.

Three Checks When Preparing Medications

Read the label:

√ When reaching for the container or unit dose package

√ Immediately before pouring or opening the medication

√ When replacing the container or before giving the unit dose to the patient

Five Rights Before Administering Medications

- Right medication
- Right patient
- Right dosage
- Right route
- Right time

### Medication Orders

A correct medication order has the patient's name and room number, the date, the name of the drug (generic or trade), the dose of the drug, the route of administration, and the times to administer the drug. It ends with the physician's signature.

There are several types of orders:

1. Standing order with termination

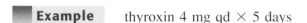 **Example**     thyroxin 4 mg qd × 5 days

2. Standing order without termination

**Example**     digoxin 0.5 mg po qd

3. A prn order

**Example**     Demerol 50 mg IM q 4 h prn

4. Single-dose order

**Example**     atropine $SO_4$ 0.3 mg SC 7:30 AM on call to OR

5. Stat order

**Example**     morphine sulfate 10 mg SC stat

Hospital guidelines provide for an automatic stop time on some classes of drugs; narcotic orders may be valid for only 3 days, antibiotics for 10 days. When the nurse first picks up and transfers the order, care must be taken to note the expiration time so that all staff who pour medications are alerted. State laws and hospital policies vary.

- Medical students may write orders on charts, but orders must be countersigned by a house physician before they are legal. Medical students are not licensed.

- In states that allow nurses or paramedical personnel to prescribe drugs, hospital guidelines must be followed in carrying out orders.

- Do not carry out an order that is not clear or that is illegible. Check with the physician who wrote the order. Do not assume anything.

- Do not carry out an order if a conflict exists with nursing knowledge; for example, Demerol 500 mg IM is above the average dose. Check with the physician who wrote the order.

- Nursing students should not accept oral or telephone orders. They should refer the physician to the nurse manager.

- Professional nurses may take oral or telephone orders in accord with institutional policy. These orders must be written on the chart by the nurse and signed by the physician within 24 hours. Two nurses should listen to and verify the order.

## Knowledge Base

- Nurses should know generic and trade names of drugs to be administered, class, average dose, routes of administration, use, side and adverse effects, contraindications, and nursing implications in administration. Nurses should also know what signs of effectiveness to look for and what drug interactions are possible. New or unfamiliar drugs should be researched.

- The nurse should be aware of the patient's diagnosis and medical history especially relative to drugs taken. Be especially alert to over-the-counter (OTC) drugs, which the patient often does not consider important. Check for allergies.

- Assess the patient's need for drug information. Be prepared to implement and evaluate a nursing care plan in drug therapy.

## Pouring Medications

- The patient has a right to considerate and respectful care and the right to refuse a medication. The patient also has a right to know the name of the medication, what it is supposed to do, any side effects that may occur, and what to do should these occur.

- In the ticket system, the Kardex is the main check against the medication ticket. If the ticket does not agree with the Kardex, go to the chart and find the original order. Check through every order to the current date to identify changes in orders.

- In the unit-dose, mobile cart system, the nurse has the medication sheets of each patient together in a folder or on a computer printout. If unsure of an order, take the sheet to the patient's chart and check from the date ordered to the current date.

- Do not pour and administer a drug about which any doubt exists. Check further with the physician, the pharmacist, or a supervising nurse.

- Quiet and concentration are needed to pour drugs. Follow a routine in pouring. *Methodology is the best safeguard in preventing error.*

- Keys are needed to obtain controlled drugs (eg, narcotics) and to prevent others' access to medications.

- Pour oral medications first, then injections. Medical asepsis (clean technique) is used for oral administration. Injections require sterile technique.

- Read labels three times: (1) when removing the drug from storage, (2) when calculating the dose, and (3) after pouring the drug.

- Orders issued as "stat" take precedence and must be carried out immediately.

- Perform indicated nursing actions before administering certain medications; for example, digitalis preparations require an apical heart rate, whereas antihypertensives require a blood pressure reading.

- Medications should be administered within 30 minutes of the time given. They may be prepared before then in the ticket system. When the mobile cart is used, medications are prepared at the patient's bed and administered.

- Keep medications within sight at all times. Never leave medications unattended. The mobile cart or the medication tray must be kept in view.

- Administer irritating oral drugs with meals or a snack to decrease gastric irritation.

- Break a tablet only if it is scored.

- Never open capsules or break enteric-coated tablets. If the patient cannot swallow them, ask the physician to order a liquid, or check with the pharmacist.

- Check tablets in a stock container. Are they the same size? Same color? If not, return them to the pharmacy.

- It is a fallacy that the nurse is no longer required to calculate or prepare drugs dispensed as unit-dose. Fractional doses may still be necessary. The pharmacy may not have the exact dose. Antibiotics must be prepared for IM or IV use. The label must still be read three times.

- Labels must be clear. If not, return them to the pharmacy.

- Never return any poured drug to a stock bottle once the drug has been taken from the preparation room.

- Never combine medications from two stock bottles. Return both bottles to the pharmacy. It is the responsibility of the pharmacists to combine drugs.

- Hydrophilic capsules are not medications. They are labeled DO NOT EAT and are placed in stock containers of tablets and capsules to absorb dampness and maintain the drug in a solid state.

- If the patient is nauseous or vomiting, hold oral medications and notify the physician or the immediate superior. Be sure to chart this action.

- A medication should not be administered if it is assessed that the drug is contraindicated or that an adverse effect may have occurred as a result of a previous dose. If a drug is withheld, notify the physician who wrote the order.

- Some liquid medications require dilution. Check references for directions.

- Some liquids may have to be administered through a straw; for example, liquid iron preparations discolor and should not come in contact with teeth.

- Liquids are poured at eye level using a medicine cup. Measure at the *center* of the meniscus. Pour with the label up to prevent soiling.

- After the patient has taken a liquid antacid, add 5–10 mL of water to the cup, mix, and have patient drink it as well. Antacids are thick and medication often remains in the cup.

- The nurse who pours medications is responsible for administering and charting.

- Do not give drugs that another nurse has poured.

## Giving Medications

- Follow the universal safeguards in administration of medication (see Chapter 13).

- *Always* check the patient's ID band before administering medications. If the patient does not have an ID band, have a responsible person identify the patient for you and be sure to notify the ward clerk to obtain an ID band for the patient.

- Listen to the patient's comments and act on them, for example, "Not mine" or "Never took this before." Check carefully, then return to the patient with the result of your investigation. Failure to do this will result in loss of the patient's trust and confidence and may also result in a medication error.

- If a patient refuses a drug, find out why. Then implement nursing action to correct the situation. Chart the reason for refusal and notify the physician who wrote the order.

- Watch to make sure the patient takes the drugs. Stay until oral drugs are swallowed.

- Keep drugs within view at all times.

- Never leave any drug at the bedside stand unless hospital policy permits this. If a medication is left, inform the patient why the drug is ordered, how to take it, and what to expect. Check to determine if the drug was taken and record findings.

## Charting

- Chart single doses, stat doses, and prn medications immediately and use the *exact time* when administered.

- Chart standing orders using *standard time* (eg, tid).

- If it was necessary to hold a drug or the drug was refused, write the reason on the nurse's notes and the name of the physician who was notified.

- Chart any nursing actions preliminary to administering drugs, for example, apical heart rate or blood pressure.

## Evaluation

- Check for the expected effect of the drug. Did side effects or adverse effects occur? Perform indicated nursing actions. Record observations.

## Error in Medication

- **Report an error immediately to the charge nurse and the physician.**

- **Primary concern must be given to the patient.**

- **Error-in-medication forms should be filled out. Follow the physician's directions in caring for the patient.**

## SELF TEST 1   Basic Information

*Give the information requested. Answers may be found at the end of the chapter.*

**1.** List at least ten kinds of information the nurse needs to know to give drugs safely.

_____     _____

_____     _____

_____     _____

_____     _____

_____     _____

**2.** List the five pregnancy categories used to identify the safety of drugs for the fetus and briefly define each.

_____

_____

_____

_____

_____

**3.** Name the major organ for these drug activities.

   **a.** Absorption _____     **c.** Biotransformation _____

   **b.** Distribution _____     **d.** Excretion _____

**4.** Define:

   **a.** Tolerance _____

_____

_____

   **b.** Cumulation _____

_____

_____

**5.** List the four elements of negligence.

_____ ,

_____ ,

_____ , and

_____

**6.** What is the standard by which a tort is judged?

_____

_____

_____

*(continued)*

**7.** List at least five positive actions to avoid liability.

_____

_____

_____

_____

**8.** List and briefly describe five ethical principles in drug therapy.

_____

_____

_____

_____

_____

**9.** What are the seven elements of a correct medication order?

_____

_____

_____

_____

_____

_____

**10.** What action should a nurse take when an order is not clear?

_____

## TEST YOUR CLINICAL SAVVY

Mr. T is a patient who is receiving a drug that is in a drug study and/or has just been released by the FDA.

**A.** What is your ethical responsibility as a nurse administering this drug?

**B.** What is an appropriate response if the patient asks "Is it safe to take this drug?" What should you do if the patient refuses to take the drug?

**C.** You are in agreement with the patient that he should not take the experimental drug. What are your ethical responsibilities? What are your legal responsibilities?

**PROFICIENCY TEST 1   Basic Drug Information**

*Name:* _____

*Choose the correct answer. Answers will be found on page 360.*

1. Two drugs are given for different reasons, but drug Y interferes with the excretion of drug X. The effect of drug X would be

   a. increased

   b. decreased

   c. unchanged

   d. stopped

2. Major biotransformation of drugs occurs in the

   a. lungs

   b. kidney

   c. liver

   d. urine

3. Toxicity to a drug is more likely to occur when

   a. elimination of the drug is rapid

   b. the drug is bound to the plasma protein, albumin

   c. the drug will not dissolve in the lipid layer of the cell

   d. the drug is free in the blood circulation

4. The term USP after a drug name indicates that the drug

   a. is made only in the United States

   b. meets official standards in the United States

   c. cannot be made by any other pharmaceutical company

   d. is registered by the U.S. Public Health Service

5. When an order is written to be administered "as needed" it is called a

   a. standing order

   b. prn order

   c. single order

   d. stat order

6. Signs of effectiveness of a drug are based on what information?

   a. Action and use

   b. Untoward effects

   c. Generic and trade names

   d. Drug interaction

*(continued)*

7. Drug classification is an aid in understanding

   a. use of the drug

   b. drug idiosyncrasy

   c. the trade name

   d. the generic name

8. Names of many drugs include

   a. several generic, several trade names

   b. several generic, one trade name

   c. one generic, one trade name

   d. one generic, several trade names

9. Which pregnancy category is considered safe for the fetus?

   a. A

   b. B

   c. C

   d. D

10. What is the primary purpose of enteric-coating medications?

    a. Improve taste

    b. Delay absorption

    c. Code the drug for identification

    d. Make the drug easier to swallow

11. Which of the following drug preparations does *not* have to be shaken before pouring?

    a. Emulsion

    b. Gel

    c. Suspension

    d. Aqueous solution

12. Most oral drugs are absorbed in the

    a. mouth

    b. stomach

    c. small intestine

    d. large intestine

*(continued)*

**13.** Nursing legal responsibilities associated with controlled substances include

   **a.** storage in a locked place

   **b.** assessing vital signs

   **c.** evaluating psychological response

   **d.** establishing automatic 24-hour stop orders

**14.** Characteristics of a Schedule II drug include

   **a.** accepted medical use with a high abuse potential

   **b.** medically accepted drug with low-dependence possibility

   **c.** no accepted use in patient care

   **d.** unlimited renewals

**15.** The responsibilities of the medication nurse in the hospital include

   **a.** prescribing drugs

   **b.** teaching patients

   **c.** regulating automatic expiration times of drugs

   **d.** preparing solutions

**16.** Under what condition does a nurse have a right to refuse to administer a drug?

   **a.** The pharmacist ordered the drug.

   **b.** The drug is manufactured by two different companies.

   **c.** The drug is prescribed by a licensed physician.

   **d.** The dose is within the range given in the *PDR*.

**17.** When administering medication in the hospital, the nurse should

   **a.** chart medications before administering them

   **b.** chart only those drugs that she or he personally gave the patient

   **c.** chart all medications given for the day at one time

   **d.** determine the best method for giving the drugs

**18.** Which of the following illustrates a medication error?

   **a.** Administering a 10 AM dose at 10:20 AM

   **b.** Giving 2 tablets of Gantrisin 500 mg when 1 g is ordered

   **c.** Pouring 5 mL of cough syrup when 1 tsp is ordered

   **d.** Giving digoxin IM when digoxin 0.25 mg is ordered

*(continued)*

19. A nurse reads a medication order that is not clear. What action is indicated?

    a. Ask the charge nurse to explain the order.

    b. Ask a doctor at the nurses' station for help.

    c. Check the *PDR* on the unit.

    d. Check with the doctor who wrote the order.

20. Which nursing action is illegal?

    a. Pouring medication from one stock bottle into another

    b. Counting control drugs in the narcotic closest each shift

    c. Labeling a vial of powder after dissolving it

    d. Refusing to carry out an order that is confusing

# Answers

## Self-Test I Basic Information

1. Generic/trade name; class; pregnancy category; dose and route; action; use; side/adverse effects; contraindications/precautions; interactions/incompatibilities; nursing implications; evaluation of effectiveness; patient teaching
2. **A.** No risk to fetus
   **B.** No adverse effects in animals, but no human studies
   **C.** Animals show adverse effects; calculated risk to fetus.
   **D.** Fetal risk exists
   **X.** Absolute fetal abnormality
3. **a.** Small intestines
   **b.** blood
   **c.** liver
   **d.** kidney
4. **a.** Repeated administration of a drug increases microsomal enzyme activity in the liver. The drug is broken down more quickly and its effectiveness is decreased.
   **b.** Biotransformation is inhibited and the drug level remains high. Adverse effects are more likely to occur.
5. A claim that a nurse–patient relationship existed
   The nurse was required to meet a standard of care
   A claim that the nurse failed to meet that standard
   A claim that this resulted in injury
6. Whether or not the nurse exercised the degree of skill and care that a reasonably prudent nurse with similar training and experience, practicing in the same community, would exercise under the same or similar circumstances
7. Know policies and practices of the institution
   Research unfamiliar drugs.
   Do not leave medicines at the bedside.
   Chart carefully.
   Listen to the patient's complaints.
   Check yourself (eg, read labels three times).
   Label anything you dilute.
   Keep up to date.
8. Autonomy: freedom to decide based on knowledge with no constraint
   Truthfulness: truth telling that can create a dilemma. Is it absolute or is there a beneficient deceit?
   Beneficence: obligation to help others
   Nonmaleficence: do no harm
   Confidentiality: keep secrets
   Justice: rights of an individual
   Fidelity: keep promises
9. Patient's name and room; date; name of drug; dose; route; times of administration; doctor's signature
10. The nurse does not administer the drug and checks with the physician who wrote the order.

# Administration Procedures

Throughout this text we calculated dosages and studied information related to drug therapy. Finally we arrive at the "how to" chapter—methods of administering drugs orally, parenterally, and topically. The adages "practice makes perfect" and "one picture is worth a thousand words" apply. Learning to administer medications is a skilled activity that requires practice, with supervision, to ensure correct technique.

Every institution has a standard procedure for administering medications, which depends on the way the drugs are dispensed—unit-dose, multidose containers, or a combination of the two. Institutional procedure may call for the use of a tray and medication tickets or for a mobile cart with medication sheets or the use of a computer printout.

Whatever the procedure is, follow it carefully. Do not look for shortcuts. *Methodology*—a step-by-step attention to detail—is the best safeguard to assure the patient's five rights. Research has proved time after time that most medication errors occur because the nurse violated procedural guidelines.

## ▶ Universal or Standard Precautions Applied to Administration of Medications

In administering drugs, there is a risk of potential exposure to hepatitis B virus (HBV), hepatitis C virus (HCV), and the immunodeficiency virus (HIV) through contact of the nurse's skin or mucous membranes with patient blood, body fluids, or tissues. The Centers for Disease Control and Prevention (CDCP) in Atlanta recommend that *Universal Precautions be employed in caring for all patients and when handling equipment contaminated with blood or blood-streaked body fluids.* In 1996 the term Standard Precautions replaced Universal Precautions; these two terms are interchangeable.

The following points that are based on CDCP guidelines are offered to aid in determining appropriate safeguards in giving medications. These points are *dependent on the type of contact you have with patients.*

## *General Safeguards in Administering Medications*

1. Oral medications: Handwashing is adequate unless there is a possibility of exposure to blood or body secretions.

2. Injections: Handwashing and gloves are required. Carefully dispose of used sharps in a puncture-proof container. Hold the sharp away from you. Never take your eyes from the sharp during the disposal process!

3. Heparin locks, intravenous catheters, and intravenous needles: Wear gloves when inserting or removing intravenous needles and catheters. The use of a clamp is recommended to hold contaminated IV needles and catheters being carried to a puncture-proof container.

4. Secondary administration sets or intravenous piggyback sets: Handwashing is adequate after removing this equipment from the main IV tubing because there is no direct exposure to blood or body secretions. Place used needles in a puncture-proof container.

5. Application of medication to mucous membranes: Wear gloves (see the following guidelines in using gowns, masks, protective eyewear).

6. Applications to skin: Exercise nursing judgment. Handwashing may be sufficient protection when applying such drug forms as transdermal patches. Use gloves when the patient's skin is not intact. Use gloves when applying lotions, ointments, or creams to areas of rash or to skin lesions.

## Hands

1. Wash hands before preparing medications and after administering medications to each patient.

2. Wash hands *after* removing gloves, gowns, masks, protective eyewear, and *before* leaving the room of any patient for whom they are used.

3. Wash hands immediately when soiled with patient blood or body fluids.

4. Wash hands *after* handling equipment soiled with blood or body fluids.

## Gloves

1. Wear gloves for any direct ("hands-on") contact with patient's blood, bodily fluids, or secretions while administering medications.

2. Wear gloves when handling materials or equipment contaminated with blood or body fluids.

3. When gloves are used, they must be changed upon completion of procedures for each patient *and* between patients.

## Gowns

When administering medications, gowns are required *only* if the nurse's clothing may become contaminated with a patient's blood or body fluids.

## Masks, Protective Eyewear, Face Shields

1. Masks are required when caring for a patient on *strict* or *respiratory* isolation procedures.

2. Masks and protective eyewear or face shields are required when a medication procedure may cause blood or body fluids to splash directly onto the nurse's face, eyes, or mucous membranes.

3. Masks and protective eyewear must be worn in a medication procedure is known to cause aerosolization of fluids containing chemicals or body fluids.

## Management of Used Needles and Sharps

1. All used needles, syringes, sharps, stylets, butterfly needles, and IV catheters must be placed in appropriate, labeled, puncture-proof containers.

2. Do not break, bend, or recap needles after use. Immediately place needles into a puncture-proof container.

3. Exercise caution in removing heparin locks, intravenous catheters, and intravenous needles. Gloves should be worn. The use of a clamp is advisable to hold the used IV needle being transported to a puncture-proof container. *Do not remove the IV needle from the IV tubing by hand: Use a clamp or use the needle unlocking device on the sharps container.*

4. If *reusable* needles and syringes are employed, the needle should be separated from the syringe with a clamp. *Never manipulate a used needle by hand.* Place the needle and synringe in appropriate puncture-proof containers for sterilization. *It is strongly recommended that disposable needles and syringes be used.*

5. Never take your eyes from the sharps container as you dispose of the sharp.

## Needleless Systems

Needleless systems are being used to reduce the risk of needlesticks and bloodborne pathogens. These devices are used in several ways. Some syringes have a needle that retracts into the syringe after it is used. There are needleless adapters for syringes to withdraw medication from vials (Fig. 13-1). Needleless systems are available for IV tubing (Fig. 13-2) and for use at the patient's intravenous site. The needleless equipment is disposed into sharp containers.

## Management of Materials Other Than Needles and Sharps

Paper cups, plastic cups, and other equipment not contaminated with blood or body fluids may be discarded according to routine hospital procedure. In cases of *strict* or *respiratory* isolation precautions, follow the protocol established by the institution.

## Management of Nurse Exposed to Blood or Body Fluids

The nurse who is exposed to blood or blood-streaked body fluids of any patient through a personal needlestick or injury or through skin laceration should immediately squeeze the area if this is indicated, wash the area with soap and copious water, and scrub the area with povidone–iodine (Betadine), alcohol 70%, or another acceptable antiseptic. If mucous membrane exposure occurs, flush the exposed areas with copious amounts of warm water. The protocol established by the health care institution for management of needlestick injury or accidental exposure to blood or body fluids should be followed.

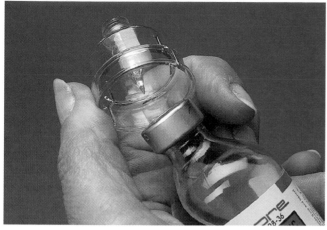

A

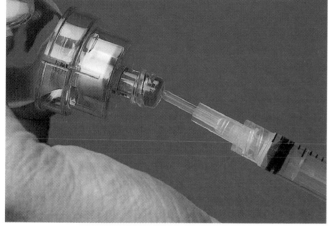

B

FIGURE 13-1

(A) Needleless system adaptor for vial. (B) Use syringe (without needle) to withdraw medication.

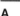

FIGURE 13-2

Needleless system for IV tubing.

# ▶ Systems of Administration

In an institutional setting, medications may be administered using tickets, the mobile cart, or computer printouts.

The ticket system is used when drugs are dispensed in multidose containers. Drugs are prepared in a medication room and carried on a tray to the patient. When unit-dose packaging is available, drugs are placed in individual patient drawers on a mobile cart. The cart is wheeled into the patient's room and medications are prepared at the bedside for administration.

## Ticket System

In this system, a medication order is transferred to three places: a medication ticket, the patient's medication sheet, and the patient's Kardex file, which contains the nursing care plan.

Tickets for all patients are kept in a central location. The nurse sorts them according to time of administration. Each ticket is compared with the Kardex entry. If there is a discrepancy, the nurse checks the original order on the patient's chart. After all tickets are verified, the nurse enters the medication room or unlocks the medication cart.

The nurse separates the first patient's tickets and places them together in a pile one on top of another, so that only one ticket is visible at a time. The nurse reads the ticket, locates the medication, and verifies the label with the ticket (first check).

The nurse compares the dose on the ticket with the label, and calculates and pours the amount of drug (second check).

Before discarding the unit dose packet or returning the container to the shelf, the nurse reads the order and the label again, and verifies the poured dose (third check).

The nurse places the medication on a tray with the ticket in front to identify it (Fig. 13-3). The nurse then dispenses the medication to the patient, identifying the patient by ID band, and keeping the medications in sight. Any required nursing assessment is completed. The nurse administers the drugs then takes the medication tray to the next patient and follows the same procedure. After medications are given, the nurse takes the medication tickets and charts the medications on each patient's chart.

There are several disadvantages to this system. Every order must be transcribed to three different places. Each time the order is rewritten an error is possible. Tickets may be lost or misplaced. An error may occur in choosing the stock. The tickets may become mixed, so that the wrong patient receives a medication. Medications that require assessment must be tagged in some way to identify them. It is time-consuming to locate the chart of each patient.

This system is rarely used because of the unit-dose system and medication carts.

### Mobile-Cart System

Compared with the ticket system, the mobile-cart system has many advantages. The pharmacist dispenses unit-dose medications directly to the patient's drawer. Each drawer is labeled with the patient's name. The cart contains all the equipment the nurse might require to administer medications.

When a drug is ordered, the nurse transcribes the order to one place—the patient's medication sheet found in a medication book on the cart. This book contains the medication sheets for every patient on the unit.

When it is time to administer medications, the nurse washes his or her hands and rolls the cart to the bedside of the first patient, greets the patient by name, unlocks the cart, and opens the medication book to the first patient's medication sheet.

The nurse checks the sheet for special nursing actions required before giving medication. The nurse carries out the orders, records the results, and decides to withhold or to administer the medication.

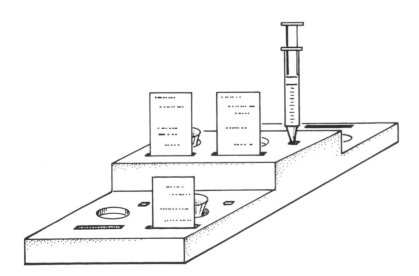

**FIGURE 13-3**

A medication tray with tickets and drugs in place.

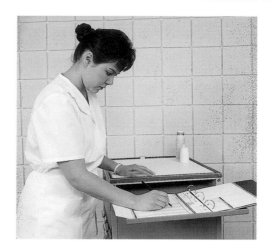

**FIGURE 13-4**
The nurse compares the medication label with the order.

The nurse places the patient's drawer on the top of the cart. The nurse reads each medication order, starting with the first medication listed. When a dose is to be given, the nurse chooses the unit dose from the drawer and compares the label with the order (first check) (Fig. 13-4).

The nurse computes the dose after comparing the order with the unit measure, opens the unit dose, and pours the amount (second check).

The nurse labels the unit dose and reads the order again and verifies the dose (third check). The nurse discards the unit-dose package in a waste receptacle on the cart. After preparing all the patient's medications, the nurse reads the name on the medicine sheet, checks the patient's ID band, and administers the drugs. The nurse remains with the patient until the medications are taken, provides any comfort measures, washes his or her hands, and returns to the cart to chart the drugs administered. The nurse replaces the patient's drawer and rolls the cart to the next patient. When all medications have been administered, the nurse returns the mobile cart to its designated area.

This system has several advantages. There are two professionals involved in checking the medication in the drawer—the pharmacist and the nurse. All the medication sheets are together on the cart. This is time-saving. Nursing assessment can be carried out and results charted before any medication is poured. The drugs can be signed for immediately after administration.

Note, however, that in both systems, the nurse checks the label three times—when choosing the drug, when calculating and pouring the dose, and before replacing the stock.

## Computer Printouts

Institutions may have computerized medication procedures. Doctors input orders directly on the computer. The order is received in the pharmacy, where it is added to the patient's drug profile. The nursing unit receives the computer printout listing the medications and times of administration. The printout replaces the medication administration record (MAR).

There are several advantages to this system. Neither the nurse nor the pharmacist has to interpret the doctor's handwriting. The nurse does not have to transfer the written orders to an MAR, thus reducing the chance for error and saving time. Moreover, a computer check will identify possible interactions among the patient's medications and alert the nurse and the pharmacist.

Figure 13-5 is an example of a computerized MAR. The patient's name, ID number, room, date of admission, age, diagnosis, sex, and attending physician are printed at the top. The administration period for this record covers 24 hours using military time.

FARLAND MEDICAL CENTER
MEDICATION ADMINISTRATION RECORD

| Patient Name | Room No. | Hospital Number | Diagnosis | |
|---|---|---|---|---|
| Velder, Chelsea | 1401 | 204452896 | CHF | |
| Allergies | Admitted | Age | Sex | Physician |
| Penicillin | 6/25/01 | 50 | F | Richardson |

DOSAGE ADMINISTRATION PERIOD: 6/26/01-6/27/01

| | 0600-1400 | 1401-2200 | 2201-0600 |
|---|---|---|---|
| Aspirin 325 mg PO qd | 0900 | | |
| Kefzol i Gm. Q 6 h IVPB | 0600 1400 | 1800 | 0200 |
| Lopressor 50 mg. PO BID | 0900 | 2100 | |
| | | | |
| | | | |
| Morphine Sulfate 4-6 mg. IV q 2-3 h prn pain | | | |
| Tylenol gr X q. 4 h prn temp > 101 | | | |

| Signature | Initials | Signature | Initials | Signature | Initials |
|---|---|---|---|---|---|
| _____ | ( ) | _____ | ( ) | _____ | ( ) |

**FIGURE 13-5**

A sample 24-hour computerized medication record. Scheduled drugs are listed at the top of the sheet and PRN orders at the bottom. Military time is used. The nurse initials the boxes to indicate the drug was administered and signs at the bottom of the sheet.

# ▶ Routes of Administration

## *Oral Route*

Regardless of the system used to pour the medications, the procedure for administering drugs contains specific steps. The nurse greets the patient orally and checks the ID band. The patient is assisted to a sitting position. The patient should be alert and able to swallow. Oral solids are given first, together with a full glass of water whenever possible, followed by oral liquid medications. Before leaving, the nurse watches to be sure the patient has swallowed all of the drugs. The paper and plastic cups may be discarded according to routine hospital procedure, unless the patient is on strict or respiratory isolation. For this, special isolation bags are utilized. The nurse makes the patient comfortable, washes his or her hands, and charts the doses given.

Special considerations for oral administration include the following:

- If the patient is NPO (nothing by mouth), check with the doctor to determine if oral medication can be administered with a small amount of water. The doctor may not wish to withhold certain drugs (for example, an anticonvulsant for a patient with epilepsy).

- When a patient refuses a drug, find out why, chart the reason, and initiate action to correct the situation.

- Solid stock medications are poured first into the container lid and then into a paper cup, using medical asepsis. The medication is not touched. Several solids may be combined in the cup, but each medication should first be poured into a separate cup until the third check is completed. Unit-dose medications should be checked three times before the package container is discarded.

- Medical asepsis is followed to break a scored tablet. This means that clean, not sterile, technique is required. One method is to place the tablet in a paper towel, fold the towel over and, with thumbs and index fingers in apposition, break the tablet along the score line. Tablets that are not scored should not be broken.

- Check expiration dates on all labels. Do not administer expired drugs.

- If the patient has difficulty swallowing solids, first determine if the medication is available in a liquid form. Enteric- and film-coated tablets should not be crushed. Ordinarily, capsules should not be opened. Check with the pharmacist for alternative forms. If a capsule can be opened, mix the drug with a small amount of applesauce, custard, or other vehicle that will make the medication more palatable and easy to swallow.

- If a medication can be crushed, it is best to use a "pill" crusher with the medication placed between two paper cups. If using a mortar and pestle, be sure they are cleaned before and after crushing so there is no residue. If no equipment is available, place the tablet in a paper towel and use the edge of a bottle or other hard surface to crush the drug. A crushed drug may be mixed with water or semisolids, such as applesauce or custard, for ease in swallowing.

- Some drugs are best taken on an empty stomach; others may be taken with food. The nurse should be aware of foods or fluids that may be ingested with the drug and of those that are contraindicated.

- Check patients for allergies to drugs. This should be a routine procedure.

- The nurse should be knowledgeable about food–drug and drug–drug interactions and act to safeguard the patient.

- Failure to shake some liquid medications can result in a wrong dose. The drug settles to the bottom and only the weak diluent is poured. Shake magmas, gels, and suspensions before pouring.

- Pour liquids at eye level, with the thumb indicating the meniscus. In pouring liquids, the label should be up so it will not be stained. Before recapping, wipe the lip of the bottle with a paper towel.

- Note the presence of an unusual color change or precipitate in a liquid. If such a change is present, do not use. Send the container to the pharmacy with a note indicating your observation.

- Check references to determine how to disguise liquids that are distasteful or irritating. Two possibilities are to mix with juice or give through a straw after diluting well. Liquid iron preparations stain the teeth and are taken through a straw placed in the back of the mouth. Tinctures are always diluted.

- Liquid cough mixtures are not diluted. They have a secondary soothing (demulcent) effect on the mucous membranes in addition to the antitussive action.

- The oral route is the least expensive, the safest, and the easiest to take.

## Parenteral Route

Medications may be given by the IM, SC, IVPB, or IV routes or intradermally. The parenteral route is used when a drug cannot be given orally, when it is necessary to obtain a rapid systemic effect, or when a drug would be rendered ineffective or destroyed by the oral route.

### Choosing the Site

The following areas should be avoided: bony prominences, large blood vessels, nerves, sensitive areas, bruises, hardened areas, abrasions, and inflamed areas. The site for IM injections should be able to accept 3 mL; rotate sites when repeated injections are given.

### Preparation of the Skin

Cleanse the site with an alcohol pad while using a circular motion from the center out. Grasp the area firmly between the thumb and forefinger and insert the needle with a dartlike motion (Fig. 13-6). If the area is obese, the skin may be spread rather than pinched together.

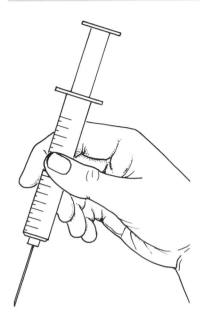

**FIGURE 13-6**

An injection is administered with a quick, dartlike motion into taut skin that has been spread or bunched together.

## Syringes for Injection

The most common syringe used for injections is a standard 3-mL size, marked in minims and in milliliters (mL or cc) to the nearest tenth. The precision (tuberculin) syringe is marked in half-minims and milliliters to the nearest hundredth. There are two insulin syringes: a regular 1-mL size marked to the U 100, and a 0.5-mL size (low-dose) insulin syringe marked to U 50.

## Needles for Injections

Needles are chosen for their gauge and their length. *Gauge* is the diameter of the needle opening. The principle is: the higher the gauge number, the finer the needle.

    The 28-gauge needle on the insulin syringe is the finest needle currently available for routine injections. Numbers 25, 26, and 28 are used for SC injections for adults and for IM injections for children and emaciated patients. Numbers 23 and 22 are used for IM injections; 20 and 21 for IV therapy; and 15 and 18 for blood transfusions.

## Angle of Insertion

*INTRAMUSCULAR.* For IM injection the syringe should be held at a right angle to the skin and the injection given at a 90-degree angle.

*SUBCUTANEOUS.* For SC injections the syringe should be held at a 45-degree angle when the needle is inserted. Some SC injections may be administered at a 90-degree angle if the subcutaneous layer of fat is thick and the needle is short. Care must be exercised to reach the correct site. When in doubt use the 45-degree angle. Intramuscular sites have a good blood supply and absorption is rapid: subcutaneous sites have a poor blood supply and absorption is prolonged.

*INTRADERMAL.* A 26-gauge or other fine needle is used for skin testing for allergy and tuberculosis.

## Preparing the Dose

Ordinarily, to prevent incompatibility of drugs only one medication should be drawn up in a syringe. When two drugs are given in one syringe, follow the procedure for mixing after determining that the drugs are compatible.

*ADDING AIR TO A SYRINGE*

Some nurses add 0.1 to 0.2 mL air to the syringe after obtaining the dose and before giving the injection. The air bubble rises to the top of the barrel and is injected last. The air acts as a seal to prevent medication oozing to the skin from the injection tract and empties the needle of medication. This procedure is required in giving a Z tract injection; otherwise it is optimal. Institutional policy should be followed.

*DRUGS THAT ARE LIQUIDS IN VIALS*

1. Cleanse the top of the vial with an alcohol sponge.

2. Draw the amount of air equivalent to the amount of solution desired into the syringe (Fig. 13-7A).

3. Inject the needle through the rubber diaphragm into the vial.

4. Expel air from the syringe into the vial. This increases the pressure in the vial and makes it easier to withdraw medication.

5. Invert the vial and draw up the desired amount into the syringe (Fig. 13-7B).

6. Withdraw the needle quickly from the vial.

7. The rubber diaphragm will seal.

*DRUGS THAT ARE POWDERS IN VIALS*

1. Cleanse the top of the vial with an alcohol sponge.

2. Draw up the amount of calculated diluent from a vial of distilled water or normal saline for injection. Follow pharmaceutical directions if another solvent is indicated.

3. Add diluent to the powder and roll the vial between your hands to dissolve the powder.

4. Label the vial with the solution made, your initials, the date and the time.

5. Cleanse the top of the vial again.

6. Draw up the amount of air equivalent to the amount of solution desired into the syringe.

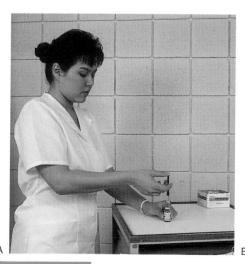
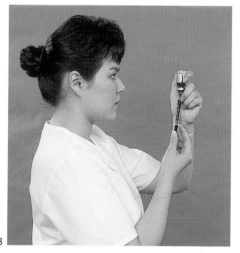

A    B

**FIGURE 13-7**

(*A*) Injecting air into the vial. (*B*) Invert the vial and draw up the desired amount of medication into the syringe.

7. Inject the needle through the rubber diaphragm into the vial.

8. Expel the air into the vial. This increases pressure in the vial and makes it easier to remove medication. Invert the vial and draw up the desired amount of medication into the syringe.

9. Check directions for storage of any remaining drug.

Note: When the whole amount of powder contained in a vial is needed for an IVPB medication, a reconstitution device may be used to dilute the powder without using a syringe.

*DRUGS IN GLASS AMPULES*

1. Tap the top of the ampule with your finger to clear out any drug.

2. Place an opened alcohol pad around the neck of the ampule.

3. Hold the ampule sideways.

4. Place thumbs in apposition above and index fingers in apposition below the ampule neck.

5. Press down with thumbs to break the ampule.

6. Invert the ampule, insert the syringe needle, and withdraw the dose (Fig. 13-8). *Important: Do not add air before removing dose.* This will cause medication to spray from the ampule.

*UNIT-DOSE CARTRIDGE AND HOLDER*
Insert the cartridge into the metal or plastic holder and screw into place. Move the plunger forward until it engages the shaft of the cartridge. Twist the plunger until it is locked into the cartridge. The holder is reusable. The cartridge is placed in a sharps container after use.

*UNIT-DOSE PREFILLED SYRINGES*
The medication is in the syringe. Some prefilled syringes are simple and require no action other than removing the needle cover; others are packaged for compactness and directions are given to prepare the syringe for use. These syringes are disposable.

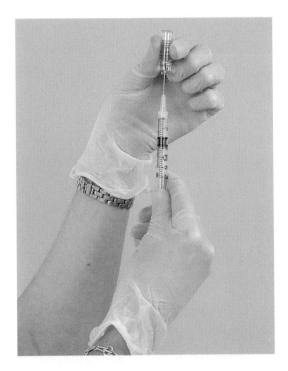

**FIGURE 13-8**

Invert the ampule for withdrawal. (© B. Proud.)

*MIXING TWO MEDICATIONS IN ONE SYRINGE*
*General Principles*

1. Determine that the drugs are compatible by consulting a standard reference.

2. When in doubt about compatibility, prepare medications separately and administer into different injection sites.

3. When medications are in a vial and an ampule, draw up the medication from the vial first then add the medication from the ampule. Discard any medication left in the ampule.

4. In preparing two types of insulin in one syringe, the vial containing *regular insulin must be drawn first* into the syringe. Regular insulin has not been adulterated with protein as have other insulins such as protamine zinc insulin.

*Method*

1. Clean both vials with an alcohol pad.

2. Choose one vial as *primary.* For example, with vials of a narcotic and a nonnarcotic, the narcotic is primary. With two insulins, regular insulin is primary.

3. Inject air into the *second* vial equal to the medication to be withdrawn. Do not permit the needle to touch the medication.

4. Inject air into the *primary* vial equal to the amount to be withdrawn and withdraw medication in the usual way. Be sure there are no air bubbles.

5. Insert the needle into the *second* vial. To avoid pushing the primary medication into the second vial, do not touch the plunger while doing this.

6. *Slowly* withdraw the needed amount of drug from the second vial. The two medications are now combined.

7. Remove the needle from the second vial and cap it. *Note:* Some authorities suggest that the needle be changed after withdrawing medication from the primary vial. Because this may result in air bubbles, be careful withdrawing the second medication to obtain an accurate dose.

## Identifying the Injection Site—Adults

*INTRAMUSCULAR*
Common sites are dorsogluteal, ventrogluteal, vastus lateralis, and deltoid muscles.

*DORSOGLUTEAL SITE.* The dorsogluteal site is composed of the thick gluteal muscles of the buttocks.

*Position:* The patient may be prone or in a side-lying position with both buttocks fully exposed.

*Location of injection site:* The area must be chosen very carefully to avoid striking the sciatic nerve, major blood vessels, or bone. The landmarks of the buttocks are the crest of the posterior ilium as the superior boundary and the inferior gluteal fold as the lower boundary. The exact site can be identified in either of two ways:

1. *Diagonal landmark* (Fig. 13-9): Find the posterior superior iliac spine and the greater trochanter of the femur. Draw an imaginary diagonal line between these two points, and give the injection lateral and superior to that line 1 to 2 inches below the iliac crest to avoid hitting the iliac bone. Should you hit the bone, withdraw the needle slightly and continue the procedure. This method is preferred because all the landmarks are bony prominences.

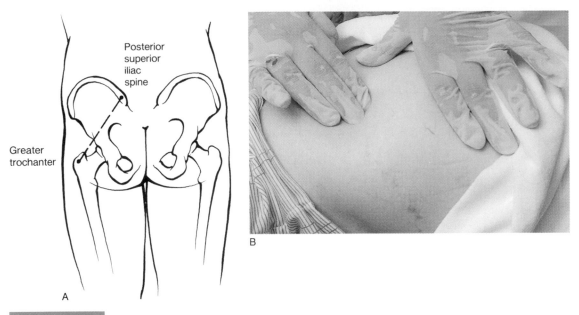

(*A*) Identification of the dorsogluteal site using a diagonal between the bony prominences. (*B*) Locating the exact location site.

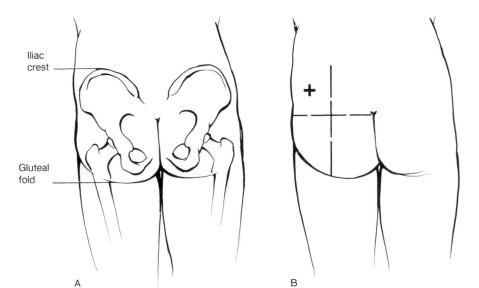

**FIGURE 13-10**

(*A*) Identification of the dorsogluteal injection site using quadrants. Draw an imaginary line from the iliac crest to the gluteal fold, and from the medial to the lateral buttock. (*B*) The *cross* indicates the injection area.

2. *Quadrant landmark* (Fig. 13-10): Divide the buttocks into imaginary quadrants. The vertical line extends from the crest of the ilium to the gluteal fold. The horizontal line extends from the medial fold of the buttock to the lateral aspect of the buttock. Locate the upper aspect of the upper-outer quadrant. The injection should be given in this area, 1 to 2 inches below the crest of the ilium, to avoid hitting bone. The crest of the ilium must be palpated for precise site selection.

*VENTROGLUTEAL SITE.* The ventral part of the gluteal muscle has no large nerves or blood vessels and less fat. It is identified by finding the greater trochanter, anterior superior iliac spine, and the iliac crest. The nurse should be standing by the patient's knee. Use the hand opposite to the patient's leg (eg, left leg, right hand). Open an alcohol pad. Place the palm of the hand on the greater trochanter.

Point the index finger toward the anterior superior iliac spine. Point the middle finger toward the iliac crest. The injection is given in the center of the triangle between the middle finger and the index finger (Fig. 13-11). Place the alcohol pad over the site. Remove the hand and proceed with the injection in the usual manner. Use the alcohol pad to prep the area from the center out.

*Position:* The patient may be supine, lying on the side, sitting, or standing.

*VASTUS LATERALIS SITE: LATERAL THIGH.* Measure one hand's width below the greater trochanter and one hand's width above the knee (Fig. 13-12). Give the injection in the lateral thigh. Ask the patient to point the big toe to the center of his body. This relaxes the vastus muscle.

*Position:* The patient may be supine, lying on the side, or standing.

*DELTOID SITE.* The deltoid muscle on the lateral aspect of the upper arm is a small muscle close to the radial and brachial arteries. *It should be used for IM injections only if specifically ordered,* and no more than 2 mL should be injected. The boundaries are the lower edge of the acromion process (shoulder bone) and the axilla (armpit) (Fig. 13-13). Give the injection into the lateral arm between these two points and about 2 inches below the acromion process.

*Position:* The patient may be sitting or lying down.

*SUBCUTANEOUS*

Common injection sites include the upper arms, anterior thighs, lower abdomen, and upper back (Fig. 13-14). Insulin SC is administered in the arm, lower abdomen, and thigh. Heparin SC is given in the lower abdomen. The injection is usually given at a 45-degree angle to avoid reaching muscle. SC injections may be given at a 90-degree angle if the subcutaneous layer of fat is thick. No more than 1 mL of medication should be injected.

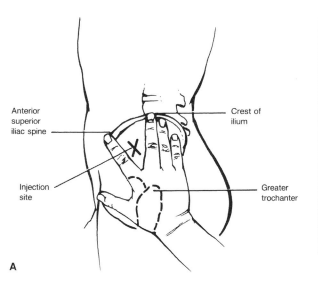

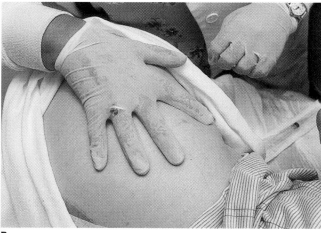

**FIGURE 13-11**

(*A*) The ventrogluteal site for IM injections; the *cross* indicates the injection site. (*B*) Locating the exact location site.

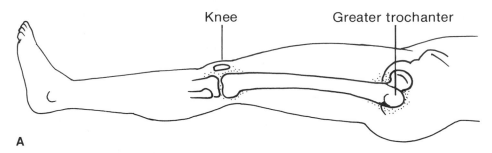

Knee    Greater trochanter

**A**

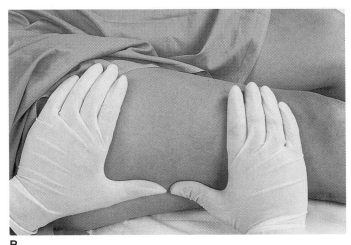

**B**

**FIGURE 13-12**

(*A*) Vastus lateralis injection site. (*B*) Locating the site.

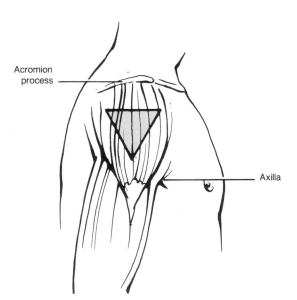

Acromion process

Axilla

**FIGURE 13-13**

The deltoid muscle site for IM injections. The *triangle* indicates the injection site.

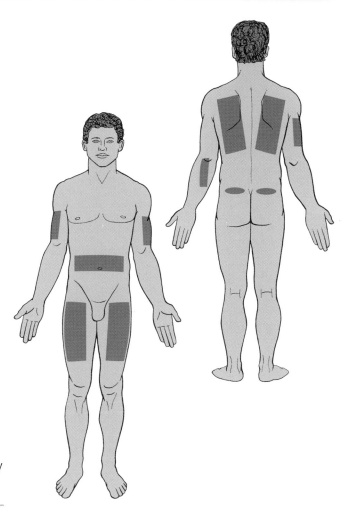

Sites for subcutaneous injection. The deltoid muscle may be used for subcutaneous injections or, when ordered, small intramuscular injections.

## INTRADERMAL (INTRACUTANEOUS)

The intradermal site is used for skin testing for allergies and diseases such as tuberculosis. Injecting an antigen causes an antigen–antibody sensitivity reaction if the individual is susceptible. If positive, the area will become raised, warm, and reddened.

The site is the inner aspect of the forearm. Prepare the skin with an alcohol pad and allow it to dry. Place your nondominant hand around the arm from below and pull the skin tightly to make the forearm tissue taut. Hold the syringe in your four fingers and thumb, with the bevel (opening) of the needle up, and insert the needle about ⅛ inch almost parallel to the skin (Fig. 13-15). The needle remains visible under the skin. Inject the solution such that it raises a small wheal (a raised bump or a blister). Remove the needle and allow the injection site to dry. *Do not massage the skin.* Place the needle and syringe in a sharps container. Make the patient comfortable. Wash your hands. Chart the procedure.

## Administering Injections

Handwashing and gloves are required.

1. Identify the patient verbally by name.

2. Check ID band.

3. Perform any assessment before injection (eg, vital signs, apical rate, site integrity).

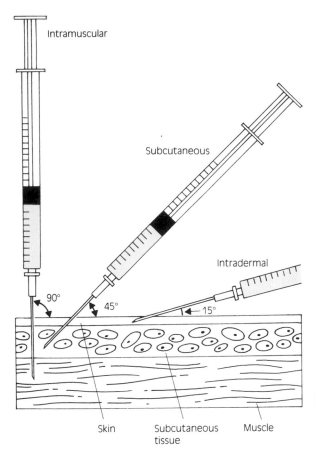

Comparison of angles of insertion for intramuscular, subcutaneous, and intradermal injection.

4. Explain the procedure to the patient.

5. Ask the patient where the last injection was given. The sites should be rotated.

6. Prepare the area with an alcohol pad, using a circular motion from the center out.

7. Place the alcohol pad between your fingers or lay it on the patient's skin above the site.

8. Remove the needle cover.

9. Make the skin taut by mounding the tissue between thumb and index finger or by spreading it firmly.

10. Dart the needle in quickly (Fig. 13-16A).

11. Hold the barrel with your nondominant hand and with your dominant hand pull the plunger back. This is termed *aspiration* and is done to be sure the needle is not in a blood vessel (Fig. 13-16B).

12. If blood enters the syringe, withdraw the needle, discard the needle and syringe into a sharps container, and prepare another injection.

13. If no blood is aspirated, inject the medication slowly (Fig. 13-16C).

14. Remove the needle quickly.

15. Press down on the area with the alcohol pad or a dry gauze pad to inhibit bleeding.

16. *Do not recap the needle.* Dispose of needle and syringe in a sharps container. Make the patient comfortable. Wash hands. Chart the medication documenting the site of injection.

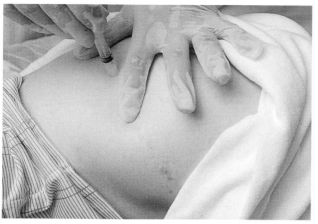

A

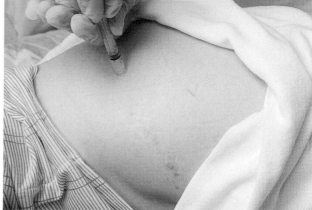

B

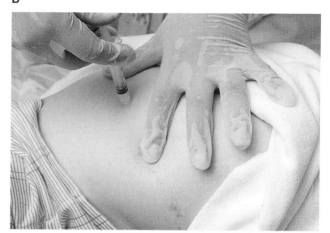

C

(A) Dart the needle into the skin; (B) aspirate slowly; (C) inject medication slowly.

## Special Injection Techniques

### SUBCUTANEOUS HEPARIN

Heparin is an anticoagulant, and care must be taken to minimize tissue trauma. Slow bleeding at the site of the injection can cause bruising. Several changes in routine injection technique are indicated. The injection is given with a fine (25-gauge) ½-inch needle into the lower abdominal fold at least 2 inches from the umbilicus. Gloves should be worn.

1. Change the needle after drawing up the dose to prevent leakage along the tract.

2. Allow the skin to dry after prepping with an alcohol pad.

3. Bunch the tissue with the nondominant hand to a depth of at least ½ inch.

4. Inject the needle at a 90-degree angle.

5. *Do not aspirate.* This minimizes tissue damage.

6. Inject the medication slowly.

7. Hold the needle in place for 10 seconds.

8. Remove the needle quickly.

9. *Do not massage the area.* If bleeding is noted, apply pressure with a dry gauze pad or alcohol pad for 1 to 2 minutes.

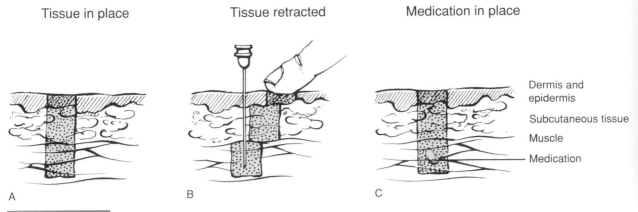

Tissue in place   Tissue retracted   Medication in place

Dermis and epidermis

Subcutaneous tissue

Muscle

Medication

A                    B                    C

**FIGURE 13-17**

Z-track technique—dorsogluteal site. The tissue is retracted to one side and held there until the injection is given. When the hand is removed, the tissue closes over the injection tract, preventing medication from rising to the surface.

*Z-TRACK TECHNIQUE FOR INTRAMUSCULAR INJECTIONS*

Some medications, such as iron dextran (Imferon) and hydroxyzine (Vistazine), are irritating to the tissues and can stain the skin. The Z-track method may be used at the dorsogluteal site to prevent medication seepage into the needle tract and onto the skin.

1. After preparing the medication, change the needle to prevent leakage along the tract.

2. Add 0.2 mL of air to the syringe. As medication is injected, the air will rise to the top of the syringe and will be administered last. This will seal off the medication and prevent its leakage to the skin.

3. Prepare the patient and the site in the usual manner.

4. Use the fingers on your nondominant hand to retract the tissue to the side. *Hold this position during the injection* (Fig. 13-17).

5. Inject as usual at a 90-degree angle. Be sure to aspirate before giving this injection (Fig. 13-18).

6. Count 10 seconds after giving the injection.

7. Remove the needle quickly.

8. Remove the hand that has been retracting the tissue.

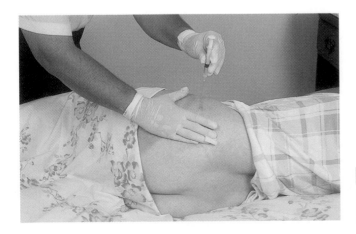

**FIGURE 13-18**

Displacing tissue in a Z-track manner and darting needle into tissue.

9. *Do not massage the site.*

10. Using an alcohol pad of dry gauze pad, press down on the site to inhibit bleeding.

## *Application to Skin and Mucous Membrane*

Drug preparations are administered for their local effect or to act systematically. To achieve a systemic effect, the drug must be absorbed into the circulation.

### Buccal Tablet (Universal Safeguard: Handwashing)

Identify the patient orally. Check the ID band. Explain the procedure and give the tablet to the patient. The patient should place the tablet between his gum and his cheek. The tablet should not be disturbed as it dissolves. Systemic absorption is rapid across mucous membranes. Doses should be alternated between cheeks to minimize irritation. Withhold food and liquids until the tablet is dissolved.

### Ear Drops (Universal Safeguard: Handwashing)

The ear drops will be labeled otic or auric. They should be warmed to body temperature. Greet the patient orally and check the ID band. Explain the procedure. Place the patient sitting in an upright position, with the head tilted toward his unaffected side or lying on his side with the affected ear up. Be sure the patient is comfortable. With a dropper, draw the medication up. *Straighten the ear canal by pulling the pinna up and back in the adult, or down and back in a child 3 years or younger.*

Place the tip of the dropper at the opening of the canal and instill the medication into the canal (Fig. 13-19). The patient should rest on his unaffected side 10 to 15 minutes. A cotton ball may be placed in the canal if the patient wishes. Make sure the patient is comfortable. Wash hands. Chart the medication.

### Eye Drops or Ointment (Universal Safeguard: Gloves)

Greet the patient and check the ID band. Explain the procedure. Hand the patient a tissue. The patient may be sitting or lying down. If exudate is present, it may be necessary to cleanse the eyelid with cotton or gauze and either normal saline or distilled water for the eye. Any medication placed in the eye must be labeled "ophthalmic" or "for the eye." Eye medications may come in a monodrop container, in a bottle with a dropper, or as an ophthalmic ointment. Gently draw the lower eyelid down to create a sac (Fig. 13-20). Instruct the patient to look up. Instill the liquid medication into the lower conjunctival sac, taking care not to touch the membrane. The ophthalmic ointment should be placed from the inner to the outer canthus of the eye.

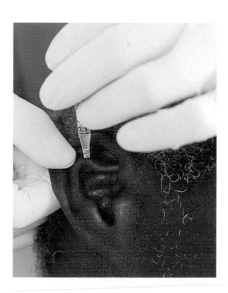

**FIGURE 13-19**

Straighten the ear canal and instill the medication.

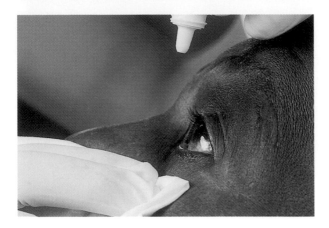

**FIGURE 13-20**

Applying eye drops: Gently draw the lower eyelid down to create a pocket. Insert the medication into this pocket.

Instruct the patient to close eyelids gently and rotate eyes. The patient may use the tissue to wipe away excess medication. After instilling eye drops, have the patient apply gentle pressure with his index finger to the inner canthus for a minute. This action inhibits the medication from entering the tear duct.

Each patient should have individual medication containers to prevent cross-contamination. Provide a safe environment if the medication impairs the patient's vision. Make the patient comfortable. Dispose of the gloves according to institutional procedure. Wash your hands and chart the medication.

## Nasogastric Route (Universal Safeguard: Gloves)

When possible, obtain the medication in liquid form. Before opening capsules or crushing tablets, check with the pharmacist for alternatives.

Dilute the medication with water. The fluid mixture should be at room temperature. Greet the patient, check the ID band, and explain the procedure. Elevate the head of the bed when possible. Put on gloves. Insert the bulb syringe into the tube. Remove the clamp on the tube. Check the position of the tube in the stomach by (1) aspirating some stomach contents or (2) placing a stethoscope on the stomach and inserting about 15 mL of air. A swishing sound indicates proper placement.

Close off the tube by bending it on itself. Hold the bulb syringe and bent tube in your nondominant hand. Remove the bulb and leave the syringe in place.

Flush the tube with at least 30 mL warm water to ensure patency. Clamp the tube. Pour the medication into the bulb syringe. Release the tubing and allow the medication to flow in by gravity. *Do not force medication to flow by using pressure on the bulb.* If the patient shows discomfort, stop the procedure and wait until he or she appears relaxed.

Before all the medication flows in, flush the tube by adding at least 30 mL of water to the syringe. Shut the tube by bending it on itself before the bulb syringe completely empties. Clamp the tube and remove the bulb syringe. Make the patient comfortable. If possible, leave the head of the bed elevated. Dispose of gloves according to institutional procedures. Wash your hands. Chart the medication.

## Nose Drops (Universal Safeguard: Gloves)

Greet the patient, check the ID band, and explain the procedure. The patient may have to blow his nose gently to clear the nasal passageway. The patient may be sitting or lying down. Have the patient tilt his head back. In bed a pillow may be placed under the shoulders to hyperextend the neck. Insert the dropper about one-third into each nostril. Do not touch the nostril. Instill the nose drops. Instruct the patient to maintain the position 1 to 2 minutes. If the patient feels the medication flowing down his throat, he may sit up and bend his head down to allow the medication to flow into the sinuses.

The patient should have his own medication container to prevent cross-contamination. Make the patient comfortable. Wash your hands. Chart the medication.

If a nasal spray is ordered, push the tip of the nose up and place the nozzle tip just inside the nares, so the spray will be directed backward when the medication is given.

## Rectal Suppository (Universal Safeguard: Gloves)

Greet the patient, check the ID band, and explain the procedure. Encourage the patient to defecate (unless the suppository is ordered for this purpose). Position the patient in the left lateral recumbent position (Fig. 13-21). Moisten the suppository with a water-soluble lubricant. Instruct the patient to breathe slowly and deeply through the mouth. Ask the patient to "bear down" as if having a bowel movement to open the anal sphincter. Using a gloved finger, insert the suppository past the sphincter. You will feel the suppository move into the canal. Wipe away excess lubricant. Encourage the patient to retain the suppository. Make the patient comfortable. Dispose of gloves according to institutional procedure. Wash your hands. Chart the medication.

The patient may insert his or her own suppository if able and wishes to do so. Provide a glove, lubricant, and suppository. Check to be sure the suppository was inserted and is not in the bed.

## Respiratory Inhaler (Universal Safeguard: Handwashing)

An inhaler is a small, pressurized metal container that holds medication. It is accompanied by a mouthpiece. *The following are general directions to teach the patient:*

1. Shake the inhaler well immediately before use.

2. Remove the cap from the mouthpiece.

3. Breathe out fully; expel as much air as you can; hold your breath.

4. Place the mouthpiece in your mouth and close your lips around it. The metal inhaler should be upright.

5. While breathing in deeply and slowly, fully depress the metal inhaler with your index finger.

6. Remove the inhaler from your mouth and release your finger. Hold your breath for several seconds.

7. Wait 1 minute and shake the inhaler again. Repeat the steps for each inhalation prescribed. (An order might read "Proventil Inhaler 2 puffs qid.")

8. Cleanse the mouthpiece and cap by rinsing in warm running water at least once a day. When dry, replace the mouthpiece and cap.

The inhaler may be left at the bedside stand if the institution's policy permits. Make the patient comfortable, wash your hands, and chart the medication.

## Skin Applications (Universal Safeguard: Gloves)

Greet the patient, check the ID band, and explain the procedure. Avoid personal contact with the medication to prevent absorption of drug. Apply the medication with a tongue blade, glove, gauze pad, or cotton-tipped applicator. Cleanse the area as appropriate before a new application.

Obtain the following information before proceeding, because many kinds of medicines are applied topically.

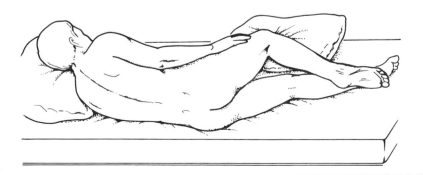

**FIGURE 13-21**
Left lateral recumbent position.

- Preparation of the skin
- Method of application
- Whether the skin should be covered or uncovered

Drug preparations include the following:

- Powders: Sprinkle on your gloved hands then apply. Use sparingly to avoid caking. Skin should be dry.
- Lotions: Pat on lightly. Use gloved hand or gauze pad.
- Creams: Rub into skin using gloves.
- Ointments: Use gloved hand or applicator. Apply an even coat and place a dressing on skin.

Make the patient comfortable. Dispose of gloves according to institutional policy. Wash your hands. Chart the medication.

### NITROGLYCERIN OINTMENT (UNIVERSAL SAFEGUARD: GLOVES)

Greet the patient, check the ID band, and explain the procedure. Take a baseline blood pressure and record. Don the gloves to protect yourself from contact with the drug, a potent vasodilator. Remove the previous dose and cleanse the skin.

Measure the prescribed dose in inches on the ruled paper that comes with the ointment. Select a nonhairy site on the trunk—chest, upper arm, abdomen, or upper back. If necessary, shave the area. (Seek advice before doing this.) Spread the measured ointment on the skin, using the ruled paper. Apply the ointment in a thin layer about 6 inches by 6 inches. *Do not rub.* Tape the ruled paper in place over the ointment. Cover the area with plastic wrap and tape the plastic in place. Check the patient's blood pressure within 30 minutes.

If a headache occurs or the blood pressure lowers, have the patient rest until the blood pressure returns to normal. Make the patient comfortable. Dispose of gloves according to institutional procedure. Wash your hands. Chart the medication.

## Transdermal Disks, Patches, and Pads (Universal Safeguard: Handwashing)

These products are unit-dose adhesive bandages consisting of a semipermeable membrane that allows medication to be released continuously over time. Some patches are effective for 24 hours, some for 72 hours, and some last as long as 1 week.

The skin should be free of hair and not subject to excessive movement; therefore, avoid distal extremities. The site should be changed with each administration. If the patch loosens with bathing, apply a new pad.

Medications that can be administered by this route include hormones, antihypertensive drugs such as clonidine (Catapres), antimotion sickness drugs such as scopolamine, and nitroglycerin.

Greet the patient, check the ID band, and explain the procedure. Select the site. The skin should be clear and dry with no signs of irritation. Open the packet. Remove the cover from the adhesive transdermal drug. *Do not touch the inside of the pad.* Apply the pad to the skin. Press firmly to be certain all edges are adherent. Make the patient comfortable, wash your hands, and chart the medication.

## Sublingual Tablets (Universal Safeguard: Handwashing)

The most common sublingual medication is nitroglycerin, which is prescribed to abort an attack of angina pectoris. If relief is not felt in 5 minutes, a second then a third tablet may be taken at 5 minute intervals. Tolerance to nitroglycerin is common. If the pain is not relieved within 15 minutes, the physician should be notified.

To administer a sublingual tablet, greet the patient, check the ID band, and explain the procedure. Instruct the patient to sit down and place the tablet under the tongue. If the patient is unable to place the tablet under his or her tongue, the nurse should wear a glove to place the tablet. The tablet should not be swallowed or chewed but allowed to dissolve. The patient should not eat or drink anything because this will interfere with the effectiveness of the medication. Stay with the patient until the pain is relieved. Consult an appropriate text for further information. Wash your hands and chart the medication.

## Vaginal Suppository or Tablet (Universal Safeguard: Gloves)

Greet the patient, check the ID band, and explain the procedure. Ask the patient to void in a bed pan. (If the perineal area has much secretion, it may be necessary to perform perineal care after the patient voids.) Insert the suppository or tablet into the applicator. Assist the patient into a lithotomy position (lying on the back with knees flexed and legs apart) and drape her, leaving the perineal area exposed. Don gloves.

Separate the labia majora and identify the vaginal opening. Insert the applicator down and back and eject the suppository or tablet into the vagina. (The patient may do this procedure herself if she wishes.) Place a pad at the opening to collect secretions. Make the patient comfortable before leaving.

Wash the applicator with soap and water, wrap it in a paper towel, and leave it at the bedside. Dispose of gloves and equipment according to institutional procedure. Chart the medication.

## Vaginal Cream or Vaginal Tablet (Universal Safeguard: Gloves)

Vaginal cream may come in a prefilled disposable syringe or in a tube with its own applicator. To fill the applicator, remove the cap from the tube and screw the top of the tube into the barrel of the applicator. Squeeze the tube to fill the barrel to the prescribed dose. Unscrew the tube from the applicator and cap it.

Prepare the patient as described above. Insert the applicator down and back and press the plunger to empty the barrel of medication (Fig. 13-22). The patient may do this herself if she wishes. Remove the applicator. Place a pad at the vaginal opening to collect secretions. Make the patient comfortable before leaving. She should remain in bed for a minimum of 20 minutes.

If the applicator is a prefilled unit dose, dispose of it according to institutional policy. If it is reusable, wash it with soap and water, and place it in a clean paper towel in the bedside stand. Dispose of gloves. Chart the medication.

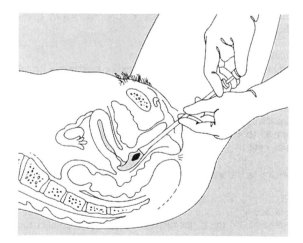

**FIGURE 13-22**

Vaginal applicator should be inserted down and back. (From Taylor, C., Lillis, C., & LeMone, P. [2001] *Fundamentals of nursing* [4th ed.]. Philadelphia: Lippincott Williams & Wilkins, p. 627.)

**SELF TEST I**    **Universal Safeguards**

*Give the information requested for universal safeguards in administering medications. Answers may be found at the end of the chapter.*

1. Universal safeguards should be applied when administering medications

    **a.** to all patients

    **b.** only to patients with HIV or hepatitis B virus

2. The type of safeguard to be used by the nurse depends on _____

    _____

3. In administering medications, gloves must be worn when

    _____ and

    _____

4. After administering an injection, the syringe should be placed _____

    _____

5. Five safeguards stressed by the Centers for Disease Control and Prevention are

    _____ , _____ , and

    _____ , _____

    _____ .

6. In administering medications, hands must be washed

    **a.** _____

    **b.** _____

    **c.** _____

    **d.** _____

7. General safeguards in administering medications advise the nurse to use a clamp to

    _____

    _____

8. A gown should be worn to protect the nurse's uniform whenever _____

    _____

9. Protective eyewear should be worn whenever _____

    _____

    _____

10. A mask should be worn when

    _____ or

    _____

## SELF TEST 2 | Medication Administration

*Supply the following information. Answers will be found at the end of the chapter.*

1. The primary reason patients should have individual eye medication is to _____

   _____

2. Two methods of checking the positioning of a nasogastric tube are _____

   _____ and

   _____

3. For administration of a rectal suppository, the patient should lie _____

   _____

4. How should each of the following be applied to a patient's skin?

   **a.** Powders _____

   **b.** Lotions _____

   **c.** Creams _____

   **d.** Ointments _____

5. How many SL nitroglycerin tablets may a patient take to relieve pain? _____

   At what time interval? _____

6. Identify these administration procedures as clean or sterile.

   **a.** SC injection _____        **f.** Nitroglycerin ointment _____

   **b.** SL tablet _____        **g.** Urethral suppository _____

   **c.** Vaginal suppository _____        **h.** Nasogastric route _____

   **d.** Nose drops _____        **i.** Intradermal _____

   **e.** IM injection _____        **j.** Rectal suppository _____

7. How should a vaginal applicator be inserted? _____

8. How should the skin be prepared for an injection? _____

   _____

9. List three reasons for administering medication by injection. _____

   _____

   _____

10. What is the difference in administering ear drops to an adult and a 2-year-old child?

    _____

    _____

## TEST YOUR CLINICAL SAVVY

A client in your outpatient clinic is to receive an IM (intramuscular) injection. The drug literature states the preferred site is the gluteus maximus or vastus lateralis.

A. When would the deltoid muscle be preferable or used over either of these sites? What are the contraindications for using the deltoid muscle?

B. The client requests the injection in the deltoid. What is your response in light of the recommended site in the drug literature?

C. If a patient is bedridden, which site would you choose for an IM injection and why?

D. Why are gloves necessary when giving IM injections, even though you are not actually touching the injection site?

*Name:* _____

*Choose the correct answer for each of these questions. There are 33 questions, each worth 0.3 credit. Aim at a grade of 90% or better. Review material you find difficult. Answers will be found on page 360.*

1. The purpose of the medication ticket in the ticket system is to identify the drug from the time the order is written until it is

   **a.** transferred to the Kardex

   **b.** poured

   **c.** administered

   **d.** charted

2. Which of the following is an appropriate action regarding medication tickets in the ticket system?

   **a.** All tickets are checked against the physician's order sheet.

   **b.** Tickets are made out only for standing orders.

   **c.** A new ticket is written each time a drug is given.

   **d.** The ticket is destroyed after charting a stat order.

3. Checking the Kardex before administering medication by ticket will enable the nurse to determine

   **a.** the name of the physician who ordered the medication

   **b.** if some tickets have been misplaced

   **c.** if a "stat" medication is to be administered

   **d.** whether the patient can have the next prn dose

4. When pouring an oral liquid medication, the nurse should

   **a.** place the cup on the tabletop and bend over to get the right level

   **b.** hold the cup in the hand and pour to the top of the meniscus

   **c.** hold the cup at eye level and pour the center of the meniscus

   **d.** rest the cup on the medication shelf and pour to the mark at the side of the cup

5. Which statement is *false* regarding injections from powders?

   **a.** Read the label twice before drawing up and once after.

   **b.** Draw up one medication at a time.

   **c.** Always use sterile water as a diluent.

   **d.** Pull back on the plunger before injecting the medication.

*(continued)*

6. Withdrawing medication from a vial is facilitated if a specific amount of air is injected into the vial beforehand. Which of these statements explains this action?

    a. It creates a partial vacuum in the vial.

    b. It makes the pressure in the vial greater than atmospheric pressure.

    c. It makes the pressure in the vial the same as atmospheric pressure.

    d. It makes the pressure in the vial less than atmospheric pressure.

7. If a patient has difficulty swallowing medications, which oral form of drug may be crushed?

    a. Sugar-coated tablet

    b. Enteric-coated tablet

    c. Buccal tablet

    d. Capsule

8. A major advantage in the unit-dose system of drug administration is that

    a. the drug supply is always available

    b. no error is possible

    c. the drugs are less expensive than stock distribution

    d. the pharmacist provides a second professional check

9. When a drug is to be administered sublingually, the patient should be instructed to

    a. drink a full glass of water when swallowing

    b. rinse the mouth with water after taking the drug

    c. chew the tablet and allow the saliva to collect under the tongue

    d. hold the medication under the tongue until it dissolves

10. Ampules differ from vials in that ampules

    a. are always glass containers

    b. contain only one dose

    c. contain solids as well as liquids

    d. are not used for injections

11. The Z-track technique for injections can be used to

    a. administer more than one drug at a single site

    b. inhibit hematoma formation by promoting drug absorption

    c. prevent skin discoloration by inhibiting drug seepage

    d. reduce allergic reactions at the injection site

*(continued)*

12. Which action is *correct* in giving a Z-track injection?

   **a.** The skin is retracted and held to one side while the medication is given.

   **b.** The skin is massaged after the injection is given.

   **c.** The plunger is not pulled back when the needle has been inserted.

   **d.** Medication is injected quickly.

13. Which angle of injection is *correctly* matched with the route of administration?

   **a.** Intradermal—45° angle

   **b.** Intramuscular—90° angle

   **c.** Subcutaneous—30° angle

   **d.** Z-track—45° angle

14. A patient asks how to put drops in his or her eye. The nurse instructs the patient to place the drops

   **a.** into the lower conjunctival sac

   **b.** under the upper lid

   **c.** directly on the cornea

   **d.** in the inner canthus

15. In administering a vaginal suppository, which statement is *false?*

   **a.** Universal safeguards should be used.

   **b.** The patient may insert the medication.

   **c.** The patient should be lying on her back.

   **d.** The applicator must be kept sterile.

16. In applying the next dose of a transdermal medication, the nurse should

   **a.** shave the new area and prepare with povidone–iodine

   **b.** cleanse the previous area and use a different site

   **c.** rotate the use of arms and legs as sites

   **d.** allow the previous patch to remain on the skin

17. Which is the muscle of choice to be used when an injection is irritating to the tissues?

   **a.** Deltoid—SC

   **b.** Dorsogluteal—Z-track

   **c.** Ventrogluteal—intradermal

   **d.** Vastus lateralis—IM

*(continued)*

18. Discomfort of an injection is reduced when the needle is inserted

    a. slowly into loose tissue

    b. slowly into firm tissue

    c. rapidly into loose tissue

    d. rapidly into firm tissue

19. After administering an injection, the nurse should

    a. immediately recap the needle

    b. break the needle off the syringe for safety

    c. place the used syringe in a nearby sharps container

    d. don gloves to carry the syringe to the utility room

20. Which statement is *incorrect* in the administration of drugs to mucous membranes?

    a. Eye medications must be labeled ophthalmic.

    b. Patients may insert their own rectal suppositories.

    c. Sublingual medications are applied to the space between the teeth and cheek.

    d. Eye medications may be left in the client's bedside stand.

*Decide whether the following actions are correct or incorrect according to the safeguards in administering medications; explain your choice.*

1. A nurse wears gloves to remove an intravenous heparin lock from a patient's arm. This action is _____

    _____

2. A nurse who has just removed a gown and gloves puts them into the disposal container in the patient's room and leaves the room. This action is _____

    _____

3. In the medication room, a nurse puts on gloves to prepare an IV for administration. This action is _____

    _____

4. A nurse puts on a mask to administer an oral medication to a patient on respiratory isolation precautions. This action is _____

    _____

5. A nurse applies universal precautions in caring for all patients on the unit. This action is

    _____

6. A nurse wears gloves to place a transdermal pad behind a patient's ear. This action is

    _____

    _____

7. A nurse puts on gloves and gown to administer 500 mL of a vaginal douche to a lethargic patient. This action is _____

    _____

8. A nurse whose finger has been stuck with a contaminated IV needle carefully washes her or his hands with soap and water and applies a Band-aid to the site. Because the patient's diagnosis is brain tumor, the nurse decides no further action is necessary. This action is

    _____

9. A nurse giving an injection to a patient makes the judgment *not* to wear gloves. This action is _____

    _____

    _____

10. A nurse puts on gloves to administer an oral tablet to an alert patient with a positive HIV blood count. This action is _____

    _____

*(continued)*

11. After administering an injection, the nurse carefully caps the needle. This action is

    _____

    _____

12. A nurse wears gloves to apply nitroglycerin ointment to a patient's chest even though there is no break in the skin. This action is _____

    _____

    _____

13. A nurse makes a judgment to omit wearing gloves in administering eye drops because they are too bulky. This action is _____

    _____

    _____

# Answers

## Self-Test 1 Universal Safeguards

1. To *all* patients. There is a risk of potential exposure to hepatitis B virus and human immunodeficiency virus that may not have been detected by standard laboratory methods.
2. The type of contact the nurse has with the patient.
3. When there is any direct "hands-on" contact with patient's blood, bodily fluids, or secretions; when handling materials or equipment contaminated with blood or body fluids
4. In a labeled puncture-proof container
5. Handwashing, gloves, gowns, masks, and protective eyewear
6. a. Before preparing medications and after administering medicines to each patient
   b. After removing gloves, gowns, masks, and protective eyewear, and before leaving each patient
   c. Immediately when soiled with the patient's blood of body fluids
   d. After handling equipment soiled with blood or body fluids
7. Hold contaminated IV needles being carried to a puncture-proof container
8. The nurse's clothing may become contaminated with a patient's blood or body fluids
9. A nurse is in extremely close contact with the patient and there is possibility of the patient's blood or blood-tinged fluids being splashed or sprayed into the nurse's eyes or mucous membranes
10. The patient is placed on *strict* or *respiratory* isolation precautions; carrying out a medication procedure may cause blood or body fluids to splash directly on the nurse's face

## Self Test 2 Medication Administration

1. Prevent cross-contamination
2. Aspirate stomach contents; *or* place a stethoscope on the stomach and insert 15 mL of air. A swishing sound indicates proper placement.
3. On the left side—left lateral recumbent position
4. a. Sprinkle on gloved hands and apply; use sparingly to prevent caking
   b. Pat on lightly with gloved hand or gauze pad
   c. Rub into skin while wearing gloves
   d. Use a gloved hand to apply an even coat and cover with a dressing
5. Three tablets; 5 minutes apart
6. a. Sterile
   b. Clean
   c. Clean
   d. Clean
   e. Sterile
   f. Clean
   g. Sterile
   h. Clean
   i. Sterile
   j. Clean
7. Back and up
8. Rub the skin with an alcohol pad in a circular motion from the center of the site out
9. The drug would be destroyed orally; a rapid effect is desired; the patient is unable to take the drug orally
10. In the adult, pull the ear back and up. In a 2-year-old child, pull the ear back and down.

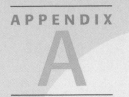

# Dimensional Analysis

In addition to the two methods discussed in Chapter 6 (Formula Method and Ratio Proportion Method), another method of solving dosage calculations can be used. This method is dimensional analysis. The following information is taken from Gloria P. Craig's, *Clinical Calculations Made Easy* (2nd ed., 2001). This method is fully explained in this text, but what follows is a simple explanation of how the problems are set up:

## ▶ Terms Used in Dimensional Analysis

**Dimensional analysis** is a problem-solving method that can be used whenever two quantities are directly proportional to each other and one quantity must be converted to the other by using a common equivalent, conversion factor, or conversion relation. All medication dosage calculation problems can be solved by dimensional analysis.

It is important to understand the following four terms that provide the basis for dimensional analysis.

- **Given quantity:** the beginning point of the problem
- **Wanted quantity:** the answer to the problem
- **Unit path:** the series of conversions necessary to achieve the answer to the problem
- **Conversion factors:** equivalents necessary to convert between systems of measurement and to allow unwanted units to be canceled from the problem
  Each conversion factor is a ratio of units that equals 1.

Dimensional analysis also uses the same terms as fractions: numerators and denominators.

- *The numerator* = the top portion of the problem
- *The denominator* = the bottom portion of the problem

Some problems will have a given quantity and a wanted quantity that contain only numerators. Other problems will have a given quantity and a wanted quantity that contain both a numerator and a denominator. This chapter contains only problems with numerators as the given quantity and the wanted quantity.

Once the beginning point in the problem is identified, then a series of conversions necessary to achieve the answer is established that leads to the problem's solution.

Below is an example of the problem-solving method, showing the placement of basic terms used in dimensional analysis.

Unit Path

| Given Quantity | Conversion Factor for Given Quantity | Conversion Factor for Wanted Quantity | Conversion Computation | Wanted Quantity |
|---|---|---|---|---|
| 1 liter (L) | 1000 mL | 1 oz | $1 \times 1000 \times 1$ | 1000 |
| | 1 liter (L) | 30 mL | $1 \times 30$ | 30 |

$$\dfrac{1000}{30} = 33.3 \text{ oz}$$

## ▶ The Five Steps of Dimensional Analysis

Once the given quantity is identified, the unit path leading to the wanted quantity is established. The problem-solving method of dimensional analysis uses the following five steps.

1. Identify the *given quantity* in the problem.

2. Identify the *wanted quantity* in the problem.

3. Establish the *unit path* from the given quantity to the wanted quantity using equivalents as *conversion factors.*

4. Set up the conversion factors to permit cancellation of unwanted units. Carefully choose each conversion factor and ensure that each factor is correctly placed in the numerator or denominator portion of the problem to allow the unwanted units to be canceled from the problem.

5. Multiply the numerators, multiply the denominators, and divide the product of the numerators by the product of the denominators to provide the numerical value of the wanted quantity.

The following examples use the five steps of dimensional analysis to solve problems.

**Example**   1 liter (L) equals how many ounces (oz)?

**Step 1.** Identify the *given quantity* in the problem.

The given quantity is *1 L.*

Unit Path

| Given Quantity | Conversion Factor for Given Quantity | Conversion Factor for Wanted Quantity | Conversion Computation | Wanted Quantity |
|---|---|---|---|---|
| 1 liter (L) | | | | = |

**Step 2.** Identify the *wanted quantity* in the problem.

The wanted quantity is the number of *ounces* (oz) in 1 L.

Unit Path

| Given Quantity | Conversion Factor for Given Quantity | Conversion Factor for Wanted Quantity | Conversion Computation | Wanted Quantity |
|---|---|---|---|---|
| 1 liter (L) | | | | = oz |

**Step 3.** Establish the *unit path* from the given quantity to the wanted quantity. You must determine what conversion factors are needed to convert the given quantity to the wanted quantity.

Given quantity: 1 L = 1000 mL

Wanted quantity: 1 oz = 30 mL

**Step 4.** Write the unit path for the problem so that each unit cancels out the preceding unit until all unwanted units are canceled from the problem except the wanted quantity.

The wanted quantity must be within the numerator portion of the problem to identify that the problem is set up correctly.

Unit Path

| Given Quantity | Conversion Factor for Given Quantity | Conversion Factor for Wanted Quantity | Conversion Computation | Wanted Quantity |
|---|---|---|---|---|
| 1 liter (L) | 1000 mL | 1 oz | | = oz |
| | 1 liter (L) | 30 mL | | |

Unit Path

| Given Quantity | Conversion Factor for Given Quantity | Conversion Factor for Wanted Quantity | Conversion Computation | Wanted Quantity |
|---|---|---|---|---|
| 1 ~~liter (L)~~ | 1000 ~~mL~~ | 1 ~~(oz)~~ | | = oz |
| | 1 ~~liter (L)~~ | 30 ~~mL~~ | | |

**Step 5.** After the unwanted units are canceled from the problem, only the numerical values remain. Multiply the numerators, multiply the denominators, and divide the product of the numerators by the product of the denominators to provide the numerical value for the wanted quantity.

One (1) times (×) any number equals that number, therefore 1s may be automatically canceled from the problem. Other factors that can be canceled from the problem include like numerical values in the numerator and denominator portion of the problem and the same number of zeroes in the numerator and denominator portion of the problem.

Unit Path

| Given Quantity | Conversion Factor for Given Quantity | Conversion Factor for Wanted Quantity | Conversion Computation | Wanted Quantity |
|---|---|---|---|---|
| 1 ~~liter (L)~~ | 1000 ~~mL~~ | 1 oz | 1000 × 1 | 1000 |
|  | 1 ~~liter (L)~~ | 30 ~~mL~~ | 1 × 30 | 30 = 33.3 oz |

33.3 oz is the wanted quantity and the answer to the problem.

Taking the first problem in Chapter 6 (page XXX), it would look like this in a dimensional analysis problem:

| Given Quantity | Conversion Factor for Given Quantity | Conversion Computation | Wanted Quantity |
|---|---|---|---|
| 0.50 ~~mg~~ |  | 0.50 |  |
|  | 0.25 ~~mg~~ | 0.25 | = 2 tablets |

Conversion Factor for Wanted Quantity

More complex calculations can also be solved using this method by adding more columns to the unit path as more conversions are needed. Again, this method is more fully explained and can be studied in the Craig text.

# Proficiency Test Answers

## Chapter 1

### Test 1: Arithmetic

**A. a)**
$$\begin{array}{r} 647 \\ \times\ \ 38 \\ \hline 5176 \\ 1941\ \ \\ \hline 24586 \end{array}$$

**b)** $\dfrac{\overset{1}{\cancel{8}}}{\underset{3}{\cancel{9}}} \times \dfrac{\overset{\cancel{4}}{\cancel{12}}}{\underset{\cancel{4}}{32}} = \dfrac{1}{3}$

**c)**
$$\begin{array}{r} 0.56 \\ \times\ 0.17 \\ \hline 392 \\ 56\ \ \\ \hline 0.0952 \end{array}$$

**B. a)**
$$\begin{array}{r} 9.670 = 9.67 \\ 82\ )\overline{793.000} \\ \underline{738}\ \ \ \ \ \ \\ 55\ 0\ \ \ \ \\ \underline{49\ 2}\ \ \ \ \\ 5\ 80\ \\ \underline{5\ 74}\ \\ 60 \end{array}$$

**b)** $5\dfrac{1}{4} \div \dfrac{7}{4} = \dfrac{\overset{3}{\cancel{21}}}{\underset{1}{\cancel{4}}} \times \dfrac{\overset{1}{\cancel{4}}}{\underset{1}{\cancel{7}}} = 3$

**c)** $0.015\ )\overline{0.300}$ overset 20.

**C. a)**
$$\begin{array}{r} 0.055\ = 0.06 \\ 18\ )\overline{1.000} \\ \underline{90}\ \ \ \\ 100 \\ \underline{90}\ \\ 100 \end{array}$$

**b)**
$$\begin{array}{r} 0.375\ = 0.38 \\ 8\ )\overline{3.000} \\ \underline{2\ 4}\ \ \ \\ 60 \\ \underline{56} \\ 40 \\ \underline{40} \end{array}$$

**D. a)** $0.35 = \dfrac{\overset{7}{\cancel{35}}}{\underset{20}{\cancel{100}}} = \dfrac{7}{20}$

**b)** $0.08 = \dfrac{\overset{2}{\cancel{8}}}{\underset{25}{\cancel{100}}} = \dfrac{2}{25}$

**E. a)** 0.4
   **b)** 0.8
   **c)** 0.83
   **d)** 0.3

**F. a)** $\dfrac{\overset{5}{\cancel{20}}}{\underset{3}{\cancel{12}}} = \dfrac{5}{3}$  $\begin{array}{r} 1.66 = 1.7 \\ 3\overline{)5.00} \\ \underline{3} \\ 2\,0 \\ \underline{1\,8} \\ 20 \\ \underline{18} \end{array}$

**b)** $\dfrac{\overset{1}{\cancel{7}}}{\underset{12}{\cancel{84}}} = \dfrac{1}{12}$  $\begin{array}{r} 0.83 = 0.8 \\ 12\overline{)1.00} \\ \underline{9\,6} \\ 40 \\ \underline{36} \end{array}$

**c)** $\dfrac{6}{13}$  $\begin{array}{r} 0.46 = 0.5 \\ 13\overline{)6.00} \\ \underline{5\,2} \\ 80 \\ \underline{78} \end{array}$

**G. a)** 5.3
   **b)** 0.63
   **c)** 0.924

**H. a)** $\dfrac{1}{3}\% =$

$\dfrac{\frac{1}{3}}{100} = \dfrac{1}{3} \div 100 =$

$\dfrac{1}{3} \times \dfrac{1}{100} = \dfrac{1}{300}$

**b)** Three ways
 **1)** $0.8\% = \underset{\curvearrowleft}{00.8} = 0.008 =$

  $\dfrac{8}{\underset{125}{\cancel{1000}}} = \dfrac{1}{125}$

 **2)** $0.8\% = \dfrac{0.8}{100}$  $\begin{array}{r} .008 \\ )0.800 \end{array} = 0.008$

  $\dfrac{8}{\underset{125}{\cancel{1000}}} = \dfrac{1}{125}$

 **3)** $0.8\% = \dfrac{\frac{8}{10}}{100} = \dfrac{8}{10} \div 100 = \dfrac{8}{10} \times \dfrac{1}{100} = \dfrac{8}{\underset{125}{\cancel{1000}}} = \dfrac{1}{125}$

**I. a)** $\dfrac{32}{128} = \dfrac{4}{x}$

$\dfrac{\overset{1}{\cancel{32}}x}{\underset{1}{\cancel{32}}} = \dfrac{\overset{4}{\cancel{128}} \times 4}{\underset{1}{\cancel{32}}}$

$x = 16$

**b)** $8 : 72 :: 5 : x$

$\dfrac{\overset{1}{\cancel{8}}}{\underset{1}{\cancel{8}}}x = \dfrac{\overset{9}{\cancel{72}} \times 5}{\underset{1}{\cancel{8}}}$

$x = 45$

**c)** $\dfrac{0.4}{0.12} \bowtie \dfrac{x}{8}$

$0.12x = 0.4 \times 8$

$\dfrac{0.12}{0.12}x = \dfrac{0.4 \times 8}{0.12}$

$x = \dfrac{3.2}{0.12}$  $\begin{array}{r} 26.66 = 26.7 \\ 0.12\overline{)3.2000} \\ \underline{2\,4} \\ 80 \\ \underline{72} \\ 80 \\ \underline{72} \\ 8 \end{array}$

$x = 27$

## Chapter 2

### Test 1: Abbreviations

1. Twice a day
2. Hour of sleep
3. When necessary
4. Both eyes
5. By mouth
6. By rectum
7. Sublingually
8. Swish and swallow
9. Three times a week
10. Milliliter
11. Every 4 hours
12. Cubic centimeters
13. Subcutaneously
14. Both ears
15. Gram
16. After meals
17. Every day
18. Immediately
19. Every 12 hours
20. Three times a day
21. Left eye
22. Kilogram
23. Every night
24. Every hour
25. Right eye
26. Milliquivalent
27. Before meals
28. Four times a day
29. Milligram
30. Intramuscularly
31. Every other day
32. Twice a week
33. Nasogastric tube
34. Every 8 hours
35. Liter
36. Microgram
37. Every 6 hours
38. Microgram
39. Unit
40. Teaspoon
41. Right ear
42. Grain
43. Intravenously
44. Suspension
45. Tablespoon
46. Intravenous piggyback
47. Minim
48. Gram
49. Every 2 hours
50. Every 3 hours

### Test 2: Reading Prescriptions

1. Nembutal one hundred milligrams at the hour of sleep, as needed, by mouth (eg, 10 PM)
2. Propranolol hydrochloride forty milligrams by mouth twice a day (eg, 10 AM, 6 PM)
3. Ampicillin one gram intravenous piggyback every 6 hours (eg, 6 AM, 12 noon, 6 PM, 12 midnight)
4. Demerol fifty milligrams intramuscularly every 4 hours as needed for pain
5. Tylenol three hundred twenty-five milligrams, two tablets by mouth immediately. (Give two tablets of Tylenol. Each tablet is 325 mg.)
6. Pilocarpine drops two in both eyes every 3 hours (eg, 3 AM, 6 AM, 9 AM, 12 noon, 3 PM, 6 PM, 9 PM, 12 midnight)
7. Scopolamine eight-tenths milligram subcutaneously immediately
8. Elixir of digoxin twenty-five hundredths of a milligram by mouth every day (eg, 10 AM)
9. Kaochlor thirty milliequivalents by mouth twice a day (eg, 10 AM and 6 PM)
10. Liquaemin sodium six thousand units subcutaneously every 4 hours (eg, 2 AM, 6 AM, 10 AM, 2 PM, 6 PM, 10 PM)
11. Tobramycin seventy milligrams intramuscularly every 8 hours (eg, 6 AM, 2 PM, 10 PM)
12. Prednisone ten milligrams by mouth every other day (eg, even days of the month at 10 AM). You might substitute qod, "odd days of the month."
13. Milk of magnesia one tablespoon by mouth at the hour of sleep every night (eg, 10 PM)
14. Septra one double-strength tablet every day by mouth (eg, 10 AM)
15. Morphine sulfate fifteen milligrams subcutaneously immediately and ten milligrams every 4 hours as needed. The stat time given determines when the next dose can be administered. (Next dose must be *at least 4 hours later.*)

### Test 3: Interpreting Written Prescription Orders

1. Colace one hundred milligrams by mouth three times a day (eg, 10 AM, 2 PM, 6 PM)
2. Ativan one milligram intravenous push times one dose now.
3. Ten milliequivalents potassium chloride in one hundred cubic centimeters of normal saline over one hour, times one dose.
4. Tylenol number three two tablets by mouth every four hours as needed for pain.
5. Heparin twenty-five thousand international units in two hundred fifty cubic centimeters dextrose five percent in water at five hundred units per hour.
6. Ticlid two hundred fifty milligrams one tablet by mouth twice a day (eg, 10 AM, 6 PM)
7. Lopressor 25 milligrams by mouth twice a day (eg, 10 AM, 6 PM)
8. Benadryl 25 milligrams by mouth every hour of sleep (ie, every night at 10 PM)

## Chapter 3

### Test 1: Labels and Packaging

1. **a.** **1.** Individually wrapped and labeled drugs
      **2.** Large stock containers of drugs
   **b.** **1.** Glass container holding a singe dose. Container must be broken to reach the drug. Any portion not used must be discarded.
      **2.** Glass or plastic container with a sealed top that allows medication to be kept sterile
   **c.** **1.** Drug applied to skin or mucous membranes to achieve a local effect. May be absorbed into the circulation and cause a systemic effect.
      **2.** Drugs given by injection include SC, IM, IV, IVPB.
   **d.** **1.** Brand or proprietary name of manufacturer. Identified by symbol ®
      **2.** Official name of a drug as listed in the USP
   **e.** **1.** Liquid sterile medication ready to administer
      **2.** Powder or crystals diluted according to specific directions. Date and time of preparation must be written on the label and expiration date noted.

2. **a.** 4        **c.** 2        **e.** 1
   **b.** 2        **d.** 1

3. **1.** g        **4.** i        **7.** j        **9.** c
   **2.** e        **5.** d        **8.** a        **10.** b
   **3.** h        **6.** f

### Test 2: Interpreting a Label

1. Fortaz
2. Ceftazidime
3. Intravenous, intramuscular
4. Varies: 1.8 mL, 3.6 mL, 5.3 mL, 10.6 mL
5. 500 mg, 1 gram
6. Reconstitute with sterile water for injection, bacteriostatic water for injection, or 0.5% or 1% lidocaine hydrochloride injection. Dilute with 1.5 mL, approximate available volume 1.8 mL to equal 500 mg (intramuscular route); add 3.0 mL, approximate available volume 3.6 mL to equal 1 gram (intramuscular route); add 5.0 mL, approximate available volume 5.3 mL to equal 500 mg (intravenous route); add 10.0 mL, approximate available volume 10.6 mL to equal 1 gram (intravenous infusion). Shake well.
7. Powder
8. Protect from light. Maintains satisfactory potency for 24 hours at room temperature or for 7 days under refrigeration. Solutions in sterile water for injection that are frozen immediately after constitution in the original container are stable for 3 months when stored at −20° C. Once thawed, solutions should not be refrozen. Thawed solutions may be stored for up to 8 hours at room temperature or for 4 days in a refrigerator.
9. Not shown
10. 500 mg or 1 gram (adults)
11. Federal law prohibits dispensing without prescription. This vial is under reduced pressure. Addition of diluent generates a positive pressure. Color changes do not affect potency.

## Chapter 4

### Test 1: Solid and Liquid Equivalents

| | | | |
|---|---|---|---|
| **1.** 0.1 | **11.** 30 | **21.** 100 | **31.** 10 |
| **2.** 30 | **12.** 16 | **22.** 1 | **32.** 1 |
| **3.** 1000 | **13.** 15 | **23.** 0.6 | **33.** 1000 |
| **4.** 5 | **14.** 2.2 | **24.** 0.01 | **34.** .6 mg |
| **5.** 15 | **15.** 1000 | **25.** 1000 | **35.** gr ½ |
| **6.** 0.01 | **16.** 0.06 | **26.** 0.0005 mg | **36.** 120 mg |
| **7.** 1 | **17.** 1 | **27.** 0.0006 | **37.** gr 4 |
| **8.** 200 | **18.** 1 | **28.** 0.25 mg | **38.** .48 mg |
| **9.** 0.03 | **19.** 8 | **29.** 0.001 | **39.** gr 17 |
| **10.** 0.5 | **20.** 1 | **30.** 125 | **40.** .3 mg |

## Chapter 5

### Test 1: Drug Preparations and Equipment

1. Diabetes mellitus; alcholism
2. Two teaspoons or less
3. SC, IM, IVPB, and IV
4. a. the date; b. the nurse's initials; c. the dilution made
5. Sterile technique is required in preparing and administering drugs parenterally (IM, SC, IV, IVPB).
6. Milk of magnesia
7. Before an oral suspension is poured, the liquid must always be shaken.
8. Aerosol powders; creams; ointments; pastes; suppositories; transdermal medications
9. Ease in administering; prolonged action
10. An ointment is a semisolid preparation in a petroleum or lanolin base for topical use.
11. 1. Pour to a line. Never estimate a dose.
    2. Pour liquids at eye level.

12. a. The natural curve of the surface of a liquid in a container
    b. Diameter or width of a needle. The higher the gauge number, the finer the needle.
13. Route of administration; size and condition of the patient; amount of adipose tissue present at the site
14. 1. When the last number is 5 or more, add 1 to the previous number.
    2. When the last number is 4 or less, drop the number.
15. The equipment used
    3 mL syringe—nearest $10^{th}$ in mL
    precision syringe—nearest $100^{th}$ in mL
    medicine cup—metric, apothecary, or househould lines

## Chapter 6

### Test 1: Calculation of Oral Doses

**Formula Method**

1. $\dfrac{\overset{10}{\cancel{20\text{ mEq}}}}{\underset{\underset{1}{2}}{\cancel{30\text{ mEq}}}} \times \overset{1}{\cancel{15}}\text{ mL} = 10\text{ mL}$

**Ratio Proportion Method**

$\dfrac{15\text{ mL}}{30\text{ mEq}} = \dfrac{x}{20\text{ mEq}}$

$\dfrac{300}{30} = x$

$10\text{ mL} = x$

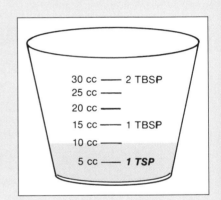

30 cc —— 2 TBSP
25 cc ——
20 cc ——
15 cc —— 1 TBSP
10 cc ——
5 cc —— *1 TSP*

**Formula Method**

2. $\dfrac{\overset{2}{\cancel{150\text{ mg}}}}{\underset{1}{\cancel{75\text{ mg}}}} \times 7.5\text{ mL} = 15\text{ mL}$

**Ratio Proportion Method**

$\dfrac{\overset{.1}{\cancel{7.5}}\text{ mL}}{\underset{1}{\cancel{75}}\text{ mg}} = \dfrac{x}{150\text{ mg}}$

$\dfrac{150 \times .1}{1} = x$

$15\text{ mL} = x$

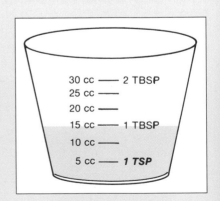

30 cc —— 2 TBSP
25 cc ——
20 cc ——
15 cc —— 1 TBSP
10 cc ——
5 cc —— *1 TSP*

*Formula Method*

3. $\dfrac{\overset{1}{\cancel{0.125}\text{ mg}}}{\underset{\underset{1}{\cancel{2}}}{\cancel{0.250}\text{ mg}}} \times \overset{5}{\cancel{10}} = 5\text{ mL}$

Alternate arithmetic

$0.25\,\overline{)0.12\,5} \times 10\text{ mL} = 5\text{ mL}$
$\phantom{0.25\,)}\underset{12\,5}{\overset{.5}{}}$

*Ratio Proportion Method*

$\dfrac{10\text{ mL}}{0.25\text{ mg}} = \dfrac{x}{0.125\text{ mg}}$

$\dfrac{1.25}{0.25} = x$

$5\text{ mL} = x$

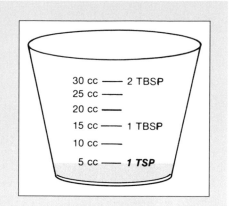

*Formula Method*

4. $\dfrac{\overset{2}{\cancel{150}\text{ mg}}}{\underset{1}{\cancel{75}\text{ mg}}} \times 6\text{ mL} = 12\text{ mL} = 3\text{ drams}$

*Ratio Proportion Method*

$\dfrac{6\text{ mL}}{75\text{ mg}} = \dfrac{x}{150\text{ mg}}$

$\dfrac{900}{75} = x$

$12\text{ mL} = x$

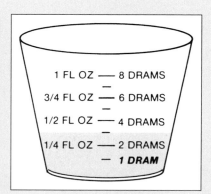

*Formula Method*

5. $\dfrac{\overset{5}{\cancel{10}\text{ mg}}}{\underset{1}{\cancel{2}\text{ mg}}} \times 5\text{ mL} = 25\text{ mL}$

*Ratio Proportion Method*

$\dfrac{5\text{ mL}}{2\text{ mg}} = \dfrac{x}{10\text{ mg}}$

$\dfrac{50}{2} = x$

$25\text{ mL} = x$

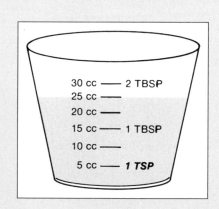

*Formula Method*

6. Rule: $\dfrac{D}{H} \times S = A$

$\dfrac{0.50\text{ mg}}{0.25\text{ mg}} \times 1\text{ tab} = 0.25\,\overset{2.}{\overline{)0.50}}\ 2\text{ tablets}$

*Ratio Proportion Method*

$\dfrac{1\text{ tab}}{0.25\text{ mg}} = \dfrac{x}{0.50}$

$\dfrac{0.50}{0.25} = x$

$2\text{ tab} = x$

*Formula Method*                    *Ratio Proportion Method*

**7.** Equivalent 0.02 mg = 20 μg (mcg)

$$\frac{\overset{1}{\cancel{10\ mcg}}}{\underset{2}{\cancel{20\ mcg}}} \times 1\ tab = \frac{1}{2}\ tablet$$

$$\frac{1\ tab}{20\ mcg} = \frac{x}{10\ mcg}$$

$$\frac{10}{20} = x$$

$$.5\ tab = x$$

*Formula Method*                    *Ratio Proportion Method*

**8.** $\dfrac{\overset{5}{\cancel{250\ mg}}}{\underset{2}{\cancel{100\ mg}}} \times 1\ tab = \dfrac{5}{2} = 2\dfrac{1}{2}$ tablets.

$$\frac{1\ tab}{100\ mg} = \frac{x}{250\ mg}$$

$$\frac{250}{100} = x$$

$$2.5\ tab = x$$

**9.** Equivalent 0.5 g = 500 mg

*Formula Method*                    *Ratio Proportion Method*

$$\frac{\overset{2}{\cancel{500\ mg}}}{\underset{1}{\cancel{250\ mg}}} \times 1\ tab = 2\ tablets$$

$$\frac{1\ tab}{250\ mg} = \frac{x}{500\ mg}$$

$$\frac{500}{250} = x$$

$$2\ tab = x$$

**10.** Equivalent 0.3 mg = 300 μg (mcg)

*Formula Method*                    *Ratio Proportion Method*

$$\frac{\overset{1}{\cancel{300\ \mu g}}}{\underset{1}{\cancel{300\ \mu g}}} \times 1\ tab = 1\ tablet$$

$$\frac{1\ tab}{300\ mcg} = \frac{x}{300\ mcg}$$

$$\frac{300}{300} = x$$

$$1\ tab = x$$

## Test 2: Calculation of Oral Doses (Test 2)

*Formula Method*                    *Ratio Proportion Method*

**1.** Rule: $\dfrac{D}{H} \times S = A$

$$\frac{1\ tablet}{400\ mg} = \frac{x}{800\ mg}$$

Equivalent 0.8 gm = 800 mg

$$\frac{800}{400} = x$$

$$\frac{\overset{2}{\cancel{800\ mg}}}{\underset{1}{\cancel{400\ mg}}} \times 1\ tab = 2\ tablets$$

$$2\ tablets = x$$

*Formula Method*                    *Ratio Proportion Method*

**2.** Equivalent 0.3 Gm = 300 mg

$$\frac{\overset{1}{\cancel{300\ mg}}}{\underset{1}{\cancel{300\ mg}}} \times 1\ tab = 1\ tablet$$

$$\frac{1\ tablet}{300\ mg} = \frac{x}{300\ mg}$$

$$\frac{300}{300} = x$$

$$1\ tab = x$$

*Formula Method*

3. $\dfrac{\overset{3}{\cancel{600\ mg}}}{\underset{2}{\cancel{400\ mg}}} \times 1\ \text{tablet} = \dfrac{3}{2} = 1.5\ \text{or}\ 1\frac{1}{2}\ \text{tablets}$

*Ratio Proportion Method*

$$\dfrac{1\ \text{tablet}}{400\ mg} = \dfrac{x}{600\ mg}$$

$$\dfrac{600}{400} = x$$

$$1.5\ \text{tablets} = x$$

*Formula Method*

4. $0.65\ Gm = 650\ mg$

$\dfrac{\overset{2}{\cancel{650\ mg}}}{\underset{1}{\cancel{325\ mg}}} \times 1\ \text{tablet} = 2\ \text{tablets}$

*Ratio Proportion Method*

$$\dfrac{1\ \text{tablet}}{325\ mg} = \dfrac{x}{650\ mg}$$

$$\dfrac{650}{325} = x$$

$$2\ \text{tablets} = x$$

*Formula Method*

5. $\dfrac{\overset{1}{\cancel{250\ mg}}}{\underset{2}{\cancel{500\ mg}}} \times 1\ \text{tablet} = \dfrac{1}{2}\ \text{tablet}$

*Ratio Proportion Method*

$$\dfrac{1\ \text{tablet}}{500\ mg} = \dfrac{x}{250\ mg}$$

$$\dfrac{250}{500} = x$$

$$.5\ \text{tablet} = x$$

*Formula Method*

6. Equivalent 1 tsp = 5 mL

$\dfrac{\overset{16}{\cancel{80\ mg}}}{\underset{5}{\cancel{25\ mg}}} \times \overset{1}{\cancel{5}}\ mL = 16\ mL = 4\ \text{drams}$

Alternate arithmetic

$80 \times 5 = 400$

$$\begin{array}{r} 16. \\ 25\overline{)400.} \\ \underline{25\phantom{0}} \\ 150 \\ \underline{150} \\ 0 \end{array}$$

*Ratio Proportion Method*

$$\dfrac{5\ mL}{25\ mg} = \dfrac{x}{80\ mg}$$

$$\dfrac{400}{25} = x$$

$$16\ mL = 4\ \text{drams}$$

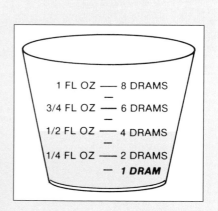

1 FL OZ —— 8 DRAMS
—
3/4 FL OZ —— 6 DRAMS
—
1/2 FL OZ —— 4 DRAMS
—
1/4 FL OZ —— 2 DRAMS
— *1 DRAM*

*Formula Method*

7. Equivalent 0.75 Gm = 750 mg

$\dfrac{\overset{3}{\cancel{750\ mg}}}{\underset{1}{\cancel{250\ mg}}} \times 5\ mL = 15\ mL$

*Ratio Proportion Method*

$$\dfrac{5\ mL}{250\ mg} = \dfrac{x}{750}$$

$$\dfrac{3750}{250} = x$$

$$15\ mL = x$$

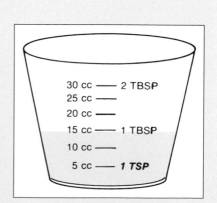

30 cc —— 2 TBSP
25 cc ——
20 cc ——
15 cc —— 1 TBSP
10 cc ——
5 cc —— *1 TSP*

*Formula Method*

8. $\dfrac{\overset{12}{\cancel{600 \text{ mg}}}}{\underset{\underset{1}{50}}{\cancel{250 \text{ mg}}}} \times \overset{1}{\cancel{5}}\text{ mL} = 12 \text{ mL}$

Alternate arithmetic

$600 \times 5 = 3000$

$\begin{array}{r} 12. \\ 250\,\overline{)3000.} \\ \underline{250}\phantom{0} \\ 500 \\ \underline{500} \\ 0 \end{array}$   $12 \text{ mL} = 3 \text{ drams}$

*Ratio Proportion Method*

$\dfrac{5 \text{ ml}}{250 \text{ mg}} = \dfrac{x}{600 \text{ mg}}$

$\dfrac{3000}{250} = x$

$12\text{mL} = x$

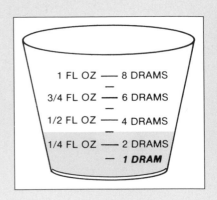

1 FL OZ —— 8 DRAMS
3/4 FL OZ —— 6 DRAMS
1/2 FL OZ —— 4 DRAMS
1/4 FL OZ —— 2 DRAMS
—— *1 DRAM*

9. No arithmetic necessary. Compounded drug.
   Pour 30 mL.

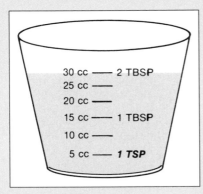

30 cc —— 2 TBSP
25 cc ——
20 cc ——
15 cc —— 1 TBSP
10 cc ——
5 cc —— *1 TSP*

*Formula Method*

10. $\dfrac{\overset{2}{\cancel{160 \text{ mg}}}}{\underset{1}{\cancel{80 \text{ mg}}}} \times 15 \text{ mL} = 30 \text{ mL}$

*Ratio Proportion Method*

$\dfrac{15 \text{ mL}}{80 \text{ mg}} = \dfrac{x}{160 \text{ mg}}$

$\dfrac{2400}{80} = x$

$30\text{mL} = x$

## Test 3: Calculation of Oral Doses (Test 3)

*Formula Method*

1. $\dfrac{\overset{10}{\cancel{20 \text{ mEq}}}}{\underset{\underset{1}{2}}{\cancel{30 \text{ mEq}}}} \times \overset{1}{\cancel{15}}\text{ mL} = 10 \text{ mL}$

*Ratio Proportion Method*

$\dfrac{\overset{1}{\cancel{15}} \text{ mL}}{\underset{2}{\cancel{30}} \text{ mEq}} = \dfrac{x}{20 \text{ mEq}}$

$\dfrac{20}{2} = x$

$10\text{mL} = x$

*Formula Method*

2. $\dfrac{\overset{16}{\cancel{80}} \text{ mg}}{\underset{25}{\cancel{125} \text{ mg}}} \times \overset{1}{\cancel{5}} \text{ mL} = \dfrac{\overset{16}{\cancel{80}}}{\underset{5}{\cancel{25}}} = \dfrac{\cancel{16}}{5} = 5\overline{)16.0}\;\overset{3.2}{} = 3.2 \text{ mL}$

If you do not have a dropper bottle, you could use a syringe without the needle to obtain the dose.

*Ratio Proportion Method*

$\dfrac{\dfrac{1}{\cancel{5} \text{ mL}}}{\underset{25}{\cancel{125} \text{ mg}}} = \dfrac{x}{80 \text{ mg}}$

$\dfrac{80}{25} = x$

$3.2 \text{ mL} = x$

*Formula Method*

3. $0.02 \text{ g} = 20 \text{ mg}$

$\dfrac{\overset{2}{\cancel{20} \text{ mg}}}{\underset{1}{\cancel{10} \text{ mg}}} \times 1 \text{ tab} = 2 \text{ tablets}$

*Ratio Proportion Method*

$\dfrac{1 \text{ tab}}{10 \text{ mg}} = \dfrac{x}{20 \text{ mg}}$

$\dfrac{20}{10} = x$

$2 \text{ tablets} = x$

*Formula Method*

4. $0.5 \text{ g} = 500 \text{ mg}$

$\dfrac{\overset{2}{\cancel{500} \text{ mg}}}{\underset{1}{\cancel{250} \text{ mg}}} \times 1 \text{ cap} = 2 \text{ capsules}$

*Ratio Proportion Method*

$\dfrac{1 \text{ capsule}}{250 \text{ mg}} = \dfrac{x}{500 \text{ mg}}$

$\dfrac{500}{250} = x$

$2 \text{ capsules} = x$

*Formula Method*

5. $\dfrac{\overset{2}{\cancel{0.50} \text{ mg}}}{\underset{1}{\cancel{0.25} \text{ mg}}} \times 1 \text{ tab} = 2 \text{ tablets}$

*Ratio Proportion Method*

$\dfrac{1 \text{ tablet}}{0.25 \text{ mg}} = \dfrac{x}{0.5 \text{ mg}}$

$\dfrac{0.5}{0.25} = x$

$2 \text{ tablets} = x$

*Formula Method*

6. $100 \text{ mcg} = 0.1 \text{ mg}$

$\dfrac{\overset{}{\cancel{0.1} \text{ mg}}}{\underset{1}{\cancel{0.2} \text{ mg}}} \times \overset{5}{\cancel{10}} \text{ mL} = 5 \text{ mL}$

*Ratio Proportion Method*

$\dfrac{10 \text{ ml}}{.2 \text{ mg}} = \dfrac{x}{.1 \text{ mg}}$

$50 \times .1 = x$

$5 \text{ mL} = x$

*Formula Method*

7. $\dfrac{\overset{3}{\cancel{75} \text{ mg}}}{\underset{2}{\cancel{50} \text{ mg}}} \times 1 \text{ tab} = \dfrac{3}{2}\overline{)3.0}\;\overset{1.5}{} = 1\tfrac{1}{2} \text{ tablets}$

*Ratio Proportion Method*

$\dfrac{1 \text{ tablet}}{50 \text{ mg}} = \dfrac{x}{75 \text{ mg}}$

$\dfrac{75}{50} = x$

$1.5 \text{ tabs} = x$

*Formula Method*                                    *Ratio Proportion Method*

8. $\dfrac{\overset{1}{\cancel{40 \text{ mg}}}}{\underset{2}{\cancel{80 \text{ mg}}}} \times 1 \text{ tab} = \dfrac{1}{2} \text{ tablet}$     $\dfrac{1 \text{ tablet}}{80 \text{ mg}} = \dfrac{x}{40 \text{ mg}}$

$\dfrac{40}{80} = x$

$.5 \text{ tablet} = x$

*Formula Method*                                    *Ratio Proportion Method*

9. $0.125 \text{ mg} = 1.25 \ \mu g$

$\dfrac{\overset{1}{\cancel{1.25 \ \mu g}}}{\underset{4}{\underset{2}{\cancel{500 \ \mu g}}}} \times \overset{5}{\cancel{10}} \text{ mL} = \dfrac{5}{2} \overset{2.5}{\overline{)5.0}} = 2.5 \text{ mL}$     $\dfrac{10 \text{ mL}}{500 \text{ mcg}} = \dfrac{x}{125}$

$\dfrac{1250}{500} = x$

$2.5 \text{ mL} = x$

*Formula Method*                                    *Ratio Proportion Method*

10. $\dfrac{\overset{3}{\cancel{75 \text{ mg}}}}{\underset{2}{\underset{1}{\cancel{50 \text{ mg}}}}} \times \overset{5}{\cancel{10}} \text{ mL} = 15 \text{ mL}$     $\dfrac{10 \text{ mL}}{50 \text{ mg}} = \dfrac{x}{75 \text{ mg}}$

$\dfrac{750}{50} = x$

$15 \text{ mL} = x$

*Formula Method*                                    *Ratio Proportion Method*

11. $\dfrac{5 \text{ mg}}{2 \text{ mg}} \times 1 \text{ tab} = \dfrac{5}{2} \overset{2.5}{\overline{)5.0}} = 2\dfrac{1}{2} \text{ tablets}$     $\dfrac{1 \text{ tablet}}{2 \text{ mg}} = \dfrac{x}{5 \text{ mg}}$

$\dfrac{5}{2} = x$

$2.5 \text{ tablets} = x$

*Formula Method*                                    *Ratio Proportion Method*

12. $0.15 \text{ mg} = 150 \ \mu g \text{ (mcg)}$

$\dfrac{\overset{1}{\cancel{150 \ \mu g}}}{\underset{2}{\cancel{300 \ \mu g}}} \times 1 \text{ tab} = \dfrac{1}{2} \text{ tablet}$     $\dfrac{1 \text{ tab}}{300 \text{ mcg}} = \dfrac{x}{150 \text{ mcg}}$

$\dfrac{150}{300} = x$

$.5 \text{ tablet} = x$

*Formula Method*                                    *Ratio Proportion Method*

13. $\dfrac{\overset{3}{\cancel{375 \text{ mg}}}}{\underset{2}{\cancel{250 \text{ mg}}}} \times 1 \text{ tab} = \dfrac{3}{2} \overset{1.5}{\overline{)3.0}} = 1\dfrac{1}{2} \text{ tablets}$     $\dfrac{1 \text{ tablet}}{250 \text{ mg}} = \dfrac{x}{375 \text{ mg}}$

$\dfrac{375}{250} = x$

$1.5 \text{ tablets} = x$

*Formula Method*    *Ratio Proportion Method*

**14.** 0.6 g = 600 mg

$$\frac{\overset{2}{\cancel{600\ mg}}}{\underset{1}{\cancel{300\ mg}}} \times 1\ tab = 2\ tablets$$

$$\frac{1\ tablet}{300\ mg} = \frac{x}{600}$$

$$\frac{600}{300} = x$$

2 tablets = x

*Formula Method*    *Ratio Proportion Method*

**15.** $\frac{\overset{3}{\cancel{1.5\ mg}}}{\underset{2}{\cancel{1.0\ mg}}} \times \overset{4}{8}\ mL = 12\ mL$; pour 3 drams!

$$\frac{8\ mL}{1\ mg} = \frac{x}{1.5\ mg}$$

12 mL or 3 drams = x

*Formula Method*    *Ratio Proportion Method*

**16.** $\frac{\overset{2}{\cancel{25.0\ mg}}}{\underset{1}{\cancel{12.5\ mg}}} \times 5\ mL = 10\ mL$

$$\frac{5\ mL}{12.5\ mg} = \frac{x}{25\ mg}$$

$$\frac{125}{12.5} = x$$

10 mL = x

*Formula Method*    *Ratio Proportion Method*

**17.** $\frac{\overset{3}{\cancel{60\ mg}}}{\underset{2}{\cancel{40\ mg}}} \times 0.6\ mL = \frac{1.8}{2} = 0.9\ mL$

$$\frac{.6\ mL}{40\ mg} = \frac{x}{60\ mg}$$

$$\frac{36}{40} = x$$

.9 mL = x

*Formula Method*    *Ratio Proportion Method*

**18.** 0.5 g = 500 mg

$$\frac{\overset{2}{\cancel{500\ mg}}}{\underset{1}{\cancel{250\ mg}}} \times 5\ mL = 10\ mL$$

$$\frac{5\ mL}{250\ mg} = \frac{x}{500\ mg}$$

$$\frac{2500}{250} = x$$

10 mL = x

*Formula Method*    *Ratio Proportion Method*

**19.** $\frac{\overset{3}{\cancel{15\ mg}}}{\underset{10}{\cancel{50\ mg}}} \times 5\ mL = 1.5\ mL$

$$\frac{5\ mL}{50\ mg} = \frac{x}{15\ mg}$$

$$\frac{75}{50} = x$$

1.5 mL = x

*Formula Method*    *Ratio Proportion Method*

**20.** $\frac{\overset{3}{\cancel{7.5\ mg}}}{\underset{4}{\cancel{10.0\ mg}}} \times 5\ mL = \frac{\overset{15}{15}}{4} \overset{3.75}{\overline{)15.00}} = 3.8\ mL$

$$\frac{5\ mL}{10\ mg} = \frac{x}{7.5}$$

$$\frac{37.5}{10} = x$$

3.8 mL = x

If you do not have a dropper, use a syringe minus the needle to get the dose.

## Chapter 7

### Test 1: Calculations of Liquid Injections (Test 1)

*Formula Method*         *Ratio Proportion Method*

**1.** Equivalent 0.1 Gm = 100 mg

$$\frac{\overset{1}{\cancel{100 \text{ mg}}}}{\underset{2}{\cancel{200 \text{ mg}}}} \times 3 \text{ mL} = \frac{3\overline{)3.0}}{2}^{1.5}$$

Give 1.5 mL IM.

$$\frac{3 \text{ mL}}{200 \text{ mg}} = \frac{x}{100 \text{ mg}}$$

$$\frac{300}{200} = x$$

$$1.5 \text{ mL} = x$$

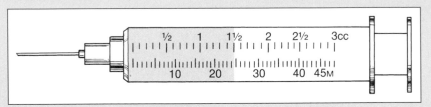

*Formula Method*         *Ratio Proportion Method*

**2.**
$$\frac{\overset{1}{\cancel{5 \text{ mg}}}}{\underset{3}{\cancel{15 \text{ mg}}}} \times 1 \text{ mL} = \frac{1}{3\overline{)1.000}}^{.333}$$

Give 0.33 mL SC.

$$\frac{1 \text{ mL}}{15 \text{ mg}} = \frac{x}{5 \text{ mg}}$$

$$\frac{5}{15} = x$$

$$.333 \text{ mL} = x$$

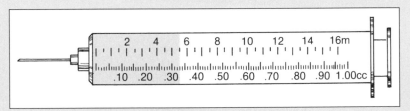

*Formula Method*         *Ratio Proportion Method*

**3.**
$$\frac{\overset{1}{\cancel{25 \text{ mg}}}}{\underset{\underset{1}{2}}{\cancel{50 \text{ mg}}}} \times \overset{1}{\cancel{2}} \text{ cc} = 1 \text{ cc}$$

Give 1 cc IM.

$$\frac{2 \text{ cc}}{50 \text{ mg}} = \frac{x}{25 \text{ mg}}$$

$$\frac{50}{50} = x$$

$$1 \text{ cc} = x$$

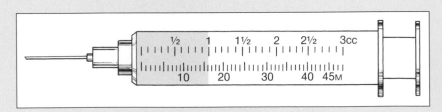

**4.** 20 units. Remember that Humulin insulin is a type of regular insulin and so must be drawn up first into the syringe!

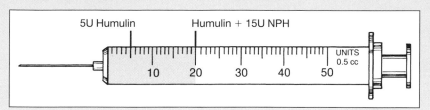

**Formula Method**

**5.** $\dfrac{\overset{1}{\cancel{20}\text{ mEq}}}{\underset{2}{\cancel{40}\text{ mEq}}} \times \overset{10}{\cancel{20}} \text{ mL} = 10 \text{ mL}$

Add 10 mL to IV.

**Ratio Proportion Method**

$\dfrac{\overset{1}{\cancel{20}}\text{ mL}}{\underset{2}{\cancel{40}}\text{ mEq}} = \dfrac{x}{20\text{ mEq}}$

$\dfrac{20}{2} = x$

$10 \text{ mL} = x$

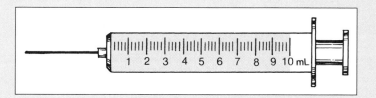

**Formula Method**

**6.** $\dfrac{\overset{3}{\cancel{0.6}\text{ mg}}}{\underset{2}{\cancel{0.4}\text{ mg}}} \times 1 \text{ mL} = \begin{array}{r} 1.5 \\ 2\overline{)3.0} \end{array} \begin{array}{l} 3 \end{array}$

Give 1.5 mL SC.

**Ratio Proportion Method**

$\dfrac{1 \text{ mL}}{0.4 \text{ mg}} = \dfrac{x}{0.6 \text{ mg}}$

$\dfrac{0.6}{0.4} = x$

$1.5 \text{ mL} = x$

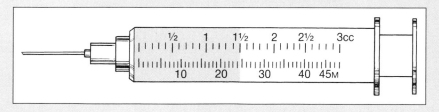

*Formula Method*

**Ratio Proportion Method**

7.
$$\frac{\overset{2}{\cancel{0.8}\text{ mg}}}{\underset{1}{\cancel{0.4}\text{ mg}}} \times 1\text{ mL} = 2\text{ mL}$$

$$\frac{1\text{ mL}}{0.4\text{ mg}} = \frac{x}{0.8\text{ mg}}$$

$$\frac{0.8}{0.4} = x$$

Give 2 mL IM.

$$2\text{ mL} = x$$

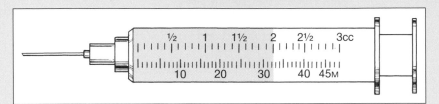

8. Equivalent 0.5 Gm = 500 mg

**Ratio Proportion Method**

$$\frac{1\text{ mL}}{250\text{ mg}} = \frac{x}{500\text{ mg}}$$

*Formula Method*

$$\frac{\overset{2}{\cancel{500}\text{ mg}}}{\underset{1}{\cancel{250}\text{ mg}}} \times 1\text{ mL} = 2\text{ mL}$$

$$\frac{500}{250} = x$$

Add 2 mL to IV. Were you confused by the 25%? No reason to use it to solve this problem!

$$2\text{ mL} = x$$

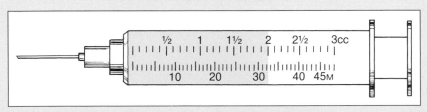

*Formula Method*

**Ratio Proportion Method**

9.
$$\frac{\cancel{200}\text{ mg}}{\cancel{500}\text{ mg}} \times 2\text{ mL} = \frac{4}{5}\overset{.8}{)4.0}$$

$$\frac{2\text{ mL}}{500\text{ mg}} = \frac{x}{200\text{ mg}}$$

$$\frac{400}{500} = x$$

Give 0.8 mL IM.

$$0.8\text{ mL} = x$$

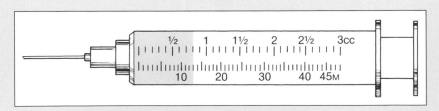

**10.** Equivalent 1:100 means    1 g in 100 mL

1 g = 1000 mg

Hence, the solution is 1000 mg/100 mL.

*Ratio Proportion Method*

$$\frac{\dfrac{1}{\cancel{100}\text{ mL}}}{\dfrac{\cancel{1000}\text{ mg}}{10}} = \frac{x}{7.5\text{ mg}}$$

*Formula Method*

$$\frac{7.5\text{ mg}}{\cancel{1000}\text{ mg}} \times \cancel{100}\text{ mL} = \frac{7.5}{10}$$

$$10\,)\overline{\begin{array}{r}.75 \\ 7.50 \\ \underline{7\ 0} \\ 50 \\ \underline{50}\end{array}}$$

$$\frac{7.5}{10} = x$$

$$.75 \text{ or } 0.8\text{ mL} = x$$

Give 0.8 mL SC.

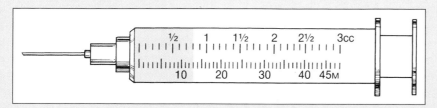

## Test 2: Calculations of Liquid Injections (Test 2)

*Formula Method*

**1.** $\dfrac{\overset{2}{\cancel{10}}\text{ mg}}{\underset{3}{\cancel{15}}\text{ mg}} \times 1\text{ mL} = \dfrac{2}{3}$

$$3\,)\overline{\begin{array}{r}.66 \\ 2.00\end{array}}$$

Give 0.7 mL SC.

*Ratio Proportion Method*

$$\frac{1\text{ mL}}{15\text{ mg}} = \frac{x}{10\text{ mg}}$$

$$\frac{10}{15} = x$$

$$0.66 \text{ or } 0.7\text{ ml} = x$$

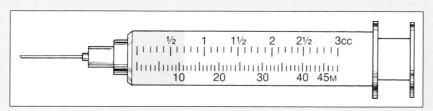

*Formula Method*

2. $\dfrac{\overset{1}{\cancel{25\ mg}}}{\underset{4}{\cancel{100\ mg}}} \times 1\ mL = \dfrac{1}{4}\overset{.25}{\overline{)1.00}}$

Give 0.25 mL. You are using a 1-mL precision syringe; therefore, the answer is the nearest hundredth.

*Ratio Proportion Method*

$$\dfrac{1\ mL}{100\ mg} = \dfrac{x}{25\ mg}$$

$$\dfrac{25}{100} = x$$

$$0.25\ mL = x$$

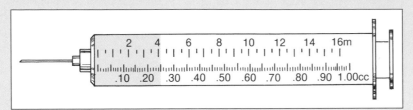

3. Equivalent 0.1 g = 100 mg

*Formula Method*

$\dfrac{\overset{1}{\cancel{100\ mg}}}{\underset{2}{\cancel{200\ mg}}} \times 3\ mL = \dfrac{3}{2}\overset{1.5}{\overline{)3.0}}$

Give 1.5 mL IM.

*Ratio Proportion Method*

$$\dfrac{3\ mL}{200\ mg} = \dfrac{x}{100\ mg}$$

$$\dfrac{300}{200} = x$$

$$1.5\ mL = x$$

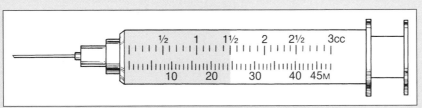

*Formula Method*

4. $\dfrac{\overset{1}{\cancel{1000\ \mu g}}}{\underset{5}{\cancel{5000\ \mu g}}} \times 1\ mL = \dfrac{1}{5}\overset{.2}{\overline{)1.0}}$

Give 0.2 mL IM.

*Ratio Proportion Method*

$$\dfrac{1\ mL}{5000\ mcg} = \dfrac{x}{1000\ mcg}$$

$$\dfrac{1000}{5000} = x$$

$$0.2\ mL = x$$

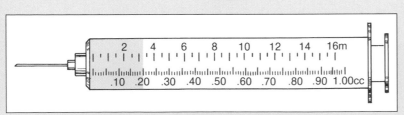

**5.** Equivalent 1% means   1 g in 100 mL
                                    1 g = 1000 mg

Hence, the solution is 1000 mg in 100 mL.

*Ratio Proportion Method*

$$\frac{\overset{1}{\cancel{100}} \text{ mL}}{\underset{10}{\cancel{1000}} \text{ mg}} = \frac{x}{25 \text{ mg}}$$

$$\frac{25}{10} = x$$

$$2.5 \text{ mL} = x$$

*Formula Method*

$$\frac{\overset{5}{\cancel{25} \text{ mg}}}{\underset{\underset{2}{10}}{\cancel{1000} \text{ mg}}} \times \overset{1}{\cancel{100}} \text{ mL} = \frac{5}{2} \quad 2\overline{)5.0}^{\,2.5}$$

Prepare 2.5 mL for the physician.

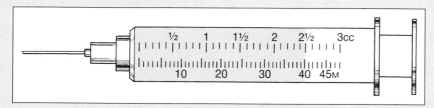

*Formula Method*

**6.** $\dfrac{0.5 \text{ mg}}{0.4 \text{ mg}} \times 1 \text{ mL} = \dfrac{5}{4} \quad 4\overline{)5.00}^{\,1.25}$

Give 1.3 mL SC.

*Ratio Proportion Method*

$$\frac{1 \text{ mL}}{0.4 \text{ mg}} = \frac{x}{0.5 \text{ mg}}$$

$$\frac{0.5}{0.4} = x$$

$$1.25 \text{ or } 1.3 \text{ mL} = x$$

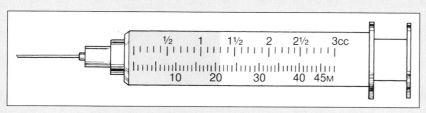

**7.** 13 units. Remember that Humulin insulin is a type of regular insulin and so must be drawn up first into the syringe!

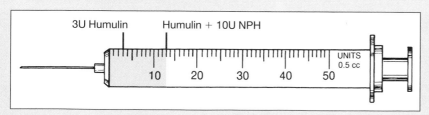

*Formula Method*

*Ratio Proportion Method*

8. $\dfrac{1.2 \ \text{mEq}}{0.5 \ \text{mEq}} \times 1 \ \text{mL} = \dfrac{1.2}{0.5} \overline{)1.20}^{\ 2.4}$

$\dfrac{1 \ \text{mL}}{0.5 \ \text{mEq}} = \dfrac{x}{1.2 \ \text{mEq}}$

Add 2.4 mL to the IV stat.

$\dfrac{1.2}{0.5} = x$

$2.4 \ \text{mL} = x$

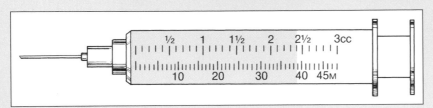

*Formula Method*

*Ratio Proportion Method*

9. $\overset{3}{\dfrac{75 \ \text{mg}}{\underset{2}{50 \ \text{mg}}}} \times 1 \ \text{mL} = \dfrac{3}{2} \overline{)3.0}^{\ 1.5}$

$\dfrac{1 \ \text{mL}}{50 \ \text{mg}} = \dfrac{x}{75 \ \text{mg}}$

Give 1.5 mL IM.

$\dfrac{75}{50} = x$

$1.5 \ \text{mL} = x$

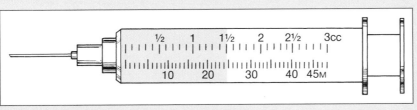

10. Equivalent 1:1000 means   1 g in 1000 mL

$\qquad\qquad\qquad\qquad\qquad$ 1 g = 1000 mg

Hence, the solution is 1000 mg in 1000 mL.

500 $\mu$g = 0.5 mg

*Formula Method*

*Ratio Proportion Method*

$\dfrac{0.5 \ \text{mg}}{\underset{1}{1000 \ \text{mg}}} \times \overset{1}{1000} \ \text{mL} = 0.5 \ \text{mL}$

$\dfrac{\overset{1}{1000} \ \text{mL}}{\underset{1}{1000} \ \text{mg}} = \dfrac{x}{0.5 \ \text{mg}}$

Give 0.5 mL SC stat.

$0.5 \ \text{mL} = x$

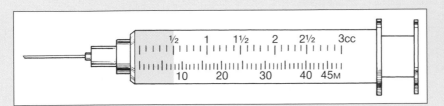

## Test 3: Calculations of Liquid Injections (Test 3)

**Formula Method**

1. $\dfrac{\overset{1}{\cancel{0.25 \text{ mg}}}}{\underset{2}{\cancel{0.50 \text{ mg}}}} \times \overset{1}{2} \text{ mL} = 1 \text{ mL}$

**Ratio Proportion Method**

$\dfrac{2 \text{ mL}}{0.5 \text{ mg}} = \dfrac{x}{0.25 \text{ mg}}$

$\dfrac{0.50}{0.50} = x$

$1 \text{ mL} = x$

**Formula Method**

2. $\dfrac{40 \text{ mg}}{50 \text{ mg}} \times 2 \text{ cc} = \overset{8}{5} \overset{1.6}{\overline{)8.0}} = 1.6 \text{ mL}$

**Ratio Proportion Method**

$\dfrac{2 \text{ cc}}{50 \text{ mg}} = \dfrac{x}{40 \text{ mg}}$

$\dfrac{80}{50} = x$

$1.6 \text{ mL} = x$

**Formula Method**

3. $\dfrac{8 \text{ mg}}{15 \text{ mg}} \times 1 \text{ mL} = \overset{8}{15} \overset{.53}{\overline{)8.00}} = 0.5 \text{ mL}$
$\qquad \qquad \qquad \qquad \underline{7\,5}$
$\qquad \qquad \qquad \qquad \ \ 50$
$\qquad \qquad \qquad \qquad \ \ \underline{45}$

**Ratio Proportion Method**

$\dfrac{1 \text{ mL}}{15 \text{ mg}} = \dfrac{x}{8 \text{ mg}}$

$\dfrac{8}{15} = x$

$0.53 \text{ or } 0.5 \text{ mL} = x$

**Formula Method**

4. $\dfrac{\overset{1}{25 \text{ mg}}}{\underset{4}{100 \text{ mg}}} \times 1 \text{ mL} = \overset{1}{4} \overset{.25}{\overline{)1.00}} = 0.3 \text{ mL}$

You could use the 1-mL precision syringe (0.25 mL).

**Ratio Proportion Method**

$\dfrac{1 \text{ mL}}{100 \text{ mg}} = \dfrac{x}{25 \text{ mg}}$

$\dfrac{25}{100} = x$

$0.3 \text{ or } 0.25 \text{ mL} = x$

**Formula Method**

5. $\dfrac{200 \text{ mg}}{500 \text{ mg}} \times 2 \text{ mL} \ \overset{4}{5} \overset{.8}{\overline{)4.0}} = 0.8 \text{ mL}$

**Ratio Proportion Method**

$\dfrac{2 \text{ mL}}{500 \text{ mg}} = \dfrac{x}{200 \text{ mg}}$

$\dfrac{400}{500} = x$

$0.8 \text{ mL} = x$

**Formula Method**

6. $\dfrac{\overset{3}{1500 \text{ }\mu g}}{\underset{10}{5000 \text{ }\mu g}} \times 1 \text{ mL} = \overset{3}{10} \overset{.3}{\overline{)3.0}} = 0.3 \text{ mL}$

**Ratio Proportion Method**

$\dfrac{1 \text{ mL}}{5000 \text{ mcg}} = \dfrac{x}{1500 \text{ mcg}}$

$\dfrac{1500}{5000} = x$

$0.3 \text{ mL} = x$

*Formula Method*

7. $\dfrac{\overset{3}{\cancel{0.6\ mg}}}{\underset{2}{\cancel{0.4\ mg}}} \times 1\ mL = \dfrac{3}{2}\overset{1.5}{\overline{)3.0}} = 1.5\ mL$

*Ratio Proportion Method*

$\dfrac{1\ mL}{0.4\ mg} = \dfrac{x}{0.6\ mg}$

$\dfrac{0.6}{0.4} = x$

$1.5\ mL = x$

*Formula Method*

8. 0.1 gm = 100 mg

$\dfrac{\cancel{100\ mg}}{\cancel{200\ mg}} \times 3\ mL = \dfrac{3}{2}\overset{1.5}{\overline{)3.0}} = 1.5\ mL$

*Ratio Proportion Method*

$\dfrac{3\ mL}{200\ mg} = \dfrac{x}{100\ mg}$

$\dfrac{300}{200} = x$

$1.5\ mL = x$

*Formula Method*

9. $\dfrac{\overset{3}{\cancel{1.5\ mg}}}{\underset{4}{\cancel{2.0\ mg}}} \times 1\ mL = \dfrac{3}{4}\overset{.75}{\overline{)3.00}} = 0.8\ mL$

You could use a 1-mL precision syringe (0.75 mL).

*Ratio Proportion Method*

$\dfrac{1\ mL}{2\ mg} = \dfrac{x}{1.5\ mg}$

$\dfrac{1.5}{2} = x$

0.75 or 0.8 mL = x

*Formula Method*

10. $\dfrac{\cancel{600,000\ units}}{\cancel{500,000\ units}} \times 1\ mL = \dfrac{6}{5}\overset{1.2}{\overline{)6.0}} = 1.2\ mL$

*Ratio Proportion Method*

$\dfrac{1\ ml}{500,000\ units} = \dfrac{x}{600,000\ units}$

$\dfrac{\cancel{600,000}}{\cancel{500,000}} = x$

$1.2\ mL = x$

11. 200 μg = 0.2 mg

*Formula Method*

$\dfrac{\overset{1}{\cancel{0.2\ mg}}}{\underset{4}{\cancel{0.8\ mg}}} \times 1\ mL = \dfrac{1}{4}\overset{.25}{\overline{)1.00}} = 0.3\ mL$

You could use a precision syringe (0.25 mL).

*Ratio Proportion Method*

$\dfrac{1\ mL}{0.8\ mg} = \dfrac{x}{0.2\ mg}$

$\dfrac{0.2}{0.8} = x$

0.25 or 0.3 mL = x

12. 1:4000 means 1 g in 4000 mL

1 g = 1000 mg

500 mcg = 0.5 mg

*Formula Method*

$\dfrac{0.5\ mg}{\cancel{1000}\ mg} \times \cancel{4000}\ mL = \dfrac{\overset{0.5}{\times 4}}{2.0\ mL}$

*Ratio Proportion Method*

$\dfrac{\cancel{4000}\ mL}{\cancel{1000}\ mg} = \dfrac{x}{0.5\ mg}$

2.0 mL = x

**Formula Method**

13. $\dfrac{3 \text{ mg}}{2 \text{ mg}} \times 1 \text{ mL} = \dfrac{3}{2}\overline{)\dfrac{1.5}{3.0}} = 1.5 \text{ mL}$

**Ratio Proportion Method**

$$\dfrac{1 \text{ mL}}{2 \text{ mg}} = \dfrac{x}{3 \text{ mg}}$$

$$\dfrac{3}{2} = x$$

$$1.5 \text{ mL} = x$$

14. 1:1000 means   1 g = 1000 mL
     1 g = 1000 mg

**Formula Method**

$\dfrac{0.4 \text{ mg}}{\cancel{1000} \text{ mg}} \times \overset{1}{\cancel{1000}} \text{ mL} = 0.4 \text{ mL}$

**Ratio Proportion Method**

$$\dfrac{\cancel{1000} \text{ mL}}{\cancel{1000} \text{ mg}} = \dfrac{x}{0.4 \text{ mg}}$$

$$0.4 \text{ mL} = x$$

15. 50% means   50 g in 100 mL
     500 mg = 0.5 g

**Formula Method**

$\dfrac{0.5 \text{ g}}{\underset{1}{\cancel{50} \text{ g}}} \times \overset{2}{100} \text{ mL} = 1.0 \text{ mL}$

**Ratio Proportion Method**

$$\dfrac{\overset{2}{\cancel{100}} \text{ mL}}{\underset{1}{\cancel{50} \text{ g}}} = \dfrac{x}{0.5 \text{ g}}$$

$$1.0 \text{ mL} = x$$

**Formula Method**

16. $\dfrac{0.75 \text{ mg}}{\underset{2}{1.50 \text{ mg}}} \times 1 \text{ mL} = \tfrac{1}{2} \text{ mL or } 0.5 \text{ mL}$

**Ratio Proportion Method**

$$\dfrac{1 \text{ mL}}{1.5 \text{ mg}} = \dfrac{x}{0.75 \text{ mg}}$$

$$\dfrac{0.75}{1.5} = x$$

$$0.5 \text{ mL} = x$$

17. 20% means   20 g in 100 mL
     100 mg = 0.1 g

**Formula Method**

$\dfrac{0.1 \text{ g}}{\underset{1}{\cancel{20} \text{ g}}} \times \overset{5}{\cancel{100}} \text{ mL} = 0.5 \text{ mL}$

**Ratio Proportion Method**

$$\dfrac{\overset{5}{\cancel{100}} \text{ mL}}{\underset{1}{\cancel{20} \text{ g}}} = \dfrac{x}{0.1 \text{ g}}$$

$$0.5 \text{ mL} = x$$

**Formula Method**

18. $\dfrac{0.125 \text{ mg}}{\underset{1}{\overset{}{0.250 \text{ mg}}}} \times \overset{1}{\cancel{2}} \text{ mL} = 1 \text{ mL}$

**Ratio Proportion Method**

$$\dfrac{2 \text{ mL}}{0.25 \text{ mg}} = \dfrac{x}{0.125 \text{ mg}}$$

$$\dfrac{0.250}{0.250} = x$$

$$1 \text{ mL} = x$$

*Formula Method*

19. $\dfrac{\overset{6}{\cancel{12}\text{ mg}}}{\underset{5}{\cancel{10}\text{ mg}}} \times 1\text{ mL} = \dfrac{6}{5 \,\overline{)6.0}} \;\overset{1.2}{} = 1.2\text{ mL}$

*Ratio Proportion Method*

$\dfrac{1\text{ mL}}{10\text{ mg}} = \dfrac{x}{12\text{ mg}}$

$\dfrac{12}{10} = x$

$1.2\text{ mL} = x$

*Formula Method*

20. $\dfrac{\overset{5}{\cancel{10}\text{ mEq}}}{\underset{2}{\cancel{40}\text{ mEq}}} \times \overset{1}{\cancel{20}}\text{ mL} = 5\text{ mL}$

This is correct because the route is IV.

*Ratio Proportion Method*

$\dfrac{\overset{1}{\cancel{20}}\text{ mL}}{\underset{2}{\cancel{40}}\text{ mEq}} = \dfrac{x}{10\text{ mEq}}$

$\dfrac{10}{2} = x$

$5\text{ mL} = x$

## Test 4: Mental Drill in Liquids for Injection Problems

1. 2 mL IM
2. 5 mL IV
3. 2 mL IM
4. 1 mL IM
5. 0.5 mL IM
6. 1 mL IM

7. 0.75 mL or 0.8 mL SC
8. 1 cc SC
9. 20 mL IV
10. 2.5 mL IM
11. 0.8 mL IM
12. 2 mL IM

13. 2 mL IV
14. 1.5 mL IM
15. 1.5 mL IM
16. 0.35 mL or 0.4 mL IM
17. 1.5 mL SC
18. 1.5 mL IM

## Chapter 8

## Test 1: Injections From Powders

1. a. 1.5 mL, sterile water
   b. 280 mg/mL

   c. *Formula Method*

   $\dfrac{250\text{ mg}}{280\text{ mg}} \times 1\text{ mL} = A$

   $.89 \times 1\text{ mL} = A$

   $.89$ or $.90\text{ mL} = A$

   *Ratio Proportion Method*

   $\dfrac{1\text{ mL}}{280\text{ mg}} = \dfrac{x}{250\text{ mg}}$

   $\dfrac{250}{280} = x$

   $.89\text{ cc} = x$

   or $.9\text{ cc} = x$

   d. 0.9 mL
   e. 280 mg/mL; date; initials
   f. Refrigerate. Stable for 7 days

2. a. 2 mL sterile water for injection
   b. 1 g/2.6 mL

   c. *Formula Method*

   $\dfrac{\cancel{1}\text{ g}}{\cancel{1}\text{ g}} \times 2.6\text{ mL} = 2.6\text{ mL}$

   *Ratio Proportion Method*

   $\dfrac{2.6\text{ mL}}{1\text{ g}} = \dfrac{x}{1\text{ g}}$

   $2.6\text{ mL} = x$

   d. 2.6 mL
   e. Nothing is left in the vial.
   f. Discard the vial in a proper receptacle.

**3. a.** 1.8 mL sterile water for injecion
   **b.** 250 mg/mL

   **c.** *Formula Method*

$$\frac{D}{H} \times S = A \qquad \frac{\cancel{300}^{\;6} \text{ mg}}{\cancel{250}_{\;5} \text{ mg}} \times 1 \text{ mL} = \frac{6}{5} \quad 5 \overline{\smash{\big)}6.0}^{\;1.2}$$

   *Ratio Proportion Method*

$$\frac{1 \text{ mL}}{250 \text{ mg}} = \frac{x}{300 \text{ mg}}$$

$$\frac{300}{250} = x$$

$$1.2 \text{ mL} = x$$

   **d.** 1.2 mL/m
   **e.** Nothing! Discard the vial. Directions say solution must be used within 1 hour.
   **f.** No. Discard the vial in an appropriate receptacle.

**4. a.** 2 mL sterile water for injection
   **b.** 400 mg/mL

   **c.** *Formula Method*

$$\frac{D}{H} \times S = A \qquad \frac{\cancel{300} \text{ mg}}{\cancel{400} \text{ mg}} \times 1 \text{ mL} = \frac{3}{4} \quad 4 \overline{\smash{\big)}3.00}^{\;.75}$$

   *Ratio Proportion Method*

$$\frac{1 \text{ mL}}{400 \text{ mg}} = \frac{x}{300 \text{ mg}}$$

$$\frac{300}{400} = x$$

$$.75 = x$$

   **d.** 0.8 mL/m
   **e.** 400 mg/mL; date; initials
   **f.** Refrigerate. Stable for 1 week

**5. a.** 2.5 mL sterile water for injection.
   **b.** 330 mg/mL

   **c.** *Formula Method*

$$\frac{D}{H} \times S = A \qquad 0.33 \text{ g is } 330 \text{ mg.}$$

   *Ratio Proportion Method*

$$\frac{1 \text{ mL}}{330 \text{ mg}} = \frac{x}{330 \text{ mg}}$$

$$\frac{330}{330} = x$$

$$1 = x$$

   **d.** 1 mL IM
   **e.** 330 mg/mL; date; initials
   **f.** Refrigerate. Stable for 96 hours

## Chapter 9

### Test 1: Basic IV Problems

**1. a.** You have 1000 mL running at 150 mL/hr; therefore

$$\frac{\overset{20}{\cancel{1000}}}{\underset{3}{\cancel{150}}} = \overset{20}{\cancel{3}} \; 3\overline{)20.0}^{\,6.6} = \text{approximately 6.6 hours}$$

$$\begin{array}{r} 18 \\ \hline 2\,0 \\ 1\,8 \end{array}$$

**b.** $\dfrac{\text{\# ML} \times \text{TF}}{\text{\# min}} = \text{gtt/min}$

$\dfrac{150 \times 10}{60} = 25 \text{ gtt/min macro}$

$\dfrac{150 \times 60}{60} = 150 \text{ gtt/min micro}$

Choose macrotubing.

**c.** 25 gtt/min macro

*Note:* You could choose microtubing; however, the drip rate is hard to count.

**2. a.** Because the amount is small and will run over 6 hours, choose *microdrip tubing.*

**b.** Step 1.

$$\frac{\text{\# mL}}{\text{hr}} = \text{mL/hr} = \overset{\cancel{100}}{6}\; 6\overline{)100.0}^{\,16.6} = 17\text{mL/hr}$$

$$\begin{array}{r} 6 \\ \hline 40 \\ 36 \\ \hline 40 \\ 36 \end{array}$$

Step 2. $\dfrac{\text{\# mL/hr} \times \text{TF}}{\text{\# min}} = \dfrac{17 \times \cancel{60}}{\cancel{60}} = 17 \text{ gtt/min}$

**3. a.** Because the stock bag is 250 mL NS, you would aseptically allow 100 mL to run off. This will leave 150 mL NS.

**b.** *Microdrip* because:

Step 1. $\dfrac{\text{\# mL}}{\text{\# hr}} = \text{mL/hr} \; \dfrac{\overset{50}{\cancel{150}} \text{ mL}}{3 \text{ hr}} = 50 \text{ mL/hr}$

Step 2. $\dfrac{\text{\# mL/hr} \times \text{TF}}{\text{\# min}} = \text{gtt/min}$

With microdrip, the # mL/hr = gtt/min; hence, microdrip would be 50 gtt/min.

Proof: $\dfrac{50 \times \cancel{60}}{\cancel{60}} = 50 \text{ gtt/min}$

*Macrodrip* would be $\dfrac{50 \times \overset{1}{\cancel{15}}}{\underset{4}{\cancel{60}}}$

$$= \overset{\cancel{50}}{4}\; 4\overline{)50.0}^{\,12.5} = 13 \text{ gtt/min}$$

$$\begin{array}{r} 4 \\ \hline 10 \\ 8 \\ \hline 2\,0 \\ 2\,0 \end{array}$$

**c.** 50 gtt/min

*Note:* It would not be incorrect to choose the macrodrip. However, 50 gtt/min provides a better flow.

**4.** 21 mL/hr

Logic: Step 1. $\dfrac{\text{\# mL}}{\text{\# hr}} = \text{mL/hr}$

$$\frac{\cancel{500} \text{ mL}}{24 \text{ hr}} = 24\overline{)500.0}^{\,20.8} = 21 \text{ mL/hr}$$

$$\begin{array}{r} 48 \\ \hline 20\,0 \\ 19\,2 \end{array}$$

Step 2 is not necessary because you have an infusion pump that delivers mL/hr.

**5.** Use a reconstitution device to add 100 mg powder to 250 mL D5W and give IVPB over 1 hr (60 min); TF = 10 gtts/mL.

$\dfrac{\text{\# mL} \times \text{TF}}{\text{\# min}} = \text{gtt/min}$

$\dfrac{250 \times 10}{60} = \overset{\cancel{250}}{6}\; 6\overline{)250.0}^{\,41.6} = 42 \text{ gtt/min}$

Label the IVPB.

Set the rate at 42 gtt/min.

**6.** Order is 500 mg. Stock is 1 g in 10 mL.
   1 g = 1000 mg

| *Formula Method* | *Ratio Proportion Method* |
|---|---|
| $\dfrac{D}{H} \times S = A \quad \dfrac{500 \text{ mg}}{1000 \text{ mg}} \times 10 \text{ mL} = 5 \text{ mL}$ | $\dfrac{10 \text{ mL}}{1000 \text{ mg}} = \dfrac{x}{500}$ |
| | $\dfrac{5000}{1000} = x$ |
| | $5 \text{ mL} = x$ |

Add 5 mL aminophylline to make 500 mg in 250 mL D5W.

$$\dfrac{\# \text{ mL}}{\# \text{ hr}} = \text{mL/hr} \qquad \dfrac{\cancel{250} \text{ mL}}{8 \text{ hr}} = 31.2 = 31 \text{ mL/hr}$$

mL/hr = microgtt/min
No math necessary.
31 mL/hr = 31 gtt/min
Label IV.
Set the rate at 31 gtt/min.

**7.** 3300 mL
   Logic: The patient gets 125 mL/hr and there are 24 hours in a day; hence

$$\begin{array}{r} 125 \\ \times\ 24 \\ \hline 500 \\ 250 \\ \hline 3000 \text{ mL} \end{array}$$

The patient gets 75 mL q6h and, therefore, is receiving 75 mL four times in 24 hours.

$$\text{So} \quad \begin{array}{r} 75 \\ \times\ 4 \\ \hline 300 \end{array}$$

$$\begin{array}{r} 3000 \text{ mL} \\ +300 \text{ mL} \\ \hline 3300 \text{ mL} \end{array}$$

**8. a.** 90 mL/hr—no math necessary—pump

   **b.** $\dfrac{\text{total \# mL}}{\text{mL/hr}} = \text{hr}$

$$\begin{array}{r} 11.1 \\ 90\ \overline{)1000.0} \\ \underline{90}\phantom{00.0} \\ 100\phantom{.0} \\ \underline{90}\phantom{0.0} \\ 10\ 0 \end{array}$$

Approximately 11 hours

**9.** 50 mg
   Logic: Have 0.5 g in 500 mL. Substitute milligrams for grams: 0.5 g = 500 mg. The solution is 500 mg in 500 mL. Reducing this means 1 mg in 1 mL. As the patient is receiving 50 mL/hr, he is receiving 50 mg of aminophylline per hour.

**10. a.** Need 75 mL D5W. Take a 100 mL bag of D5W and aseptically remove 25 mL. Add 5 mL Bactrim to the 75 mL. Time is 60 min. The order is 75 mL/hr. No math is necessary. You have a pump in mL/hr.
   Label the IVPB.

   **b.** Set the pump:
   Secondary volume (mL): 75
   Secondary rate (mL/hr): 75

## Chapter 10

### Test 1: Special IV Calculations

**1.** *Formula Method*

$$\frac{D}{H} \times S = A$$

$$\frac{\overset{3}{\cancel{15 \text{ units/hr}}}}{\underset{\underset{1}{25}}{\cancel{125 \text{ units}}}} \times \overset{10}{\cancel{250} \text{ cc}} = A$$

30 cc/hr on a pump

Set the pump:

Total # cc: 250

mL or cc/hr: 30

*Ratio Proportion Method*

$$\frac{x \text{ mL}}{15 \text{ units}} = \frac{250 \text{ cc}}{125 \text{ units}}$$

$$x = 30 \text{ cc/hr}$$

**2.** *Formula Method*

$$\frac{D}{H} \times S = A$$

$$\frac{\overset{3}{\cancel{1500 \text{ units/hr}}}}{\underset{\underset{1}{50}}{\cancel{25000 \text{ units}}}} \times \overset{10}{\cancel{500}} = A$$

30 mL = hr

Set the pump:

Total # mL = 500 cc

mL/hr = 30

*Ratio Proportion Method*

$$\frac{x \text{ mL}}{1500 \text{ units}} = \frac{\overset{1}{\cancel{500}} \text{ mL}}{\underset{50}{\cancel{25000}}}$$

$$x = \frac{1500}{50}$$

$$x = 30 \text{ mL/hr}$$

**3.** Logic: Infusion pumps are set in mL/hr so multiply:

2 mg/min × 60 minutes = 120 mg/hr

2 g = 2000 mg

*Formula Method*

$$\frac{D}{H} \times S = A$$

$$\frac{\overset{30}{\cancel{120 \text{ mg/hr}}}}{\underset{\underset{1}{4}}{\cancel{2000 \text{ mg}}}} \times \overset{1}{\cancel{500} \text{ mL}} = 30 \text{ mL/hr on a pump}$$

Set the pump:

Total # mL: 500

mL/hr: 30

*Ratio Proportion Method*

$$\frac{\overset{1}{\cancel{500} \text{ mL}}}{\underset{4}{\cancel{2000} \text{ mg}}} = \frac{x}{120 \text{ mg}}$$

$$\frac{120}{4} = x$$

$$30 \text{ mL} = x$$

**4.** Addition diltiazem to the IV.

*Formula Method*

$$\frac{D}{H} \times S = A$$

$$\frac{\overset{25}{\cancel{125 \text{ mg}}}}{\underset{1}{\cancel{5 \text{ mg}}}} \times 1 \text{ mL} = 25 \text{ mL drug}$$

*Ratio Proportion Method*

$$\frac{1 \text{ mL}}{5 \text{ mg}} = \frac{x}{125 \text{ mg}}$$

$$25 \text{ mL} = x$$

Remove 25 mL of IV fluid from the IV bag and add 25 mL of diltiazem = 1000 mL altogether.

*Formula Method*

$$\frac{D}{H} \times S = A$$

$$\frac{\overset{1}{\cancel{5 \text{ mg/hr}}}}{\underset{1}{\underset{25}{\cancel{125 \text{ mg}}}}} \times \overset{4}{\cancel{100}} \text{ mL} = 4 \text{ mL/hr}$$

*Ratio Proportion Method*

$$\frac{100 \text{ mL}}{125 \text{ mg}} = \frac{x}{5}$$

$$4 \text{ mL} = x$$

Second way: If you add 25 mL of drug to the 100 mL D5W, you make 125 mL (a 1:1 solution). Since the order is 5 mg/hr, set the pump at 5 mL/hr.

*Formula Method*

Proof: $\dfrac{D}{H} \times S = A$

$$\frac{\overset{1}{\cancel{5 \text{ mg/hr}}}}{\underset{1}{\underset{25}{\cancel{125 \text{ mg}}}}} \times \overset{5}{\cancel{125}} \text{ mL} = 5 \text{ mL/hr}$$

*Ratio Proportion Method*

$$\frac{125 \text{ mL}}{125 \text{ mg}} = \frac{x}{5 \text{ mg}}$$

$$5 \text{ mL} = x$$

It is considered better to remove fluid from the IV bag so the volume remains the same.

**5.** 2 g = 2000 mg

Order calls for 4 mg/min. Pumps are set in mL/hr. Multiply 4 mg/min × 60 min = 240 mg/hr.

*Formula Method*

$$\frac{D}{H} \times S = A$$

$$\frac{\overset{60}{\cancel{240 \text{ mg/hr}}}}{\underset{1}{\underset{4}{\cancel{2000 \text{ mg}}}}} \times \overset{1}{\cancel{500}} \text{ mL} = 60 \text{ mL/hr on a pump}$$

*Ratio Proportion Method*

$$\frac{\overset{1}{\cancel{500 \text{ mL}}}}{\underset{4}{\cancel{2000 \text{ mg}}}} = \frac{x}{240}$$

$$60 \text{ mL} = x$$

Set the pump:
Total # mL: 500
# mL/hr: 60

**6. a.** Add KCl to the IV.

*Formula Method*

$$\frac{D}{H} \times S = A$$

$$\frac{\overset{2}{\cancel{40\ mEq}}}{\underset{1}{\cancel{20\ mEq}}} \times 10\ mL = 20\ mL$$

*Ratio Proportion Method*

$$\frac{10\ mL}{20\ mEq} = \frac{x}{40\ mEq}$$

$$20\ mL = x$$

**b.** Remove 20 mL of IV fluid and add the 20 mL of KCl to make 1000 mL.

*Formula Method*

$$\frac{D}{H} \times S = A$$

1 liter = 1000 mL

$$\frac{\overset{1}{\cancel{10\ mEq/hr}}}{\underset{1}{\underset{\cancel{4}}{\cancel{40\ mEq}}}} \times \overset{250}{\cancel{1000}}\ mL = 250\ mL/hr$$

*Ratio Proportion Method*

$$\frac{\overset{25}{\cancel{1000}}\ mL}{\underset{1}{\cancel{40}}\ mEq} = \frac{x}{10\ mEq}$$

$$250\ mL = x$$

Set pump at 250 mL/hr. This is a large volume and KCl is a potent electrolyte; therefore the patient must be on a cardiac monitor for safety. Check the order with the doctor.
Total # mL: 1000
mL/hr: 250

**7.** 2 g = 2000 mL
Order calls for 1 mg/min. Pumps are set in mL/hr. Multiply 1 mg/min × 60 mg = 60 mg/hr.

*Formula Method*

$$\frac{D}{H} \times S = A$$

$$\frac{\overset{15}{\cancel{60\ mg/hr}}}{\underset{1}{\underset{\cancel{4}}{\cancel{2000\ mg}}}} \times \overset{1}{\cancel{500}}\ mL = 15\ mL/hr$$

*Ratio Proportion Method*

$$\frac{\overset{1}{\cancel{500}}\ mL}{\underset{4}{\cancel{2000}}\ mg} = \frac{x}{60\ mg/hr}$$

$$\frac{60}{4} = x$$

$$15\ mL/hr = x$$

Set the pump:
Total # mL: 500
# mL/hr: 15

**8.** Use a reconstitution device (see Chapter 9) to add 50 mg of drug to 500 mL D5W.

$$\frac{\# \text{ mL}}{\# \text{ hr}} = \text{mL/hr}$$

$$\frac{500 \text{ mL}}{6 \text{ hr}} \quad \frac{83.0}{)500.0} = 83 \text{ mL/hr}$$

$$\begin{array}{r} \underline{48} \\ 20 \\ \underline{18} \\ 20 \\ \underline{18} \end{array}$$

Set pump:
Total # mL: 500
# mL/hr: 83

**9.** Add vasopressin to the IV.

***Formula Method***

$$\frac{D}{H} \times S = A$$

$$\frac{\overset{10}{\cancel{200 \text{ units}}}}{\underset{1}{\cancel{20 \text{ units}}}} \times 1 \text{ mL} = 10 \text{ mL}$$

***Ratio Proportion Method***

$$\frac{1 \text{ mL}}{20 \text{ units}} = \frac{x}{200 \text{ units}}$$

$$10 \text{ mL} = x$$

Remove 10 mL fluid from the IV and add 10 mL of the drug = 500 mL.

***Formula Method***

$$\frac{D}{H} \times S = A$$

$$\frac{\overset{9}{\cancel{18 \text{ units/hr}}}}{\underset{1}{\cancel{200 \text{ units}}}} \times 500 \text{ mL} = 45 \text{ mL/hr}$$

***Ratio Proportion Method***

$$\frac{500 \text{ mL}}{200 \text{ units}} = \frac{x}{18 \text{ units/hr}}$$

$$\frac{90}{2} = x$$

$$45 \text{ mL} = x$$

Set pump:
Total # mL: 500
mL/hr: 45

**10.**   Order: 250 mcg/min
Solution: 500 mg in 500 mL D5W

Step 1. $\dfrac{500 \text{ mg}}{500 \text{ mL}} = 1 \text{ mg/mL}$

Step 2. 1 mg = 1000 mcg/mL
Step 3. Not needed
Step 4. 1000 mcg/60 gtt

Step 5. $\dfrac{\overset{1}{\cancel{250 \text{ mcg/min}}}}{\underset{\underset{1}{\cancel{4}}}{\cancel{1000 \text{ mcg}}}} \times \overset{15}{\cancel{60}} \text{ gtt}$

15 gtt/min = 15 mL/hr
Set pump:
Total # mL: 500
# mL/hr: 15

11.   Order: 2.5 mcg/kg/min
Solution: 400 mg in 250 mL
Weight: 60 kg
Multiply 60 kg × 2.5 mg = 150 mcg.

Step 1. $\dfrac{\overset{8}{\cancel{400}}\ mg}{\underset{5}{\cancel{250}}\ mL} = 8\ mg/5\ mL$

Step 2. 8 mg = 8000 mcg. Solution is 8000 mcg/5 mL

Step 3. $\dfrac{8000\ mcg}{5\ mL} = 1600\ mcg/mL$

Step 4. 1600 mcg/60 gtt

Step 5. $\dfrac{150\ \cancel{mcg}/min}{1600\ \cancel{mcg}} \times 60\ gtt = \dfrac{90}{16}$   $16\overline{)90.0}\phantom{0}\ = 6$
$\phantom{16)}\underline{80}$
$\phantom{16)}10\ 0$
$\phantom{16)0}\underline{9\ 6}$

6 gtt/min = 6 mL/hr
Set pump:
Total # mL: 250
# mL/hr: 6

12.   Order: 2 milliunits/min
Solution: 10 units in 1000 mL Ringers

Step 1. $\dfrac{\overset{1}{\cancel{10}}\ units}{\underset{100}{\cancel{1000}}\ mL} = 1\ unit\ in\ 100\ mL$

Step 2. 1 unit = 1000 milliunits/100 mL

Step 3. $\dfrac{1000\ milliunits}{100\ mL} = 10\ milliunits/mL$

Step 4. 10 milliunits/60 gtt

Step 5. $\dfrac{2\ \cancel{milliunits}/min}{\underset{1}{\cancel{10}}\ \cancel{milliunits}} \times \overset{12}{\cancel{60}}\ gtt = 12$

12 gtt/min = 12 mL/hr
Set the pump:
Total # mL: 1000
# mL/hr: 12

13. **a.** Correct.
**b.** Correct; 100 mg/m² × 1.7 = 170 mg
**c.** 1 L = 1000 mL

$\dfrac{\#\ mL}{\#\ hr} = mL/hr$   $\dfrac{1000}{24}$   $24\overline{)1000.0}\phantom{0}\ = 42\ mL/hr$
$\phantom{24)}\underline{96}$
$\phantom{24)}40$
$\phantom{24)}\underline{24}$
$\phantom{24)}16\ 0$
$\phantom{24)}\underline{14\ 4}$

Set the pump:
Total # mL: 1000
# mL/hr: 42

## Chapter 11
### Test 1: Infants and Children Dosage Problems

**1.** Safe dose 0.5 mg to 1 mg/dose IM. The order is safe.

*Formula Method*       *Ratio Proportion Method*

$\dfrac{D}{H} \times S = A$       $\dfrac{1\ mL}{10\ mg} = \dfrac{x}{1\ mg}$

$\dfrac{1\ mg}{10\ mg} \times 1\ mL$       0.1 mL = x

= 0.1 mL IM.
Use a precision syringe.

**2.** Safe dose is 20–40 mg/kg/24h given q8h.

*Low Range*       *High Range*
20 mg       40 mg
$\underline{\times 10}$ kg       $\underline{\times 10}$ kg
200 mg/24h       400 mg/24h

Order is 125 mg q8h (3 doses).
125 mg × 3 doses = 375. Dose is safe.
No math necessary. Stock is 125 mg/5 mL. Give 5 mL.

**3.** Safe dose: 50,000 units/kg × 1 dose.

50,000 units
× 10 kg
───────────
500,000 units

The order is safe.

*Formula Method*

$$\frac{D}{H} \times S = A \quad \frac{500,000 \text{ units}}{600,000 \text{ units}} \times 1 \text{ mL} = \frac{5}{6} = 0.83 \text{ mL}$$

*Ratio Proportion Method*

$$\frac{1 \text{ mL}}{600\,000 \text{ units}} = \frac{x}{500\,000 \text{ units}}$$

$$0.83 \text{ mL} = x$$

Give 0.83 mL IM. Use a precision syringe.

**4.** Step 1. Safe dose: 2.5 mg/kg/dose q8h

2.5 mg
× 3.6 kg
─────────
9 mg

Order is safe.

Step 2. Minimum safe dilution: 2 mg/mL

$$2 \text{ mg}\,)\overline{9 \text{ mg}}^{\,4.5 \text{ mL}} \quad \text{is the minimum safe dilution. 10 mL is safe.}$$

*Formula Method*

Step 3. $\dfrac{D}{H} \times S = A$

$$\frac{9 \text{ mg}}{40 \text{ mg}} \times 1 \text{ mL} = \frac{9}{40}\,)\overline{9.000}^{\,.225} = 0.23 \text{ mL}$$

Use a precision syringe to draw up 0.23 mL.

Step 4. Add about 5 mL D5¼NS to the Buretrol. Add the 0.23 mL drug. Add more D5¼NS to make 10 mL.

Step 5. Set the pump at 20 because 20 mL in an hr will deliver the 10 mL in 30 min.

Step 6. When the IV is completed, add a flush of 20 mL D5¼NS to the Buretrol to clear the tubing of medication.

*Ratio Proportion Method*

$$\frac{1 \text{ mL}}{40 \text{ mg}} = \frac{x}{9 \text{ mg}}$$

$$0.23 \text{ mL} = x$$

**5.** Safe dose: infants and children under 3 yr: 10–40 mg. The dose is safe.

*Formula Method*

$$\frac{D}{H} \times S = A \quad \frac{10 \text{ mg}}{20 \text{ mg}} \times 5 \text{ mL} = \frac{5}{2} = 2.5 \text{ mL po}$$

*Ratio Proportion Method*

$$\frac{5 \text{ mL}}{20 \text{ mg}} = \frac{x}{10 \text{ mg}}$$

$$\frac{10}{4} = x$$

$$2.5 \text{ mL} = x$$

6. Step 1. Safe dose: 10 mg/kg q8h IV

$$\begin{array}{r} 10 \text{ mg} \\ \times\ 5.5 \text{ kg} \\ \hline 55 \text{ mg q8h} \end{array}$$

Dose is safe.

Step 2. Minimum safe dilution: 5 mg/mL; infuse over 1 hr.

$$5 \text{ mg} \overline{)\begin{array}{c}10.8\\54 \text{ mg}\end{array}} = 11 \text{ mL}; 12 \text{ mL is safe.}$$

Step 3. To the 500 mg powder add 10 mL sterile water for injection to make 50 mg/mL.

*Formula Method*

$$\frac{D}{H} \times S = A$$

$$\frac{54 \text{ mg}}{50 \text{ mg}} \times 1 \text{ mL} = \frac{54}{50} = 50\overline{)\begin{array}{c}1.08\\54.00\\4\,00\end{array}} = 1.1 \text{ mL}$$

Withdraw 1.1 mL of the drug; label the vial; refrigerate.

*Ratio Proportion Method*

$$\frac{1 \text{ mL}}{50 \text{ mg}} = \frac{x}{54 \text{ mg}}$$

$$1.1 \text{ mL} = x$$

Step 4. Add about 5 mL D5¼NS to the Buretrol. Add 1.1 mL drug. Add more D5¼NS to make 12 mL.

Step 5. Set the pump for 12 (12 mL over 1 hr).

Step 6. When the IV is completed, add 20 mL D5¼NS as a flush to the Buretrol to clear the tubing of medication.

7. Safe dose: 50–75 mg/kg/dose

*Low Range*

$$\begin{array}{r} 50 \text{ mg} \\ \times\ 6.7 \text{ kg} \\ \hline 335 \text{ mg/dose} \end{array}$$

*High Range*

$$\begin{array}{r} 75 \text{ mg} \\ \times\ 6.7 \text{ kg} \\ \hline 502.5 \text{ mg/dose} \end{array}$$

Order of 350 mg is safe.

*Formula Method*

$$\frac{D}{H} \times S = A \qquad \frac{\overset{1}{\cancel{350 \text{ mg}}}}{\underset{100}{\cancel{500 \text{ mg}}}} \times \cancel{5} \text{ mL} = \frac{35}{10} = 3.5 \text{ mL}$$

*Ratio Proportion Method*

$$\frac{\overset{1}{\cancel{5}} \text{ mL}}{\underset{100}{\cancel{500}} \text{ mg}} = \frac{x}{350 \text{ mg}}$$

$$\frac{350}{100} = x$$

$$3.5 \text{ mL} = x$$

**8.** Safe dose: 22 mg/kg/24h given q6h

$$\begin{array}{r} 22 \text{ mg} \\ \times\ \ 9.9 \text{ kg} \\ \hline 217.8 \text{ mg/24h} \end{array}$$

Order is 65 mg qid (4 doses).

65 mg × 4 = 260 mg

The dose does not meet safe requirements. Do not prepare the medication. Consult with the physician who ordered the drug.

**9.** Step 1. Safe dose is 2 g to 6 g in a 24-hr period divided into either q8h or q12h.
The order is 2 g q8h (3 doses).
2 g × 3 doses = 6 g. The order is safe.

Step 2. Minimum safe dilution is 50 mg/mL over 30 min.

$$50 \text{ mg} \overline{)\begin{array}{l} 40 \text{ mL} \\ \hline 2000 \text{ mg} \end{array}}$$

is the minimum safe dilution: 50 mL is safe.

Step 3. Order is 2 g. Stock is a 2-g powder. Directions say to dilute initially with 10-mL sterile water for injection. Draw the total amount into a syringe.

Step 4. Add about 20 mL D5⅓NS to the Buretrol. Add the medication from the syringe. Then add more D5⅓NS to make 50 mL.

Step 5. Set the pump for 100. It will deliver 50 mL in 30 min.

Step 6. When the IV is completed, add 20 mL D5⅓NS as a flush to the Buretrol to clear the tubing of medication.

**10.** Usual dose is 0.5 mg/lb to 1 mg/lb.

*Low Range*

$$\begin{array}{r} 35 \text{ lb} \\ \times\ \ 0.5 \text{ mg} \\ \hline 17.5 \text{ mg} \end{array}$$

*High Range*

$$\begin{array}{r} 35 \text{ lb} \\ \times\ \ 1 \text{ mg} \\ \hline 35 \text{ mg} \end{array}$$

20 mg is a safe dose.

*Formula Method*

$$\frac{D}{H} \times S = A \quad \frac{20 \text{ mg}}{50 \text{ mg}} \times 1 \text{ mL} = \frac{2}{5} = 0.4 \text{ mL IM.}$$

*Ratio Proportion Method*

$$\frac{1 \text{ mL}}{50 \text{ mg}} = \frac{x}{20 \text{ mg}}$$

$$\frac{2}{5} = 0.4 \text{ mL} = x$$

Use a precision syringe.

## Chapter 12

### Test 1: Basic Drug Information

| | | | | |
|---|---|---|---|---|
| **1.** a | **5.** b | **9.** a | **13.** a | **17.** b |
| **2.** c | **6.** a | **10.** b | **14.** a | **18.** d |
| **3.** d | **7.** a | **11.** d | **15.** b | **19.** d |
| **4.** b | **8.** d | **12.** c | **16.** a | **20.** a |

## Chapter 13

### Test 1: Administration Procedures

#### Part A

| | | | | |
|---|---|---|---|---|
| **1.** d | **5.** c | **9.** d | **13.** b | **17.** b |
| **2.** d | **6.** b | **10.** a | **14.** a | **18.** d |
| **3.** b | **7.** a | **11.** c | **15.** d | **19.** c |
| **4.** c | **8.** d | **12.** a | **16.** b | **20.** c |

#### Part B

1. Correct. As the needle or catheter is removed, there is a possibility of bleeding at the site. In addition, the nurse should use a clamp to carry the needle or catheter to a puncture-proof container.
2. Incorrect. The nurse must wash his or her hands before leaving the room.
3. Incorrect. It is not necessary to wear gloves to prepare an IV because there is no contact at this time with the patient's blood or body fluids.
4. Correct. Universal safeguards state that a mask must be worn when the patient is on strict or respiratory isolation precautions.
5. Correct. There is a potential risk of exposure to hepatitis B virus and human immunodeficiency virus. Laboratory testing may not show the presence of the virus or antibodies to the virus.
6. Incorrect. Transdermal pads are applied to intact skin. There is no danger of contact with the patient's blood or body fluids.
7. Correct. In carrying out the vaginal douche there is a possibility of exposure to vaginal secretions.
8. Incorrect. The nurse should squeeze the finger and, after washing hands with soap and water, scrub the area with povidone–iodine (Betadine) or another accepted antiseptic. In addition, the needlestick should be reported to the proper authority and the protocol for exposure to blood should be carried out. Universal safeguards apply to all patients regardless of the diagnosis.
9. Incorrect. There is always a possibility or risk when doing an invasive procedure such as an injection.
10. Incorrect. Because the patient is alert and can take the medicine cup from the nurse, handwashing is adequate.
11. Incorrect. The CDCP guidelines advise the nurse not to recap a needle but to place it immediately in a puncture-proof container.
12. Correct. Nitroglycerin ointment is a potent vasodilator. Wearing gloves protects the nurse against the drug's effect.
13. Incorrect. The nurse's fingers may come in contact with mucous membrane in administering eye drops.

# Glossary

**Absorption**   the passing of a drug in the body across tissue into the general circulation and becomes active in the body

**Adverse effects**   nontherapeutic effects that may be harmful

**Ampule (ampoule)**   sealed glass container for powdered or liquid drugs

**Antagonism**   interaction between two drugs in which the combined effect is less than the sum of the effects of the drugs acting separately

**Apothecary system**   measurement system using grains and minims, introduced into the U.S. from England in colonial times

**Avoirdupois system**   measurement system using ounces and pounds; used for patients' weights and some drugs

**Bactericidal**   drug action that kills an organism

**Bacteriostatic**   drug action that inhibits an organism's ability to grow and reproduce

**bid**   twice a day

**Bioavailability**   availability of a drug once it is absorbed and transported in the body to the site of its action

**Biotransformation**   conversion of an active drug to an inactive compound

**Body Surface area (BSA)**   calculation of meters squared ($m^2$) based on height and weight, as shown in a nomogram

**Buccal**   route of administration in which a drug is placed in the pouch between the teeth and cheek

**C**   Centigrade, Celsius

**Capsule**   a gelatin container that holds a drug in a solid or liquid form

**CDC**   Centers for Disease Control

**Chemical name**   drug name that is derived from its chemical structure

**Civil law**   statutes concerned with the rights and duties of individuals

**Clark's Rule**   a way to determine dosage of medications for children over age 2; based on weight

**Common factor**   a number that is a factor of two different numbers, i.e., 3 is a factor of 6 and 9

**Common fraction**   fraction with a whole number in the numerator and denominator, i.e., 7/9

**Concentration**   amount of drug in a solution, in fraction, decimal or percentage form

**Contraindication**   situation in which a drug should be avoided

**Controlled drug**   drug controlled by federal, state, and local law; a drug that may be lead to drug abuse or dependence

**Cream**   semisolid drug preparation applied externally to the skin or mucous membrane

**CR**   controlled release

**Criminal law**   statutes that protect the public again actions harmful to society

**CSF**   cerebrospinal fluid

**Cumulation (Accumulation)**   the inability of the body to metabolize one dose of a drug before another dose is administered; cumulation leads to increased concentration of the drug in the body and possible toxicity

**d**   day

**DEA**   U.S. Drug Enforcement Administration

**Denominator** bottom number in a fraction

**Dermal route** topical application of a drug to the skin

**Diluent** a liquid used to dissolve a solid, usually a powder, into a solution

**Displacement** the increase in the volume of fluid added to a powder, when the powder dissolves and goes into solution

**Distribution** the movement of a drug through body fluids, chiefly blood, to cells

**Dividend** the number to be divided, 40 divided by 5, 40 is the dividend

**Divisor** the number by which the dividend is divided; in the example above, 5 is the divisor

**dL** deciliter (100 mL)

**Dose** amount of drug to be administered at one time or the total amount to be given

**DR** delayed release

**Drop** a minute sphere of liquid

**Drip or Drop factor** number of drops of an IV fluid in 1 cc or mL; listed on the IV tubing set or package

**Drip rate** the number of drops of an IV solution to be infused per minute

**Drug** a chemical agent used in the treatment, diagnosis, or prevention of disease

**Elixir** a clear aromatic, sweetened alcoholic preparation

**Emulsion** suspension of a fat or oil in water with the aid of an agent to reduce surface tension

**Enteral** refers to the small intestine

**Enteric coating** a layer placed over a tablet or capsule to prevent dissolution in the stomach; used to protect the drug from gastric acid or to protect the stomach from drug irritation

**Epidural route** medication is administered into the space around the dura mater of the spinal column

**ER** extended release

**Ethics** a system of values and morals

**Excretion** the physiologic elimination of substances from the body

**Expiration date** a drug cannot be administered after the last day of the month stamped on the label

**F** Fahrenheit

**FDA** Food and Drug Administration

**Film coated tablets** compressed powdered drugs that are smooth and easy to swallow because of their outer shell covering

**First pass effect** drugs that are administered orally that pass from the intestine to the liver and are partially metabolized before entering the circulation

**Flow rate** number of cc or mL per hour of IV fluid to be infused

**Fluid extract** potent alcoholic liquid concentration of a drug

**Fraction** division of one number by another

**Fried's rule** rule to calculate drug dosages for infants under 1; based on age

**g or Gm** gram

**Gauge** the diameter or width of a needle; the higher the gauge number, the finer the needle

**Gel** aqueous suspension of small particles of an insoluble drug in a hydrated form

**Generic name** official name of a drug as listed in the U.S. or other pharmacopoeia

**Gram** weight of one cubic centimeter of water at 4 degrees C; basic unit of weight in metric system

**gtt** drop

**h** hour

**Half life** time that the drug is metabolized by 50% in the body

**Hepatotoxic** a drug or side effects of the drug that may affect the liver

**Household system** measurement system based on household items of measurement; uses teaspoon, tablespoon, cups

**hs** hour of sleep, at bedtime

**I & O** intake and output

**IM** intramuscular

**Improper fraction** fraction with the numerator larger or equal to the denominator

**Incompatibility** mixture of two or more drugs that results in a harmful chemical or physical interaction

**Inhalant** vapors that are inhaled via the nose, lungs, or trachea

**Inhaler**   a device used to spray liquid or powder in a fine mist into the lungs during inspiration

**inj**   injection

**Interaction**   either desirable or undesirable effects produced by giving two or more drugs together

**Intra-articular**   medication injected into the joints

**Intradermal**   injection given into the upper layers of the skin

**Intramuscular**   injection given into the muscle

**Intrathecal**   administration into the cerebrospinal fluid via the subarachnoid space

**Intravenous**   medication given by injection or infusion into a vein

**Isotonic**   solutions that have the same osmotic pressure as physiological body fluids

**IV**   intravenous

**IVPB**   intravenous piggyback; a medication placed in an infusion set and attached to the main line IV for delivery to the patient

**kg**   kilogram

**lbs**   pounds

**Liter (L)**   unit of fluid volume in the metric system; equal to 1/10 of a cubic meter

**Lotion**   liquid suspension intended for external use

**Lowest Common Denominator**   smallest number that is a multiple of all denominators

**Lowest terms**   smallest numbers possible in the numerator and denominator of a fraction; reducing a fraction to lowest terms means the numerator and denominator cannot be reduced further

**Lozenge**   flat, round, or rectangular preparation held in the mouth until it dissolves

**Magma**   bulky suspension of an insoluble preparation in water, which must be shaken before pouring

**MDI**   metered dose inhaler; an aerosol device that consists of two parts: a canister under pressure and a mouthpiece. Finger pressure on the mouthpiece opens a valve that discharges one dose

**Meniscus**   the curved surface of a liquid in a container

**Metabolism**   the chemical biotransformation of a drug to a form that can be excreted

**Meter (m)**   unit of length in the metric system; equals 39.27 inches

**Metric System**   measurement system that uses meter, liter, gram; common system used worldwide except in the U.S. widely used system in dosages of drugs; based on units of 10

**$\mu$g or mcg**   microgram

**mg**   milligram

**Military time**   time based on a 24-hour clock rather than the traditional 12-hour clock

**Milliequivalent (mEq)**   number of grams of solute in a 1 mL solution; used to measure electrolytes and some medications

**min**   minute

**Mixed Number**   a whole number and a fraction, i.e., 1 1/2

**ML**   milliliter

**mo**   month

**Multidose**   large stock containers of medication

**NDC**   National Drug Code; a number used by the pharmacist to identify the drug and the packaging method

**Nephrotoxic**   a drug or side effects of the drug that may affect the renal system

**Nomogram**   tabular illustration of body surface area based on height and weight

**Nonparenteral drugs**   drugs administered by topical, rectal, or oral route

**Nonprescription drug**   drug obtained without a prescription; also called over the counter (OTC)

**NPO**   nothing by mouth

**Numerator**   top number in a fraction

**Official name**   a drug's official name as listed in the *United States Pharmacopoeia* and the National Formulary

**Ointment**   semisolid preparation in a petroleum or lanolin base for external use

**Ophthalmic**   pertaining to the eye

**Oral Route (PO)**   drugs given through the mouth

**OTC**   over the counter

**Otic**   pertaining to the ear

**Ototoxic**   a drug or side effects of the drug that may affect the ear

**oz**   ounces

**Parenteral** a general term that means administration by injection (IV, IM, or SQ or SC)

**Paste** thick ointment used to protect the skin

**Pastille** disklike solid that slowly dissolves in the mouth

**Patch** small patch that releases medication over an extended period of time; applied topically

**Percentage** parts per hundred, designated by a percent sign (%)

**Percentage solution** the solid that is dissolved in a liquid represents a percentage of the total weight of the solution; measured in grams per 100 ml of solution

**Pharmacodynamics** study of the chemical and physical effects of drugs in the body

**Pharmacokinetics** science of the factors that determine how much drug reaches the site of action in the body and is excreted

**Pharmacology** study of the origin, nature, chemistry effects, and uses of drugs

**Pharmacotherapeutics** study of the use of drugs to treat, prevent, diagnose diseases

**Piggyback** medication placed in an intravenous infusion set and attached to the mainline IV for delivery to the patient

**Placebo** an inert substance used in place of a drug for its psychological effect and the physiological changes caused by the psychological response

**PO** by mouth, oral

**Powder** a finely ground solid drug or mixture of drugs for internal or external use

**Prefilled cartridge** a small vial with a needle attached that fits into a metal or plastic holder for injection

**Prefilled syringe** a liquid, sterile medication that is ready to administer without further preparation

**Prescription** order for medication written by an authorized prescriber

**Prescription drug** drug that requires a prescription; regulated usually by state laws

**Prime Number** whole number only divisible by 1 and itself; whole number that cannot be reduced any further; i.e., 3, 5, 7

**PR** per rectum

**PRN** when required

**Product** answer in multiplication

**Prolonged-release or slow-release tablet** powdered, compressed drug that disintegrates more slowly and has a longer duration of action

**Proper fraction** fraction with the numerator smaller than the denominator

**Proportion** set of ratios or fractions

**q** each, every

**qd** every day

**qid** four times a day

**qod** every other day

**Quotient** answer in division

**Ratio** way to compare numbers; numbers are separated by a colon, i.e., 1:5 which reads 1 is to 5.

**Reconstitution** dissolving a powder to a liquid form

**Rectal Route (PR)** medication administered through the rectum

**Reduce** simplify

**Rounding** reducing decimal places in a number. A number may be rounded off to the nearest tenth, nearest hundredth, nearest thousandth, etc. A number may also be reduced to the nearest whole number

**SC** subcutaneous

**Score tablet** compressed powdered drug with a line down the center so that the tablet can be broken in half

**SI units** System International d'Unites; measurement adapted from the metric system used in most developed countries to provide a standard language

**Solution** a clear liquid that contains a drug dissolved in water

**Spansule** long-acting capsule that contains drug particles coated to dissolve at different times

**Spirits** concentrated alcoholic solutions of volatile substances

**SR** sustained release

**Subcutaneous (SC or SQ)** the tissue between the skin and muscle

**Sublingual tablet** powdered drug compressed or molded into a solid shape that dissolves quickly under the tongue

**Suppository** mixture of a drug with a firm base molded into a shape to be inserted into a body cavity

**Suspension**  solid particles of a drug dispersed in a liquid that must be shaken to obtain an accurate dose

**Syrup**  a solution of sugar in water to disguise the unpleasant taste of a medication

**Tablet**  a powdered drug that is compressed or molded into solid shape and may contain additives that bind the powder or aid in its absorption

**tid**  three times a day

**Timed release**  small beads of drug in a capsule coated to delay absorption

**Tincture**  alcoholic or hydroalcoholic solution of a drug

**Tolerance**  decreased responsiveness to a drug after repeated exposure

**Topical**  route of administration in which a drug is applied to the skin or mucous membrane

**Toxicity**  nontherapeutic effect that may result in damage to tissues or organs

**Trade name**  a brand or proprietary name identified by the symbol ® that follows the name

**Transcribe**  rewriting; in nursing and hospitals, a drug order is transcribed usually to another form that is used to record and document administration of medications

**Transdermal**  medication drug molecules contained in a unique polymer patch applied to the skin for slow absorption

**Troche**  flat, round, or rectangular preparation held in the mouth (or placed in the vagina) until it dissolves

**U**  units

**Unit dose**  individually wrapped and labeled dose of a drug

**Unit System**  a measurement system using units (U) to measure amounts of drugs; drugs that use this system include Heparin, Penicillin, insulin

**Universal precautions**  procedures to protect against infection that are employed in caring for all patients and when handling contaminated equipment

**Vaginal route**  medication inserted or injected into the vagina

**Vial**  glass container with a rubber stopper containing one or more doses of a drug

**Young's Rule**  rule used to calculate drug dosages for children ages 1 to 12; based on age of the child

# Index

# CD-ROM to Accompany Henke's Med-Math,
## *4th Edition*

## SYSTEM REQUIREMENTS

### Windows:

Windows 95, 98, 2000 or NT
200 MHz processor or higher
32MB or RAM (64MB recommended)
10MB free hard disk space
8× or faster CD-ROM drive
640 × 480 monitor with thousands colors or better
Netscape 4.78 or higher with Java settings enabled
OR
Internet Explorer 5.0 or higher with Java settings enabled
Browser Cookies should be enabled

### Macintosh:

PowerPC (200 MHz or higher recommended)
MAC OS 8.0 or higher
32 MB of RAM (64MB recommended)
10 MB free hard disk space
8× or faster CD-ROM drive
640 × 480 monitor with thousands colors or better
Netscape 4.78 or higher with Java settings enabled
OR
Internet Explorer 5.0 or higher with Java settings enabled
Browser Cookies should be enabled

## INSTALLATION INSTRUCTIONS

### Windows:

1. From Windows 95, 98, 2000, NT Start menu, select Run.
2. Type D:\setup. (Where D is the CD-ROM drive letter.)
3. Follow the on-screen instructions.
   Note: This software is designed to run with Netscape Communicator 4.78 or higher; or Internet Explorer 5.0 or higher and comes with Netscape 6.2.3 and Internet Explorer 5.5. If you do not have Netscape 6.2.3 or higher; or have Internet Explorer 5.0 or higher, choose to install either Netscape 6.2.3 or Internet Explorer 5.5.
4. To start the program after installation, select "Henke's Med-Math" from the "Henke's Med-Math" folder in the Programs option in the Start menu.

### Macintosh:

1. Double click the "Henke's Med-Math CD-ROM" icon on the desktop.
2. Double click the "Install Henke's Med-Math" icon.
3. Follow the on-screen instructions.
   Note: This software is designed to run with Netscape Communicator 4.78 or higher; or Internet Explorer 5.0 or higher and comes with Netscape Communicator 4.78 and Internet Explorer 5.5. If you do not have Netscape Communicator 4.78 or higher; or have Internet Explorer 5.0 or higher, choose to install either Netscape 6.2.3 or Internet Explorer 5.5.
4. To start the program after installation, double click the "Start Henke's Med-Math" icon in the "Henke's Med-Math" folder on the hard drive.